Cancer Screening

CURRENT ◊ CLINICAL ◊ PRACTICE

Cancer Screening: A Practical Guide for Physicians, edited by KHALID AZIZ AND GEORGE Y. WU, 2002

Hypertension Medicine, edited by MICHAEL A. WEBER, 2001

Allergic Diseases: Diagnosis and Treatment, 2nd Edition, edited by PHIL LIEBERMAN AND JOHN A. ANDERSON, 2000

Parkinson's Disease and Movement Disorders: Diagnosis and Treatment Guidelines for the Practicing Physician, edited by CHARLES H. ADLER AND J. ERIC AHLSKOG, 2000

Bone Densitometry in Clinical Practice: Application and Interpretation, SYDNEY LOU BONNICK, 1998

Sleep Disorders: Diagnosis and Treatment, edited by J. STEVEN POCETA AND MERRILL M. MITLER, 1998

Diseases of the Liver and Bile Ducts: A Practical Guide to Diagnosis and Treatment, edited by GEORGE Y. WU AND JONATHAN ISRAEL, 1998

The Pain Management Handbook: A Concise Guide to Diagnosis and Treatment, edited by M. ERIC GERSHWIN AND MAURICE E. HAMILTON, 1998

Osteoporosis: Diagnostic and Therapeutic Principles, edited by CLIFFORD J. ROSEN, 1996

CANCER SCREENING
A PRACTICAL GUIDE FOR PHYSICIANS

Edited by

KHALID AZIZ, MBBS, MRCP (UK),
MRCP (IRE), FACG
*Newington VA Medical Center,
Newington, CT*

and

GEORGE Y. WU, MD, PhD
*University of Connecticut School of Medicine,
Farmington, CT*

Foreword by
PRAMOD SRIVASTAVA, MD, PhD

*University of Connecticut Health Center,
Farmington, CT*

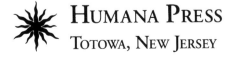

HUMANA PRESS
TOTOWA, NEW JERSEY

© 2002 Humana Press Inc.
Softcover reprint of the hardcover 1st edition 2002
999 Riverview Drive, Suite 208
Totowa, New Jersey 07512

humanapress.com

For additional copies, pricing for bulk purchases, and/or information about other Humana titles, contact Humana at the above address or at any of the following numbers: Tel.: 973-256-1699; Fax: 973-256-8341, E-mail: humana@humanapr.com; or visit our Website: http://humanapr.com

All rights reserved.

No part of this book may be reproduced, stored in a retrieval system, or transmitted in any form or by any means, electronic, mechanical, photocopying, microfilming, recording, or otherwise without written permission from the Publisher.

All articles, comments, opinions, conclusions, or recommendations are those of the author(s), and do not necessarily reflect the views of the publisher.

Due diligence has been taken by the publishers, editors, and authors of this book to assure the accuracy of the information published and to describe generally accepted practices. The contributors herein have carefully checked to ensure that the drug selections and dosages set forth in this text are accurate and in accord with the standards accepted at the time of publication. Notwithstanding, as new research, changes in government regulations, and knowledge from clinical experience relating to drug therapy and drug reactions constantly occurs, the reader is advised to check the product information provided by the manufacturer of each drug for any change in dosages or for additional warnings and contraindications. This is of utmost importance when the recommended drug herein is a new or infrequently used drug. It is the responsibility of the treating physician to determine dosages and treatment strategies for individual patients. Further it is the responsibility of the health care provider to ascertain the Food and Drug Administration status of each drug or device used in their clinical practice. The publisher, editors, and authors are not responsible for errors or omissions or for any consequences from the application of the information presented in this book and make no warranty, express or implied, with respect to the contents in this publication.

Production Editor: Jason S. Runnion
Cover design by Patricia F. Cleary

This publication is printed on acid-free paper. ∞
ANSI Z39.48-1984 (American National Standards Institute) Permanence of Paper for Printed Library Materials.
Photocopy Authorization Policy:
Authorization to photocopy items for internal or personal use, or the internal or personal use of specific clients, is granted by Humana Press Inc., provided that the base fee of US $10.00 per copy, plus US $00.25 per page, is paid directly to the Copyright Clearance Center at 222 Rosewood Drive, Danvers, MA 01923. For those organizations that have been granted a photocopy license from the CCC, a separate system of payment has been arranged and is acceptable to Humana Press Inc.

10 9 8 7 6 5 4 3 2 1

Library of Congress Cataloging-in-Publication Data

Cancer screening: a practical guide for physicians, edited by Khalid Aziz and George Y. Wu.
    p.   cm.—(Current clinical practice)
   Includes bibliographical references and index.
   ISBN 978-1-61737-229-2   e-ISBN 978-1-59259-191-6
   RC669.9.N58 2001
   616.1'07—dc21   99-054493

DEDICATION

To the memory of my parents, whose guidance has provided me with inspiration for all my accomplishments in life (KA).

To my family, who have supported me in spite of the time away from them necessitated by completion of this book; to my mentors Irwin Arias and Sam Seifter, who have been role models and inspirations for me throughout my career (GYW).

FOREWORD

The "war on cancer" has lead to remarkable collateral gains in understanding the cell and molecular biology of normal and cancer cells, even as there has been little measurable progress in a main goal of that war, treatment of the most common solid cancers of adults. An understanding of the mechanisms of carcinogenesis has not automatically translated into better clinical treatment of cancers, at least in the immediate term. Immunotherapy and antiangiogenesis approaches that rely on the host response to cancer, rather than on studies of cancers themselves, are believed today to be the most promising modalities of treatment of cancer. Pending fulfillment of that promise, prevention and early detection are the two most fruitful avenues of action open to us in the war on cancer. *Cancer Screening: A Practical Guide for Physicians* addresses itself eloquently to the latter avenue.

Screening for cancer has seen rapid progress during the last two decades and this has had a direct influence on the clinical course of the disease in selected solid cancers. However, there has been a gap in the availability of this information in one place. *Cancer Screening: A Practical Guide for Physicians*, edited by Professor George Wu and Dr. Khalid Aziz of the University of Connecticut School of Medicine, and with contributions from 19 sets of authors, ably addresses that lacuna. The scope of this volume is suitably broad as it deals with aspects ranging from common issues on screening for malignancies in general to issues specific for various cancer types, to emerging technologies in cancer screening and ethical and legal aspects of such screening. *Cancer Screening: A Practical Guide for Physicians* should be a valuable resource for a broad spectrum of users including internists, epidemiologists, primary care physicians, students, residents, and those responsible for development of public health policies.

Pramod Srivastava, MD, PhD
Professor of Immunology,
Center for Immunotherapy of Cancer
and Infectious Diseases,
University of Connecticut Health Center,
Farmington, CT

PREFACE

Cancer remains a major killer throughout the world. It is estimated that approximately one in three persons living in the United States will develop cancer during his or her lifetime, and one in four will die because of it. Despite major advances in the treatment of cancer, prevention remains the best method of cancer control. New techniques for early detection of precancerous conditions have been developed and new guidelines for cancer screening have been established. *Cancer Screening: A Practical Guide for Physicians* provides an up-to-date text on cancer screening, including epidemiology and biology of various cancers, rationale for the use of screening techniques, sensitivity and specificity of the methods, and algorithms for an overview at a glance. Discussions on cost-effectiveness, indication for consulting subspecialists, and a summary of key principles are also included.

Some countries have very high incidences of certain types of cancers, e.g., stomach cancer in Japan and esophageal cancer in China. Physicians in these countries have developed several innovative and simple, but cost-effective, methods for cancer screening. These methods may be of interest to readers in the United States as the incidence of some of these cancers is increasing. International experts have been invited to write chapters covering the major issues in cancer screening and prevention in their respective countries.

Recently several advances have been made in molecular genetics and imaging technology. One section of *Cancer Screening: A Practical Guide for Physicians* is devoted to the future prospects in cancer screening, including present and future application of molecular genetics and new radiological methods in cancer screening.

Cancer Screening: A Practical Guide for Physicians will provide a quick review of cancer screening for primary care physicians, internists, and various subspecialists, and will be a valuable reference book in the offices of all the physicians involved with cancer screening on a regular basis.

The editors are indebted to the invaluable assistance of Mrs. Rosemary Pavlick and Jocelynn Albert. This project would not have been possible without their dedication and organizational skills. Also, we would like to express our gratitude to Natasha Aziz who, despite a busy schedule, worked diligently to review the chapters in this book.

Khalid Aziz, MBBS, MRCP (UK), MRCP (IRE), FACG
George Y. Wu, MD, PhD

CONTENTS

Foreword v

Preface vii

Contributors xi

Algorithms xvii

PART I   INTRODUCTION

    1   Principles of Cancer Screening 3
        Maurie Markman

PART II   SCREENING FOR BREAST AND GYNECOLOGICAL CANCERS

    2   Screening for Breast Cancer 13
        Kristen Zarfos and Peter J. Deckers

    3   Screening for Cervical Cancer 27
        Amreen Husain and William J. Hoskins

    4   Screening for Ovarian Cancer 43
        Beth E. Nelson and Allan R. Mayer

    5   Screening for Endometrial Cancer 63
        Allan R. Mayer and Beth E. Nelson

PART III   SCREENING FOR GASTROINTESTINAL CANCERS

    6   Screening for Colorectal Cancer 87
        Kittichai Promrat, Khalid Aziz, and George Y. Wu

    7   Screening for Hepatocellular Carcinoma 111
        Kirti Shetty, Khalid Aziz, and George Y. Wu

    8   Screening for Oropharyngeal Cancer 129
        Krishnamoorthy Srinivasan and Mohan Kameswaram

PART IV   SCREENING FOR UROGENITAL CANCERS

    9   Screening for Prostate Cancer 141
        Peter C. Albertsen

   10   Screening for Testicular Cancer 161
        Charles G. Petrunin and Craig R. Nichols

PART V DERMATOLOGICAL CANCERS

11 Screening for Skin Cancer 173
Marti J. Rothe, Tracy L. Bialy,
and Jane M. Grant-Kels

PART VI SCREENING FOR RESPIRATORY CANCERS

12 Screening for Lung Cancer 195
Michael J. McNamee

PART VII SCREENING FOR CANCERS IN HIGH-RISK GROUPS

13 Screening for Esophageal Cancer in High Risk
Groups: *Barrett's Esophagus* 211
Elisabeth I. Heath and Marcia I. F. Canto

14 Screening for Esophageal Cancer in China 227
You-Lin Qiao and Guoqing Wang

15 Screening for Liver Cancer in China 241
Boheng Zhang and Binghui Yang

16 Screening for Gastric Cancer in Japan 255
Masao Ichinose, Naohisa Yahagi, Masashi Oka,
Hitoshi Ikeda, Kaumasa Miki, and Masao Omata

PART VIII FUTURE PROSPECTS IN CANCER SCREENING

17 Advanced Imaging Technology
for Future Cancer Screening 271
Jeff L. Fidler

18 Molecular Genetics and Cancer Screening:
Current Status and Future Prospects 285
Zhong Ling, Khalid Aziz, and George Y. Wu

PART IX MEDICOLEGAL ASPECTS OF CANCER SCREENING

19 Medicolegal Issues in Cancer Screening 303
Charlotte Brooks

Index 315

CONTRIBUTORS

PETER C. ALBERTSEN, MD • *Associate Professor, Chief, Division of Urology, University of Connecticut Health Center, Farmington, CT*

KHALID AZIZ, MBBS, MRCP (UK), MRCP (IRE), FACG • *Assistant Clinical Professor of Medicine, University of Connecticut Health Center, Acting Chief, Division of Gastroenterology and Hepatology, Newington VA Medical Center, Newington, CT*

TRACY L. BIALY, BA • *Department of Dermatology, University of Connecticut Health Center, Farmington, CT*

CHARLOTTE BROOKS, BS, RN • *Medical Legal Consultant, Avon, CT*

MARCIA I. F. CANTO, MD, MHS • *Division of Gastroenterology, Director, Therapeutic Endoscopy and Endoscopic Ultrasonography, Johns Hopkins University School of Medicine, Baltimore, MD*

PETER J. DECKERS, MD • *Dean, School of Medicine, Murray-Heilig Professor of Surgery, University of Connecticut Health Center, Farmington, CT*

JEFF L. FIDLER, MD • *Assistant Professor of Radiology, Department of Radiology, Mayo Clinic, Rochester, MN*

JANE M. GRANT-KELS, MD • *Professor and Chairperson, Clinic Chief of Dermatology, Department of Dermatology, University of Connecticut Health Center, Farmington, CT*

ELISABETH I. HEATH, MD • *Department of Oncology, Johns Hopkins Oncology Center, John Hopkins University School of Medicine, Baltimore, MD*

WILLIAM J. HOSKINS, MD • *Chief, Gynecology Division, Department of Surgery, Avon Chair, Gynecologic Oncology Research, Memorial Sloan-Kettering Cancer Center, New York, NY*

AMREEN HUSAIN, MD • *Gynecology Service Academic Office, Memorial Sloan-Kettering Cancer Center, New York, NY*

MASAO ICHINOSE, MD, PhD • *First Department of Internal Medicine, University of Tokyo, Tokyo, Japan*

HITOSHI IKEDA, MD • *First Department of Internal Medicine, University of Tokyo, Tokyo, Japan*

MOHAN KAMESWARAM, MS, FRCS, MAMS • *Sree Kamachandra Medical College and Research Institute, Deemed University, Madras, India*

ZHONG LING, MD, PHD • *Department of Obstetrics and Gynecology, University of Connecticut Health Center, Farmington, CT*

MAURIE MARKMAN, MD • *Director, Cleveland Clinic Taussig Cancer Center, Chairman, Department of Hematology and Medical Oncology, The Lee and Jerome Bukons Research Chair in Oncology, Cleveland Clinic Foundation, Cleveland, OH*

xiii

ALLAN R. MAYER, DO • *Co-Director of GYN Oncology, Associate Professor of Obstetrics and Gynecology, University of Connecticut Health Center, St. Francis Hospital and Medical Center, Hartford, CT*

MICHAEL J. MCNAMEE, MD, FCCP • *Director of Pulmonary Medicine, Director of Intensive Care, Associate Professor of Clinical Medicine, University School of Medicine, New Britain General Hospital, New Britain, CT*

KAUMASA MIKI, MD • *First Department of Internal Medicine, University of Tokyo, Tokyo, Japan*

BETH E. NELSON, MD • *Co-Director of GYN Oncology, Associate Professor of Obstetrics and Gynecology, University of Connecticut Health Center, St. Francis Hospital and Medical Center, Hartford, CT*

CRAIG R. NICHOLS, MD • *Professor of Medicine, Department of Medicine, Division of Hematology and Medical Oncology, Oregon Health Science University, Portland, OR*

MASASHI OKA, MD • *First Department of Internal Medicine, University of Tokyo, Tokyo, Japan*

MASAO OMATA, MD • *First Department of Internal Medicine, University of Tokyo, Tokyo, Japan*

CHARLES G. PETRUNIN, MD • *Division of Hematology and Medical Oncology, Oregon Health Science University, Portland, OR*

KITTICHAI PROMRAT, MD • *Hepatology Fellow, Liver Disease Section, NIDDK, National Institutes of Health, Bethesda, MD*

YOU-LIN QIAO, MD • *Professor and Chief, Department of Cancer Epidemiology, Cancer Institute, Chinese Academy of Medical Services, Beijing, The People's Republic of China*

MARTI J. ROTHE, MD • *Associate Professor of Medicine, Department of Dermatology, University of Connecticut Health Science Center, Farmington, CT*

KIRTI SHETTY, MD • *Division of Gastroenterology, University of Connecticut Health Center, Farmington, CT*

KRISHNAMOORTHY SRINIVASAN, MS, SLO • *Associate Professor, Department of Ear, Nose and Throat, Sree Kamachandra Medical College, Deemed University, Madras, India*

GUOQING WANG, MD • *Professor of Surgery, Department of Surgery, Cancer Institute, Chinese Academy of Medical Services, Beijing, The People's Republic of China*

GEORGE Y. WU, MD • *Professor of Medicine, Chief, Division of Gastroenterology-Hepatology, Herman Lopata Chair in Hepatitis Research, University of Connecticut Health Science Center, Farmington, CT*

NAOHISA YAHAGI, MD • *First Department of Internal Medicine, University of Tokyo, Tokyo, Japan*

BINGHUI YANG, MD • *Professor of Medicine, Director, Zhong Shan Hospital, Shanghai Medical University, Shanghai, The People's Republic of China*

KRISTEN ZARFOS, MD • *Assistant Professor, Department of Surgery, University of Connecticut Health Science Center, Farmington, CT*

BOHENG ZHANG, MD, PhD, MSC • *Associate Professor of Medicine, Liver Cancer Institute, Shanghai Medical University, Shanghai, The People's Republic of China*

ALGORITHMS

Chapter 2
Algorithm 1: Evaluation of breast abnormalities in premenopausal women *17*
Algorithm 2: Evaluation of breast abnormalities in perimenopausal and postmenopausal women *17*

Chapter 3
Algorithm 1: Screening for cervical cancer *37*

Chapter 4
Algorithm 1: Screening for ovarian cancer *56*

Chapter 5
Algorithm 1: Endometrial cancer risk *73*

Chapter 6
Algorithm 1: CRC screening in average-risk patients *102*
Algorithm 2: CRC screening in high-risk patients: 1 .... *102*
Algorithm 3: CRC screening in high-risk patients: 2 .... *103*

Chapter 7
Algorithm 1: Screening for hepatocellular carcinoma *122*

Chapter 8
Algorithm 1: Patients for routine examination *135*

Chapter 9
Algorithm 1: Screening for prostate cancer *155*

Chapter 10
Algorithm 1: Screening for testicular cancer *165*

Chapter 11
Algorithm 1: New or changing skin lesion *176*
Algorithm 2: Differential diagnosis of common skin cancers *179*

Chapter 12
Algorithm 1: Lung cancer risk level in smokers vs nonsmokers .. *205*

Chapter 13
Algorithm 1: Surveillance guidelines for Barrett's esophagus *220*

Chapter 14
Algorithm 1: Screening for esophageal carcinoma in China *234*

Chapter 15
Algorithm 1: PLC screening and daignosis *250*

Chapter 16
Algorithm 1: Diagnosis of stomach cancer *260*
Algorithm 2: Stomach cancer screening with a combination of methods *265*

I INTRODUCTION

1 Principles of Cancer Screening

Maurie Markman, MD

KEY PRINCIPLES

- Cancer will surpass heart disease as the leading cause of death in this century.
- The major aim of cancer screening is to find a cancer at a point in its natural history where the opportunity for long-term disease-free survival will be optimized.
- A successful screening strategy can significantly decrease the costs associated with the management of a particular malignancy.
- For a cancer screening strategy to be successful, there must be both great specificity and sensitivity of the test for the specific malignancy.

OBJECTIVES OF CANCER SCREENING

It is an established fact that the survival of individuals with nonhematologic malignancies is strongly influenced by the stage of disease at presentation *(1)*. Cancers discovered to be localized to their site of origin following routine staging procedures (e.g., radiographic evaluation) have a significantly lower risk of experiencing relapse than disease found to have spread to regional lymph nodes or more distant locations (e.g., lung, liver, brain). Thus, the major goal of cancer screening is to find a cancer as early as possible in its natural history, optimizing the opportunity for the individual with the malignancy to experience long-term disease-free and overall survival.

Although improvement in survival is the ultimate aim of all cancer screening strategies, it must be noted that there are a number of important secondary goals of screening. First, it would be anticipated that the

From: *Cancer Screening: A Practical Guide for Physicians*
Edited by: K. Aziz and G. Y. Wu © Humana Press Inc., Totowa, NJ

earlier discovery of cancer will result in the finding of a smaller-volume disease and less local spread of the malignancy. In this clinical setting, definitive therapy to control both local and possible distant spread may be less extensive, resulting in both reduced short-term and long-term morbidity. This is an important issue independent of the overall impact of screening on long-term disease-free or overall survival. For example, the local and systemic treatment of a woman with a nonpalpable, node-negative, 0.4-cm infiltrating ductal breast cancer discovered on routine screening mammography will be vastly different from that of an individual with a 7-cm breast mass and 16 positive axillary lymph nodes detected when the local cancer begins to ulcerate. In this case, the screening will have a highly favorable impact on quality of life, even if both patients are ultimately cured of their cancers.

Second, the costs of medical care associated with the treatment of a malignancy can be significantly reduced with a successful screening strategy. The costs of caring for an individual with cancer include not only those required for the initial treatment and its complications (e.g., surgery, radiation, chemotherapy) but also for the risk of progressive disease (e.g., pain medications, home/hospice care). The issues of reduction in costs associated with screening are highly relevant to the individual/family with cancer, third-party payers responsible for payment of medical services (e.g., employers, insurance companies), and to society.

Finally, a successful screening program can increase productivity of an individual and his/her spouse or caregiver, by reducing the time/effort required for treatment of the cancer and for dealing with the complications of the disease and its therapy.

REQUIREMENTS FOR A SUCCESSFUL CANCER SCREENING TESTING STRATEGY

There are a number of important features associated with all successful cancer screening strategies (Table 1). From the public health perspective, it is imperative that the considerable resources to be expended in a screening program favorably impact the morbidity and mortality associated with a relatively common malignancy. For example, it is difficult to justify screening all adult members of society on a yearly basis for a cancer which will ultimately affect <1 in 1000 individuals over their lifetime. In contrast, breast cancer, which will be found in 1 of 9 women during their lives is an excellent target for screening. A demonstrated reduction in the morbidity and mortality associated with the discovery of breast cancer at a lower stage (e.g., stage 1 versus all other stages) may have a profound impact on public health.

Chapter 1 / Principles of Cancer Screening   5

Table 1

Features Associated with a Successful Cancer Screening Program

1. Relatively common disease (e.g., breast cancer) or ability to define a subset (e.g., age, ethnicity) of the population where the disease is a relatively important clinical entity
2. Screening procedures/techniques
   a. Relatively inexpensive
   b. Simple to perform
   c. Easy to teach
   d. Relatively easy to maintain essential quality control
3. Unambiguous interpretation of results (i.e., low rates of false-positive or false-negative testing)
4. Evidence that detecting the cancer at an earlier time-point in its natural history will significantly impact survival

To be able to successfully apply a screening strategy across a large population, it is critically important that the test be relatively inexpensive and easily transported outside the research/academic/investigative setting where the approach originally demonstrated clinical utility.

It is also important that there exists an effective method to maintain quality control, which can be successfully employed in the community setting. The fact that an academic investigative team, highly trained in the use of a screening procedure (e.g., radiography, cytology), can produce a clinically useful test does not necessarily mean that this outcome will result from the dissemination of the strategy outside this carefully controlled research setting.

The question of the incidence of false-negative and false-positive tests is a critically important issue for all cancer screening strategies. "False-positive" refers to those individuals who are found to have a positive test result but who do not have the cancer, and "false-negative" refers to the finding of a negative test result in an individual who actually has the malignancy.

The specificity of a screening test is the probability of screening negative if the disease is not present. A test, which is highly specific, will rarely be "positive" in the absence of actual disease. In this setting, there will be few individuals without disease who are incorrectly labeled as "positive" and are required to undergo subsequent additional testing and be subjected to the anxiety associated with this laboratory finding.

The sensitivity of a screening test is the probability of testing positive if the disease is actually present in an individual. A cancer screening test

Table 2

Specificity and Sensitivity of Cancer Screening Tests

Sensitivity:
$$\frac{\text{True-positive}}{\text{True-positive} + \text{false-negative}} \times 100$$

Specificity:
$$\frac{\text{True-negative}}{\text{True-negative} + \text{false-positive}} \times 100$$

is stated to be more sensitive as the number of individuals who possess the malignancy, but are called "test negative," decreases. For a screening test to be clinically useful, it must demonstrate high level of both specificity and sensitivity. The mathematical definitions of specificity and sensitivity are shown in Table 2.

Finally, in the tumor type for which the screening test is being employed, there must be evidence that finding the malignancy somewhat earlier in its natural history will exert a favorable impact on both the morbidity and mortality of the cancer. For example, breast cancer has a well-defined progression over an extended time period, which can be significantly influenced by finding smaller malignant lesions. Survival in stage 1 disease is superior to more advanced cancer, whether locally advanced or metastatic disease. In contrast, it would be highly questionable if cancer of the pancreas will be substantially influenced by any screening strategy in view of unique biological and anatomical considerations.

CONCERNS WITH SCREENING PROGRAMS FOR CANCER

There are several problems inherent in the evaluation of any approach to cancer screening. First, one must always be concerned with the potential cost of a strategy, relative to its clinical utility. For example, if it is demonstrated that the performance of an expensive radiographic test (e.g., proton-emission tomography [PET] scanning) performed yearly on all adults until age 75 can detect the presence of a particular malignancy at an early stage (e.g., endometrial cancer), a cost-effectiveness analysis will almost certainly yield a highly unfavorable result.

Second, the specific impact of a false-positive result of a screening test on the individual declared to have a "positive test" must be considered. In addition to considerable anxiety, unnecessary (e.g., radiographs) and potentially morbid procedures (e.g., surgery) may result from the

Chapter 1 / Principles of Cancer Screening 7

false test result. Again, the costs of these procedures, both monetary and time/effort, to the individual/family and society must be considered.

Third, there are also potential important implications associated with a false-negative outcome of a screening program. In addition to failing to detect the malignancy, patients who develop symptoms of the disease may assume that they cannot have the cancer because of the incorrect test results. This may delay their seeking necessary medical intervention and impact negatively on the ultimate outcome of subsequent treatment.

Finally, the issue of lead-time bias must be considered. If a screening test "discovers a cancer" at an "earlier time-point" than anticipated by traditional methods of disease detection (e.g., routine physical examination, evaluation of cancer-related symptoms), this does not necessarily mean that the test has favorably influenced the ultimate survival outcome. For example, a cancer that appears to be "small" may have already developed subclinical metastatic disease, with the outcome predetermined and not influenced by the screening strategy. However, because the period of time between detection and progression or death has increased, one might incorrectly interpret the prolongation of this time interval as a "favorable impact of screening". Similarly, even if a small cancer grows and is only found when symptoms develop, treatment of the cancer may be identical and the ultimate survival unchanged.

Therefore, the actual impact of any cancer screening strategy on survival can only be defined through the conduct of well-designed and well-conducted randomized controlled clinical trials comparing a screened population to a group of individuals not undergoing the screening procedure.

CERVIX CANCER: EXAMPLE OF A SUCCESSFUL CANCER SCREENING STRATEGY

The development of a simple and cost-effective method of cytologic screening for cervix cancer (Papanicolaou smear) and its associated premalignant and early malignant conditions (e.g., severe dysplasia, carcinoma *in situ*) has been one of the most important public health developments of the last century *(2,3)*.

In the United States in the 1940s, there were approximately 26,000 deaths each year from this malignancy. By 1996, when screening with Papanicolaou smears had long become a part of routine medical care for women in this country, the annual death toll from cervix cancer had decreased to less than 5000 *(4)*. In an analysis of survival following the diagnosis of invasive cervical cancer in Sweden, the use of cytologic screening was shown to have substantially decreased the mortality associated with this malignant condition *(3)*. For example, for women with cervix cancer under the age of 50, the 5-yr survival rate from 1960 to 1964 (before the widespread use of cytological screening) was only 70%, compared to 89% during the years 1980–1984. In addition, this strategy has been shown to be highly cost-effective, even in an elderly Medicare patient population *(5)*.

Unfortunately, despite the documented success of this simple public health measure when correctly applied in appropriate individuals, major concerns remain for the use of the test in clinical practice *(4,6)*. For example, there continue to exist large segments of the female population in this country (e.g., lower socioeconomic groups, elderly), which have not participated in routine cytological cervical screening. The reasons for this state of affairs are complex and include fear, a lack of education regarding the test, and cost.

In addition, in an effort to control medical costs, technologists in many laboratories have been required to increase the number of tests they read in an average day, with documented reduction in quality control *(4,6)*.

There is also evidence that in some settings, individuals who actually obtain the smear are inadequately trained to perform the procedure. It has been recommended that specific training and quality control measures be substantially enhanced to optimally utilize this valuable screening strategy.

Automated devices to read the cervical smears have been introduced into anatomic pathology laboratories, but concern with the added costs associated with screening employing these systems has been raised *(7)*. However, despite these issues relating to the optimal conduct of cervical cancer screening, the value of this screening strategy in significantly decreasing the risk of death from this malignancy is unquestioned.

OVARIAN CANCER: EXAMPLE OF AN UNSUCCESSFUL CANCER SCREENING STRATEGY

In contrast to the documented clinical utility of cytological screening for cervix cancer, there is currently no evidence of a benefit associated with screening for another, even more difficult gynecologic malignancy, e.g., ovarian cancer *(8)*.

Important differences between the two disease entities help explain the lack of efficacy for ovarian cancer screening. First, although the cervix is very accessible to visual inspection and routine cytological analysis, the small ovaries are protected deep in the pelvis and present a serious problem for direct visualization.

Chapter 1 / Principles of Cancer Screening 9

Second, especially in premenopausal females, the ovaries are in constant change during the menstrual cycle. Thus, "abnormalities" observed on radiographic evaluation (e.g., ultrasound) may simply represent physiologic changes and not serious pathology. Even the common finding of cysts on ultrasound examination may be viewed in most women, more as a variant of normal physiology and anatomy rather than as a cause of serious concern.

Third, although obtaining frequent cytological analysis of the cervix is quite simple and associated with minimal discomfort, the biopsy of an ovary requires a surgical procedure (e.g., laparoscopy) and is associated with a concern for surgical morbidity and small risk of loss of ovarian function.

Fourth, although cervix cancer has well-defined premalignant (i.e., severe dysplasia) and early malignant (i.e., carcinoma *in situ*) components that can be diagnosed and easily treated, there are currently no established precursor lesions for cancer of the ovary.

Finally, the natural history of cervix cancer, from precursor lesions to invasive cancer, has been well documented. It is recognized that by finding and treating premalignant and early-stage malignancy the prognosis is greatly improved.

In the case of ovarian cancer, it remains completely unknown if the finding of "stage 1" disease during the performance of any screening test (e.g., abnormal vaginal ultrasound, elevated serum CA-125 antigen level) will have a favorable impact on survival from the malignancy *(9,10)*. For example, despite the fact that the cancer appears to be confined to the organ of origin, microscopic metastatic disease may already be present at the time of diagnosis. Also, as it is known that approx 10–20% of patients with ovarian cancer currently are found to have surgically documented stage 1 ovarian cancer, without the use of any screening strategy, it remains uncertain if screening will actually favorably impact on the percentage of individuals presenting at this early stage of disease. An alternative hypothesis is that nonscreened individuals who are destined to have stage 1 ovarian cancer will be essentially the same patient population whose cancers are discovered by any screening strategy to be confined to the ovary.

In view of these considerations it should not be surprising that several analyses of the cost-effectiveness of ovarian cancer screening have concluded that, with available techniques, such screening is highly unlikely to be a useful approach to decrease the morbidity and mortality associated with this difficult malignancy in a general patient population without a family history of ovarian cancer *(11–13)*.

CONCLUSION

Cancer will ultimately affect one-third of all individuals and two-thirds of all families in the United States. Early in this new century, malignant disease will surpass heart disease as the leading cause of death in this country. Thus, it is important that we carefully and critically examine any and all strategies that have the potential to effectively lessen the morbidity and mortality associated with malignancy. Cancer screening is an obvious approach to accomplish this goal. However, despite the promise of this therapeutic strategy, we must be careful to avoid the temptation to accept the clinical usefulness of a proposed cancer screening program until it has been thoroughly tested in randomized controlled trials to document that the "costs" associated with the approach (e.g., monetary, time, inconvenience, anxiety, unnecessary procedures for false-positive testing) are justified by a favorable impact on survival. The cost-effectiveness of all proposed cancer screening strategies, as well as careful definitions of target populations, should be established before any approach is accepted as a component of routine medical care.

REFERENCES

1. Sparen P, Gustafsson L, Friberg L-G, et al. (1995) Improved control of invasive cervical cancer in Sweden over six decades by earlier clinical detection and better treatment. *J Clin Oncol* 13:715–725.
2. Cannistra SA, Niloff JM. (1996) Cancer of the uterine cervix. *N Engl J Med* 334:1030–1038.
3. Adami H-O, Ponten J, Sparen P, et al. (1994) Survival trend after invasive cervical cancer diagnosis in Sweden before and after cytologic screening. *Cancer* 73:140–147.
4. Austin RM, McLendon WW. (1997) The Papanicolaou smear. Medicine's most successful cancer screening procedure is threatened. *JAMA* 277:754,755.
5. Fahs MC, Mandelblatt J, Schechter C, et al. (1992) Cost effectiveness of cervical cancer screening for the elderly. *Ann Intern Med* 117:520–527.
6. Koss LG. (1989) The Papanicolaou test for cervical cancer detection. A triumph and a tragedy. *JAMA* 61:737–743.
7. Marshall CJ, Rowe L, Bentz S. (1999) Improved quality-control detection of false-negative pap smears using the Autopap 300 QC system. *Diag Cytopath* 20(3):170–174.
8. Cannistra SA. (1993) Cancer of the ovary. *N Engl J Med* 329:1550–1559.
9. NIH Consensus Development Panel on Ovarian Cancer. (1995) Ovarian cancer. Screening, treatment, and follow-up. *JAMA* 273:491–497.
10. DePriest PD, Gallion HH, Pavlik EJ, et al. (1997) Transvaginal sonography as a screening method for the detection of early ovarian cancer. *Gynecol Oncol* 65:408–414.
11. Schapira MM, Matchar DB, Young MJ. (1993) The effectiveness of ovarian cancer screening. A decision analysis model. *Ann Intern Med* 118:838–843.
12. Carlson J, Skates SJ, Singer DE. (1994) Screening for ovarian cancer. *Ann Intern Med* 121:124–132.
13. Mackey SE, Creasman WT. (1995) Ovarian cancer screening. *J Clin Oncol* 13:783–793.
14. Landis SH, Murray T, Bolden S, et al. (1999) Cancer statistics, 1999. *CA Cancer J Clin* 49:8–31.

II

SCREENING FOR BREAST AND GYNECOLOGICAL CANCERS

2 Screening for Breast Cancer

Kristen Zarfos, MD and Peter J. Deckers, MD

KEY PRINCIPLES

- Breast cancer is the most common cancer in women and the second most common cause of cancer death in the United States.
- Mammography, regular breasts exams, and breast self-examination are the key components of early detection and surveillance.
- Multiple risk factors for the development of breast cancer have been established; these include women: with a personal or family history of breast cancer, age over 60 yr, and atypical proliferative fibrocystic change. However, 45% of women with newly diagnosed breast cancer have no identifiable risk factor.
- Mammography, although proven to reduce the cancer death in screened women, is not a perfect screening test. It fails to detect 10–20% of cancers.
- Controversy exists regarding the age to institute mammographic screening, indeterminate findings on the breast biopsy, and genetic testing.

INTRODUCTION

One hundred eighty thousand (180,000) women were diagnosed with breast cancer in the United States in the year 2000 and about 45,000 women died of this disease *(1)*. The mortality rate and the possibility of breast conservation are linked to the size of the cancer at the time of detection. In general, the smaller the tumor at the time of diagnosis, the

From: *Cancer Screening: A Practical Guide for Physicians*
Edited by: K. Aziz and G. Y. Wu © Humana Press Inc., Totowa, NJ

lower the mortality rate for an individual woman and the more likely breast conservation will be successful (2,3).

These facts support the very important role primary care physicians have in minimizing the mortality and morbidity for their patients with breast cancer. Primary care physicians, by having the most direct contact with their patients, play a key role in early detection. By examining patients annually, ordering baseline and regular mammograms, and educating patients in breast cancer facts and self-examination, primary care physicians can make a major impact on the lives of their patients who may eventually be diagnosed with breast cancer.

EPIDEMIOLOGY

Breast cancer is the most common malignancy in women in the United States (4). It is second only to lung cancer as the most common cause of cancer death (4). The incidence of breast cancer had steadily increased in the United States over the last few decades (5). Since 1997, however, breast cancer mortality has declined each year by 1.8% (6,7).

Internationally, the incidence of breast cancer varies greatly, with the lowest rates in the eastern Asian region (China, Japan, and India) to the highest in Western Europe and the United States, where a fivefold increase is observed (8,9).

Racial variability has been observed within the United States. Whereas breast cancer incidence is higher among premenopausal African-American women, the incidence is lower among postmenopausal African-American women compared to white women of similar age (10).

Multiple risk factors for developing breast cancer have been established (Table 1). Despite this, 45% of women with newly diagnosed breast cancer have no identifiable risk factor (11). Being female is the foremost risk factor. Ninety-nine percent of all breast cancer occurs in women. Male breast cancer accounts for less than 1% of all breast cancers (12). Age is the second most critical factor. The risk of breast cancer increases steadily with age through the childbearing years until the mid-50s, and then abruptly rises into the mid-60s. Thereafter, the incidence continues to rise, but gradually (13). Whereas a physician should have a higher index of suspicion in a woman over 50 with a breast mass, breast cancer has been occasionally, although very rarely, diagnosed in women in their late teens (14).

Family history is important in assessing the risk of developing breast cancer. The risk of breast cancer doubles in patients with a family history of breast cancer in the first-degree relatives (mother, sister, daughter) (15). The risk is more than twofold if more than two first-degree

Chapter 2 / Screening for Breast Cancer

Table 1

Established Risk Factors for Invasive Breast Carcinoma

High risk (RR>4)
- First-degree relative with history of breast cancer
- Age over 60
- Patient born in North America or northern Europe
- Atypical proliferative fibrocystic change

Moderate risk (RR 2–4)
- Age over 30 at first full-term pregnancy
- Obesity
- History of breast cancer
- Any first-degree relative with history of breast cancer
- Dysplastic mammographic parenchymal pattern
- Chest-wall irradiation
- Proliferative fibrocystic change without atypia
- High socioeconomic status

Low risk (RR 1.1–1.9)
- Nulliparity
- Early menarche
- Late menopause
- Postmenopausal obesity
- History of ovarian or endometrial cancer

relatives have breast cancer and the risk is more than three times if one of those relatives had either premenopausal disease or bilateral breast cancer *(16,17)*.

Certain characteristics of a woman's reproductive history have also been shown to increase the risk of developing breast cancer. Nulliparous women and women having a first birth after the age of 30 yr have twice the risk of developing breast cancer *(18)*. Absence of breast-feeding also increases the risk *(19,20)*. Early onset of menarche, before the age of 12, and late onset of menopause, after the age of 55, each increases the risk by twofold *(21,22)*.

A diagnosis of atypical hyperplasia on a previous breast biopsy and a 65% or greater area of density on the mammogram poses a four times increased risk of developing breast cancer *(23–25)*. Having cancer in one breast increases the relative risk of developing a second cancer in the contralateral breast by a factor of 2–4. This is most marked if a woman has an associated family history of breast cancer *(26)*.

Other factors associated with increased risk are obesity, as defined by weight >200 lbs., history of endometrial and ovarian carcinoma, and prior radiotherapy to the chest or mediastinum *(27)*.

THE BIOLOGY OF BREAST CANCER

Breast cancer is both a local and a systemic disease. Breast cancer is heterogeneous in its presentation and course. Its propensity for early systemic spread is, more often than not, directly related to an overall cure rate that does not exceed 65% in the United States. Its natural history is protracted over time, making the definition of the "cure" of breast cancer difficult *(28,29)*.

We know that, in general, the smaller the tumor, the less likely there is lymph node involvement, and the better the long-term survival *(30–32)*. Yet, metastases can become apparent as late as 10–20 yr after a disease-free period from initial treatment *(33)*.

The behavior of the primary tumor within the breast starts as a single malignant cell, which is estimated to take approximately 5–8 yr to reach 1 cm *(34)*. It spreads within the breast by direct infiltration of adjacent tissue, along mammary ducts and through breast lymphatics *(35)*. The systemic problems develop from breast cancer cells metastasizing beyond the breast to regional lymph nodes and distant organs. Axillary lymph nodes are the major regional drainage site for the breast. In half the patients with a clinically palpable breast mass, axillary lymph nodes are involved *(32)*. The internal mammary lymph-node chain and supra-clavicular lymph nodes are less frequently involved *(36,37)*.

Metastases to distant organs may be recognized at the time of diagnosis or as late as 10 yr or more after initial treatment *(30)*. In general, the incidence and the time-course to distant metastases correlates with the size of the primary tumor *(30)*. Yet, it is recognized that there are subsets of patients whose tumors do not behave in this predictable manner *(28)*. Distant metastases are most frequently found in the lungs, liver, bone, adrenal glands, pleura, brain, and skin *(38–40)*.

SCREENING FOR BREAST CANCER

The purpose of breast cancer screening is to separate women who are clearly normal from those with abnormalities, with the goal of intervening in the disease process after biologic onset but before symptoms or signs develop *(41)* (*see* Algorithms 1 and 2). Mammography, regular breast exams, and breast self-examination are the key components of early detection and surveillance *(42)*. Additional radiological modalities will be mentioned as adjuncts, but they are not basic screening tools.

The use of mammography to screen asymptomatic women 40 yr of age and over for early detection of breast cancer has been shown to reduce mortality rates by 20–30% *(43–45)*. A standard screening mammogram includes two views of each breast. Additional views at differ-

Chapter 2 / Screening for Breast Cancer

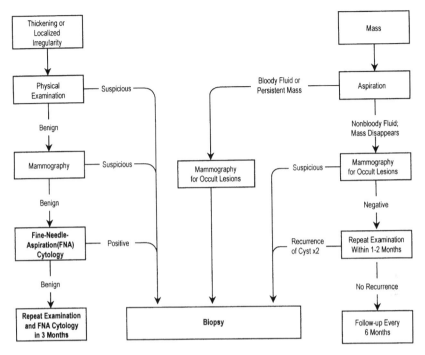

Algorithm 1. Evaluation of breast abnormalities in premenopausal women.

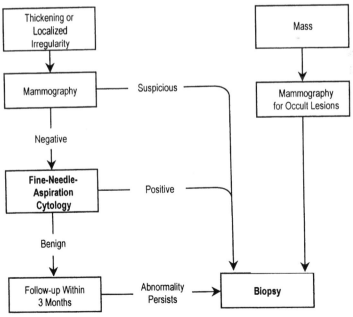

Algorithm 2. Evaluation of breast abnormalities in perimenopausal and postmenopausal women.

ent angles or increased compression of the breast tissues may be included for better definition of the character of the breast tissue *(46,47)*.

Although there has been a decade of controversy as to the timing of mammograms, the current consensus, based on recommendations of the American Cancer Society, is as follows:

1. Baseline mammogram at age 40
2. Between ages 40 and 49, a mammogram yearly or every other year
3. At age 50 or older, a mammogram yearly

Mammograms at an earlier age or more frequently are indicated for women with increased risk *(42)*.

Routine, regularly scheduled clinical breast exams by a skilled physician have been shown to play an important role in early detection of breast cancer. When combined with mammography, clinical breast exams decrease mortality from breast cancer *(48,49)*.

At the minimum, breast examination should be performed annually beginning at age 30 and become part of a woman's routine physical examination. However, physicians should practice clinical breast examinations with yearly gynecological or physical exams in younger women as well. Key elements to the success of a clinical breast exam are consistency in the examiner, regular scheduling, and attention to technique.

With a woman disrobed from the waist up, a woman should be examined in both the sitting and supine positions. The breast should be examined for symmetry of the overall appearance, nipple–areolar complexes, and skin texture, with the arms by the sides and also elevated above the head. Note of any retraction or bulging of the breast tissue, skin edema, peau d'orange, or erythema should be made. The nipples should be examined for crusting, bleeding, irregularity, or retraction. Palpation of the breast skin should follow, examining for thickening, nodules, or induration. Again, in both the sitting and supine positions and with the arms beside the torso and raised above the head, the breasts should be firmly but gently palpated in their entirety. Either a concentric circular or radial search pattern is effective, as long as it is complete. Palpation should extend to the clavicle, to the sternum, to the lower rib cage and into the axilla, in which much breast tissue is located, especially in older women. Documentation of any abnormalities should include size, location, mobility, and character.

The final portion of the exam is addressed by examining the node-bearing regions. In the sitting and supine position, the supraclavicular fossae and both axillae should be examined. The axillae are best examined while sitting with the physician supporting the flexed arm with one hand, palpating with the other.

Chapter 2 / Screening for Breast Cancer

A third and complementary component to breast surveillance is breast self-examination. Although regular breast self-examination alone cannot be linked to a decreased mortality from breast cancer, it does have a measurable impact on earlier detection when carefully practiced *(50–52)*. To be of value, physicians should teach breast self-examination carefully and consistently *(53,54)*. Women should be encouraged to participate in self-examination. Upon finding a mass on self-examination, a woman should be promptly seen and evaluated.

The most important message concerning the roles of mammography, clinical breast examination, and breast self-examination is that they complement, but do not replace, each other *(55)*. It is an important role of the primary care physician to educate his or her patients to the fact that even when a mammogram reveals no lesion in the presence of a palpable mass, a breast cancer may be present and further evaluation should be made. In either the setting of a nonpalpable mammographic lesion or a palpable lesion not seen on a mammogram, surgical consultation is imperative *(56)*.

Other radiological modalities available for breast evaluation include ultrasound and magnetic resonance imaging (MRI). Both of these can add additional information to mammographic and clinical findings, but they are incapable of detecting early-stage cancers with reliability and do not provide a screening tool *(47,57)*. Ultrasound is very useful in distinguishing cysts from solid lesions *(58,59)*.

GENETIC SCREENING

With the discovery of the autosomal dominant genes BRCA 1 and BRCA 2, which transmit a high breast cancer risk, questions arise as to the role of genetic screening. When present, these genes indicate significant susceptibility to developing breast cancer *(60,61)*. The presence of a mutated version of BRCA 1 carries a 90% lifetime risk for developing breast cancer *(62)*.

The current testing, however, is limited in its applicability. Because of technical constraints, its utility is confined to women from a large family in which a relative has been diagnosed with breast cancer and has had a gene alteration identified. Therefore, women to consider for counseling for genetic testing should include the following:

1. Women from large families with relatives with breast and/or ovarian cancer
2. Women from small families with early-onset disease or bilateral cancer, or individual women diagnosed before 40 yr of age
3. Women with male breast cancer relatives *(63)*

However, genetic testing must be approached cautiously because of the significant long-term implications to a woman. Counseling before testing is imperative and preferably is conducted as part of a research program before proceeding with genetic analysis *(64,65)*. Unexpected adverse reactions of guilt and depression, dilemmas as to treatment options (prophylactic mastectomies, prophylactic tamoxifen), and ethical dilemmas surrounding families who choose not to know their status have been experienced *(66)*. As there is no protection for privacy of genetic information, there are significant implications for discrimination and stigmatization. Insurers can deny coverage for surveillance or prevention if a high-risk gene is identified, or breast cancer care of an affected woman might be denied based on the concept that the condition was pre-existing. Furthermore, documentation of the results in the medical record may result in loss of medical or life insurance coverage and discrimination by an employer *(67)*. Therefore, consideration of genetic testing should be approached cautiously and is best handled with counseling in a research program.

COST-EFFECTIVENESS

The cost-effectiveness of screening for breast cancer in asymptomatic women usually includes the cost of the screening tests, the cost of further workup of abnormal screening tests, cost of false-positive and false-negative screening tests, and the cost of treatment in the unscreened population. The potential possibilities for the latter are multiple and are, therefore, too numerous to discuss in this setting. However, when breast cancer is found at a later stage, more involved surgery, potential radiation to the chest wall, potential reconstruction, chemotherapy and the increased risk of eventual need for metastatic treatment, and numerous resultant periodic tests are the norm. All of these require significant expenditure and increase patient suffering. Most analyses of breast cancer screening have been either mathematical models or related to clinical trials, and virtually all consider it a useful expenditure of resources *(68–70)*.

INDICATIONS FOR REFERRAL TO A SURGEON

After screening results are obtained, the following are guidelines for referral to a general surgeon for further examination.

Mammographic Findings

1. Indeterminate findings or benign findings in a woman at high risk.
2. Suspicious findings or those highly suggestive of cancer.

Physical Findings (Regardless of Mammographic Findings)

1. Palpable mass or irregular thickening in the breast.
2. Bloody nipple discharge.
3. Skin changes of erythema, thickening, or peau d'orange character.
4. Supraclavicular or axillary lymphadenopathy.

CONTROVERSIAL AREAS

Controversy exists regarding the timing of a surgical consultation in a woman with a mammographic abnormality amenable to a core or fine-needle aspiration and/or a palpable mass that is amenable to needle biopsy. Although other physicians are capable of these procedures, because the ultimate responsibility rests in the hands of the surgeon, early surgical consultation before a needle biopsy is preferable. This allows the surgeon to give the patient a full up-front discussion about the possibilities of future treatment should the needle biopsy be positive, allowing the patient a broader sense of the implications of the finding at hand, and the possible course ahead. In palpable lesions, the needle biopsy eliminates the possibility of hematoma formation obscuring physical findings at the time of the surgeon's patient examination and treatment planning.

A higher profile controversy is the age to institute mammographic screening. Multiple studies from around the world have looked at this issue. There is no question that there is a decrease in mortality in women over 50 yr of age receiving screening mammograms. The controversy is in the 40–49-yr-old age group *(43,45)*. Because of the density of breasts in the younger age group, mammograms are not as sensitive in detecting malignancies. After much discussion and review of multiple studies, the American Cancer Society and National Cancer Institute recommend that mammograms be performed in the 40–49-yr-old age group either annually or every other year *(42)*.

The controversy surrounding genetic testing has been described earlier. Presently, each physician needs to weigh the pros and cons of recommending this testing with its inherent limitations. There is no controversy that once genetic testing is discussed with a patient that counseling must be incorporated in the process, and preferably within a research program. As technology advances, legislation catches up with the technology, and future breast cancer chemopreventive agents are discovered, the controversies surrounding breast cancer genetic testing may become more manageable.

One final area of controversy is the use of hormonal replacement therapy (HRT). Although more appropriately discussed in the setting of

22   Part II / Screening for Breast and Gynecological Cancers

treatment rather than screening, the increased risk posed by HRT should be commented upon. Treatment with both estrogen replacement therapy and estrogen–progesterone combination therapy has been shown to increase the risk of developing breast cancer *(71,72)*. This risk increases directly with the duration of treatment. The risk associated with the estrogen–progesterone combination exceeds that of estrogen alone, especially in overweight women *(72)*. Thus, in perimenopausal and postmenopausal women, hormonal replacement therapy should be recognized as an increased risk factor (RR = 1.4 at a minimum) for developing breast cancer, with the risk increasing with the duration of treatment.

SUMMARY

Breast cancer is the most common cancer in women. Despite major advances in the diagnosis and treatment of this disease, it carries significant mortality and morbidity. There are about 47 million women above the age of 40 eligible for screening mammography in the United States. Currently about half of the eligible women receive regular screening. One of the most important determinants of a woman's participation in screening is the referral from her primary care physician. Hence, women's access to primary care physicians and their physicians' mammography referral practices are critical steps in the screening and prevention of this disease.

REFERENCE

1. Landis SH, Murray T, Bolden S, et al. (1998) Cancer statistics. *CA Cancer J Clin* 48(1):6–29.
2. Fisher B, Slack NH, Bruss DM, et al. (1969) Cancer of the breast: size of neoplasms and prognosis. *Cancer* 24:1071.
3. Fisher B, Anderson S, Redmond CK, et al. (1995) Reanalysis and results after 12 years of follow-up in a randomized clinical trial comparing total mastectomy and lumpectomy with or without irradiation in the treatment of breast cancer. *N Engl J Med* 333:1456–1461.
4. Boring CC, Squires TS, Tong T, et al. (1994) Cancer statistics. *CA Cancer J Clin* 44:7.
5. Miller BA, Feur EJ, Hankey BF. (1993) Recent incidence trends for breast cancer in women and the relevance of early detection: an update. *CA Cancer J Clin* 43:27.
6. Wingo PA, Ries LAG, Giovino GA, et al. (1999) Annual Report to the nation on the status of cancer, 1973-1996, with a special section on lung cancer and tobacco smoking. *J Natl Cancer Inst* 91:675–690.
7. Wingo PA, Ries LAG, Parker SL, et al. (1998) Long-term cancer patient survival in the United States. *Cancer Epidemol Biomarkers Prev* 7:271–282 .
8. Aoki K, Kurihara M, Hayakawa N, et al. (eds.) (1992) Death Rates for Malignant Neoplasm for Selected Sites by Sex and Five-Year Age Group in 33 Countries, 1953–1957 to 1983–1887. Coop Press, University of Nagoya, Japan.

Chapter 2 / Screening for Breast Cancer   23

9. Parkin DM, Muir CS, Whelan SL, et al. (eds.) (1992) Cancer Incidence in Five Continents,. IARC Scientific Publication no. 120. Lyon: IARC; vol. 6.
10. Ries LAG, Miller BA, Hankey BF, et al. (eds.) (1994) *Seer Cancer Statistics Review, 1973–1991: Tables and Graphs.* Bethesda, USDHHS National Cancer Institute.
11. Bruzzi P, Green SB, Byar DP, et al. (1985) Estimating the population attributable risk for multiple risk factors using case-control data. *Am J Epidemiol* 122:904.
12. Boreng C, Squires T, Tong T, et al. (1994) Cancer statistics 1994. *CA Cancer J Clin* 44:18.
13. Henderson IC. Breast Cancers. In: Murphy GP, Lawerence Jr WL, Lenhard Jr RE, eds., (1995) American Cancer Society Textbook of Clinical Oncology, 2nd edition, Atlanta, GA: American Cancer Society.
14. Spratt JS, Donegan WL, Greenberg RA. Epidemology and etiology. In: Donegan WC, Spratt JS, eds., *Cancer of the Breast.* 3rd edition. Saunders, 1988, Philadelphia, PA.
15. Claus EB, Risch NJ, Thompson UD. (1990) Age of onset as an indicator of a familial risk of breast cancer. *Am J Epidemiol* 131:961.
16. Hulka BS, Stark AT. (1995) Breast cancer: cause and prevention. *Lancet* 346:883–887.
17. Kelsey JL. (1993) Breast cancer epidemiology: summary and future directions. *Epidemiol Rev* 15: 256–263.
18. MacMahon B, Cole P, Lin TM, et al. (1970) Age at first birth and breast cancer risk. *Bull WHO* 43:209.
19. Newcomb PA, Storer BE, Longnecker MP, et al. (1994) Lactation and a reduced risk of premenopausal breast cancer. *N Engl J Med* 330:81.
20. Byers T, Graham S, Rzeplca T, Marshall J. (1985) Lactation and breast cancer: evidence for a negative association in premenopausal women. *Am J Epidemiol* 121:664.
21. Brinton LA, Schaier CS, Hoover RN, et al. (1988) Menstrual factors and risk of breast cancer. *Cancer Invest* 6:245.
22. Trichopoulos D, MacMahon B, Cole P. (1972) Menopause and breast cancer risk. *J Natl Cancer Inst* 48:605.
23. Dupont WD, Page DL. (1985) Risk factors for breast cancer in women with proliferative breast disease. *N Engl J Med* 312:146.
24. Krieger N, Hiatt RA. (1992) Risk of breast cancer after benign breast diseases: variation by histologic type, degree of atypia, age at biopsy, and length of follow-up. *Am J Epidemiol* 135:619.
25. Saftlas AF, Hoover RN, Brinton LA, et al. (1991) Mammographic densities and risk of breast cancer. *Cancer* 67:2833.
26. Bernstein JL, Thompson WD, Risch N, et al. (1992) The genetic epidemiology of second primary breast cancer. *Am J Epidemiol* 136:937.
27. Brinton LA, Devesa SS. (1996) Etiology and pathogenesis of breast cancer: epidemiologic factors. In: Harris JR, Lippman ME, Morrow M, Hellman S, eds., *Diseases of the Breast.* Philadelphia: Lippincott-Raven, p. 166.
28. Fox M. (1979) On the diagnosis and treatment of breast cancer. *JAMA* 241:489.
29. Hellman S. (1994) The natural history of small breast cancers. David A. Karnofsky Memorial Lecture. *J Clin Oncol* 12:2229.
30. Koscielny S, Tubiana M, Le M, et al. (1984) Breast cancer: relationship between the size of the primary tumor and the probability of metastatic dissemination. *Br J Cancer* 49:709.
31. Koscielny S, Le M, Tubiana M. (1989) The natural history of human breast cancer: the relationship between involvement of auxiliary lymph nodes and the initiation of distant metastases. *Br J Cancer* 59:775.
32. Carter C, Allen C, Henson D. (1989) Relation of tumor size, lymph node status, and survival in 24,740 breast cancer cases. *Cancer* 63:18.

24 Part II / Screening for Breast and Gynecological Cancers

33. Brinkley D, Haybittle J. (1984) Long-term survival of women with breast cancer. *Lancet* 1:1118.
34. Collins V, Loeffler R, Tivey H. (1956) Observations on growth rates of human tumors. *Am J Roentgenol* 76:988.
35. Holland R, Veling S, Mravanac M, et al. (1985) Histologic multi-focality of Tis, T1-2 breast carcinomas. *Cancer* 56:979.
36. Handley R. (1975) Carcinoma of the breast. *Ann R Coll Surg Engl* 57–59.
37. Veronesi U, Cascinelli N, Greco M, et al. (1985) Prognosis of breast cancer patients after mastectomy and dissection of internal mammary nodes. *Ann Surgery* 202:702.
38. Haagensen C. (1986) *Diseases of the Breast*, 3rd edition. Philadelphia: WB Saunders, p. 686.
39. Warren S, Witham E. (1933) Studies on tumor metastases: the distribution of metastases in cancer of the breast. *Surg Gynecol Obstet* 57:81.
40. Saphir O, Parker M. (1941) Metastases of primary carcinoma of the breast with special reference to spleen, adrenal glands and ovaries. *Arch Surg* 42:1003.
41. Rimer BK. (1996) Breast cancer screening, In: Harris JR, Lippman ME, Morrow M, Hellman S, eds., *Diseases of the Breast*. Philadelphia: Lippincott-Raven, p. 307.
42. Leitch AM, Dodd GD, Costanza M, et al. (1997) American Cancer Society guidelines for the early detection of breast cancer: update 1997. *CA Cancer J Clin* 473:150–153.
43. Fletchers S, Black W, Harris R, et al. (1993) Report of the International Workshop on Screening for Breast Cancer. *J Natl Cancer Inst* 85:1644.
44. Baines CJ. (1994) A different view on what is known about breast screening and the Canadian National Breast Screening Study. *Cancer* 74(4):1207–1211.
45. Nystrom L, Rutquist LE, Wall S, et al. (1993) Breast cancer screening with mammography: overview of Swedish randomized trials. *Lancet* 341:973 .
46. Sickles EA, Weber WN, Galvin HB, et al. (1986) Mammographic screening: how to operate successfully at low cost. *Radiology* 160:95.
47. Swan CA, Kopans DB, McCarthy KA, et al. (1987) Practical solutions to problems of triangulation and preoperative localization of breast lesions. *Radiology* 163:577.
48. Morrison A, Brisson J, Khalid N. (1988) Breast cancer incidence and mortality in the Breast Cancer Detection Demonstration Project. *J Natl Cancer Inst* 80:1540.
49. Sox Jr HC. (1993) Preventive health services in adults. *N Eng J Med* 330:1589.
50. Foster RS, Costanza MC. (1984) Breast self-examination practices and breast cancer survival. *Cancer* 53:999.
51. Gastrin G, Miller AB, To T, et al. (1994) Incidence and mortality from breast cancer in the MA–MA Program for Breast Screening in Finland, 1973–1986. *Cancer* 73:2168.
52. Grady KE. (1992) The efficacy of breast self-examination. *J Gerontol* 47:69.
53. Champion V. (1992) The role of breast self-examination in breast cancer screening. *Cancer* 69:1985.
54. McKenna Sr RJ, Greene P, Winchester DP, et al. (1992) Breast self-examination and breast physical examination. *Cancer* 69(7):2003.
55. Foster RS, Worden JK, Costanza MC, et al. (1992) Clinical breast examination and breast self-examination. *Cancer* 69:1992.
56. Kopans DB, Meyer JE, Cohen AM, et al. (1981) Palpable breast masses: the importance of preoperative mammography. *JAMA* 246:2819.
57. Heywang-Kobranner SH. (1994) Contrast-enhanced magnetic resonance imaging of the breast. *Invest Radiol* 29:9.
58. Bassett LW, Kimme-Smith C. (1991) Breast sonography. *Am J Roentgenol* 156:449.
59. Jackson VP. (1990) The role of US in breast imaging radiology. *Radiology* 177(2):305–311.

Chapter 2 / Screening for Breast Cancer

60. Miki Y, Swensen J, Shattuck-Eidens D, et al. (1994) A strong candidate for the breast and ovarian cancer susceptibility gene BRCA 1. *Science* 266:66.
61. Wooster R, Neuhausen S, Mangion J, et al. (1994) Localization of a breast cancer susceptibility gene, BRCA 2, to chromosome 13q12-13. *Science* 265:2088.
62. Easton D, Bishop D, Ford D, et al. (1993) Genetic linkage analysis in familial breast and ovarian cancer: results from 214 families. *Am J Hum Genet* 52:678.
63. Garber JE, Smith BL. (1996) Management of the high-risk and the concerned patient. In: Harris JR, Lippman ME, Morrow M, Hellman S, eds. *Diseases of the Breast.* Philadelphia: Lippincott-Raven, pp. 327,328.
64. Biesecker B, Boehnke M, Calzone K, et al. (1993) Genetic counseling for families with inherited susceptibility to breast and ovarian cancer. *JAMA* 269:1970.
65. Lynch HT, Watson P, Conway T, et al. (1993) DNA screening for breast/ovarian cancer susceptibility based on linked markers: a family study. *Arch Intern Med* 153:1979.
66. Benjamin CM, Adam S, Wiggins S, et al. (1994) Proceed with care: direct predictive testing for Huntington disease. *Am J Hum Genet* 55:606.
67. Ostrer H, Allen W, Crandall LA, et al. (1993) Insurance and genetic testing: where are we now? *Am J Hum Genet* 552:65.
68. Clark RA. (1992) Economic issues in screening mammography. *Am J Roentgenol* 158(3):527–534.
69. Brown, ML, Fintor L. (1993) Cost effectiveness of breast cancer screening. *Breast Cancer Res Treat* 25(2):113–118.
70. Greenwald P. (1986) Cancer control objectives for the nation. *Natl Cancer Inst Monogr* 2:1.
71. Colditz GA, Hankinson SE, Hunter DJ, et al. (1995) The use of estrogens and progestins and the risk of breast cancer in postmenopausal women. *N Engl J Med* 332:1589–1593.
72. Schairer C, Lubin J, Troisi R, et al. (2000) Menopausal estrogen and estrogen-progestin replacement therapy and breast cancer risk. *JAMA* 283(4):485–491.

3 Screening for Cervical Cancer

Amreen Husain, MD
and William J. Hoskins, MD

KEY PRINCIPLES

- Cervical cancer continues to be a major health problem in the developing world, where screening is not universal.
- Exfoliative cervical cytology or the Pap test is the primary tool in screening for cervical cancer.
- The Pap smear is effective in the diagnosis of preinvasive cervical carcinoma.
- The incidence of invasive cervical carcinoma has been reduced by 75% from 1950 to 1990 as a result of cervical cancer screening.
- The Pap smear is recommended annually for all women starting at age 18 or the age at the onset of sexual activity.
- Cervical cancer is associated with human papillomavirus infection and is considered a sexually transmitted disease.
- There is a strong correlation between cervical cancer and high-risk behaviors such as multiple sexual partners and early onset of sexual activity. Immunosuppressed status confers increased risk of cervical neoplasia and more frequent screening is recommended in these patients.
- Patients with an abnormal Pap smear should be referred to a physician with expertise in colposcopy.
- Cervical cancer when diagnosed in early stages is 90% curable and such patients should be referred to a gynecologic oncologist for appropriate management.

From: *Cancer Screening: A Practical Guide for Physicians*
Edited by: K. Aziz and G. Y. Wu © Humana Press Inc., Totowa, NJ

INTRODUCTION

Cervical cancer and preinvasive neoplasia, thought to be caused by infection with human papillomavirus (HPV), is a major public health problem worldwide. In the developed world, where women have good access to health care and cancer screening, the incidence of deaths from cervical cancer has declined. In the developing world, however, cervical cancer remains one of the top causes of cancer deaths in women.

Squamous-cell carcinoma constitutes the majority of cervical cancers (90%), with the remainder being adenocarcinoma. Most of the epidemiological and screening data relates to the squamous-cell carcinoma. This chapter will review the epidemiology and pathophysiology, with an emphasis on screening techniques and mechanisms of prevention of cervical carcinoma.

EPIDEMIOLOGY

In the United States, it is estimated that in the year 2000, there will be about 12,800 new cases of invasive cervical cancer and 4600 deaths from this disease. The incidence of invasive cervical cancer has steadily declined since the 1950s, and indirect evidence suggests that this decline is the result of the institution of screening with cervical smears. From 1947 through 1984, cervical cancer mortality declined more than 70% *(1)*. Worldwide, however, cervical cancer remains one of the major causes of death among women in developing countries. In the United States, it is the seventh leading cause of cancer-related death.

The history of screening for cervical cancer dates back to the 1940s, when Dr. George Papanicoloau first proposed evaluation of the cells obtained from the cervix as a method of direct screening for cervical cancer and its precursors.

Cervical cancer is believed to result from the progression of dysplasia or cervical intraepithelial neoplasia (CIN). There is a gradient from mild to more severe grades of dysplasia. The gradient is characterized by increasing nuclear atypia and failure of cellular differentiation. Support for a continuum of the disease is based on the knowledge that cervical dysplasia is most often diagnosed among women in their 20s, carcinoma *in situ* between the ages of 25 and 35 yr, and invasive cancer after the age of 40. Because of this presumed continuum of cervical disease from CIN to invasive cancer, there is little doubt that exfoliative cytology of the Pap smear can alter rates of morbidity and mortality from cervical cancer. The best demonstration of this has been in the Scandinavian countries, where screening has been widespread and prolonged and where the institution of

Chapter 3 / Screening for Cervical Cancer 29

organized screening dramatically reduced the incidence as well as mortality from cervical cancer within 6–10 yr *(2)*.

ETIOLOGIC AGENTS

Epidemiologists and virologists now regard infection with HPV as the major risk factor for cervical cancer *(3)*. Human papillomavirus is a double-stranded DNA virus of approximately 8000 basepairs. There are over 70 types of HPV known. Human papillomavirus types 2 and 4 mainly cause skin warts, whereas types 6 and 11 are the most common agents for venereal warts (condyloma acuminata). Types 16 and, to a lesser degree, 18, 31, and 45 are predominantely considered to be associated with cancer. The vast majority of women with cervical cancer have detectable HPV DNA. A case study of 1000 cervical cancers from over 20 countries found that over 85% of these tumors tested positive for HPV types by the PCR tests *(4)*. HPV infection precedes cytologic atypia in exfoliated cervical cells and may predict the progression rate of CIN.

Other agents have been examined in the etiology of cervical cancer, and HSV2 and chlamydia have been investigated the most. The association with these two agents and cervical cancer is weak and inconsistent. Other infections that have been studied include syphilis, gonorrhea, cytomegalovirus, and Epstein–Barr virus. There has been no significant association between any of these agents and cervical cancer *(3)*.

PREDISPOSING FACTORS

The major risk factors predisposing women to the development of invasive cervical cancer are strongly correlated with sexual behavior. Numerous studies support the theory that this cancer is a sexually transmitted disease, particularly given the close association between increased sexual activity and HPV. This theory is supported further by the discovery of HPV DNA in up to 90% of squamous-cell carcinoma of the cervix.

Age

The peak incidence of cervical cancer is between 45 and 60 yr of age. Sexual activity at a younger age is one of the most consistently found risk factors for the development of cervical cancer *(5)*. Other factors that are frequently found in association and are most likely related to the age at first intercourse are a high number of sexual partners and high parity *(6)*. An important risk factor may be a short time interval between onset of menses and first sexual intercourse. Studies on intervals of less than

30 Part II / Screening for Breast and Gynecological Cancers

1 yr increased the relative risk of cervical cancer to 26.4, and the interval between 1 and 5 yr increased the relative risk to 6.9. This relative risk is probably significantly associated with multiple sexual partners. The disease is rare in societies where marriages occur at an earlier age but monogamy is more common *(7)*.

Cigaret Smoking

Studies have found cigaret smoking to be an independent risk factor for the development of invasive cervical cancer *(8)*. In most studies, the excessive risk for smokers has been found to be around twofold, with the highest risk conferred by heavy, long-term smoking. However, these studies have not adjusted for the HPV status of the patients. The specific biologic mechanisms leading to the carcinoma are unknown but may be related to the carcinogenic effect of nicotine present in cervical mucus.

Socioeconomic Status

Low socioeconomic status is often cited as a risk factor for the development of cervical cancer, although whether it is an independent factor or, more likely, associated with a higher incidence of cigaret smoking and sexual risk factors along with a lower rate of screening remains undetermined *(6–9)*.

Contraceptive Methods

The use of barrier methods of contraception may be associated with a decreased risk of cervical cancer, or this association may be related to the antiviral properties found in spermicides used in conjunction with contraception. Several studies have suggested an increased risk of cervical cancer with all contraceptive use, but the presence of confounding factors such as HPV infections continue to exist in all of these studies. There does seem to be increasing incidence of adenocarcinoma in young women, possibly associated with oral contraceptive use. A role for HPV DNA regulation by hormones has been postulated but remains unproven *(10,11)*.

BIOLOGY OF CERVICAL CANCER

Human papillomavirus plays a critical role in cervical carcinogenesis and conclusive evidence from studies has allowed investigators to define it as an oncogene. It has been demonstrated that, in turn, oncogenic subtypes of HPV encode proteins that inactivate the products of critical cellular-growth regulatory genes. Human papillomavirus DNA has been

Chapter 3 / Screening for Cervical Cancer

detected in host cells in both integrated and nonintegrated states. Invasive carcinoma almost always contains integrated viral DNA. Human papillomavirus DNA integrates and produces HPV E6 and E7 proteins which participate in the processes of immortalization and transformation of the host cell to a malignant cell.

An important property of the E6 and E7 oncoproteins, as they are called, is their biochemical interactions with tumor-suppressor gene products. Both have been shown to bind the retinoblastoma gene product and the P53 gene product. Inactivation of these genes by HPV-produced proteins probably disrupts control of cellular proliferation and this furthers the malignant transformation process (Fig. 1) *(12–14)*.

PATHOGENESIS AND DIAGNOSIS OF PREINVASIVE LESIONS OF THE CERVIX

Squamous Lesions

The normal squamous epithelium consists of a basal layer with palisading cells that have small uniform nuclei and three to four layers of parabasal cells that undergo occasional mitosis. Most of the squamous lesions arise from the transformation zone, which is the junction between the normal columnar epithelium and the squamous metaplasia.

Cervical intraepithelial neoplasia is a spectrum of intraepithelial changes. The severity of these lesions is based on alterations in the cellular maturation, cellular organization, polarity, nuclear features, and mitotic activity. Worsening grades of CIN (1–3) are defined by the thickness of the epithelium occupied by cytologically abnormal cells and invasive cancer by the extension of abnormal cells beyond the basement membrane (Fig. 2A–D). In an effort to standardize the reporting of cervical cytology, the Bethesda system was introduced in 1988. This system introduced the cytologic terms "low-grade" and "high-grade" squamous intraepithelial lesion (LSIL and HSIL) (Table 1) *(15)*.

Glandular Lesions

Glandular lesions arise in the mucin-producing endocervical glands of the cervix. Current classification of these lesions includes endocervical glandular dysplasia, adenocarcinoma *in situ*, and microinvasive and invasive adenocarcinoma. To date, premalignant changes have not been well defined. In adenocarcinoma *in situ* the dominant abnormalities are cytological while the general characteristics of the endocervical epithelium are retained, making these lesions difficult to identify and making it hard to distinguish *in situ* from early invasive cancers. There has been an increase in the incidence of cervical adenocarcinoma, and

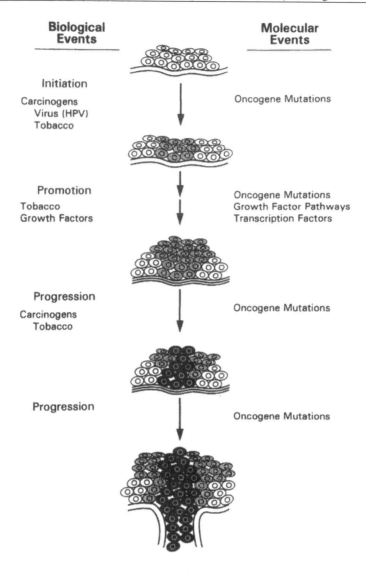

Fig. 1. Multistage model for the development of cervical carcinoma. (From ref. *14*.)

worldwide registries have reported an absolute increase in the incidence of invasive adenocarcinoma in women aged 35 or younger *(16–19)*.

SCREENING

Papanicolaou Smear

The Pap smear has proven to be the most efficacious and cost-effective method for cervical cancer screening *(20)*. Traditional cervical

Chapter 3 / Screening for Cervical Cancer 33

cancer control programs rely on Pap smear screening and destruction or surgical removal of histopathologically verified neoplastic lesions. Pap screening, however, has a sensitivity of 50–60% and a specificity of 90%, and thus can lead to overtreatment or failed screening.

One of the most controversial issues regarding cervical cancer screening relates to the frequency of screening. Studies have shown a decreased relative risk in patients screened within 3–5 yr with a single negative cervical smear. The degree of protection is even greater after two negative smears *(21–23)*. Currently, the American College of Obstetricians and Gynecologists recommend that all women who have been sexually active or who have reached 18 yr of age should undergo an annual Pap test and pelvic examination. After a woman has had three or more consecutive, satisfactory, annual cytological examinations with normal findings, the Pap test may be performed less frequently in a low-risk woman at the discretion of her physician *(24)*. The American Cancer Society screening recommendations suggest that asymptomatic low-risk women 20 yr of age and older and those under 20 yr of age who are sexually active have a Pap smear performed annually for two consecutive years, at least one every 3 yr, until the age of 65 *(25)*.

Studies on the natural history of cervical cancer suggest that not all cervical neoplasia progress from dysplasia to invasive carcinoma (*see* Algorithm 1). Cervical dysplasia indicates morphologic changes in the cells of the squamous epithelium of the cervix. The thickness of the epithelium involved determines the degree of dysplasia as mild, moderate, or severe. Carcinoma *in situ* indicates the involvement of the full thickness of the epithelium by neoplastic cells. When there is an invasion by malignant cells beyond the epithelial basement membrane, the neoplasia is classified as invasive cancer. There is a very high percentage of spontaneous regression of cytologic atypia. The risk of progression to carcinoma *in situ* and invasive cancer from low-grade dysplasia is relatively small (11 and 1%, respectively). However, the rate of progression to invasive carcinoma is higher with high-grade lesions (5 and 15%) *(26)* (Table 2).

HPV Typing

There is controversy as to whether testing for specific papillomavirus DNA can increase the efficiency of screening for lesions that are more likely to progress to invasive cancer. Low-risk HPV types, which are 6, 11, 42, 43, and 44, are found principally in benign condyloma or low-grade dysplasia, whereas high-risk HPV subtypes, 16, 18, 31, 33, 35, 39, 45, 51, 52, 56, and 58, are found mainly in high-grade dysplasia and invasive cancers. The current role of HPV testing, however, is as an

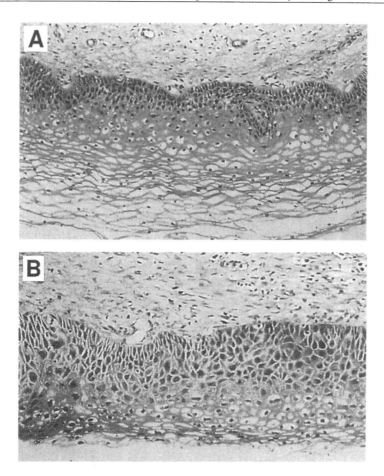

Fig. 2. (A) Normal squamous epithelium; (B) low-grade dyplasia (CIN 1).

adjunct diagnostic tool that occasionally helps in the management of equivocal lesions.

Cervicography

Cervicography is a photographic screening technique in which a 35-mm photo is taken of the cervix after staining with acetic acid. Studies have found cervicography to be more sensitive but significantly less specific than cytologic screening.

MANAGEMENT OF THE ABNORMAL PAP SMEAR

A patient with an abnormal Pap smear should be referred to a trained gynecologist or a physician trained in the use of colposcopy.

Chapter 3 / Screening for Cervical Cancer 35

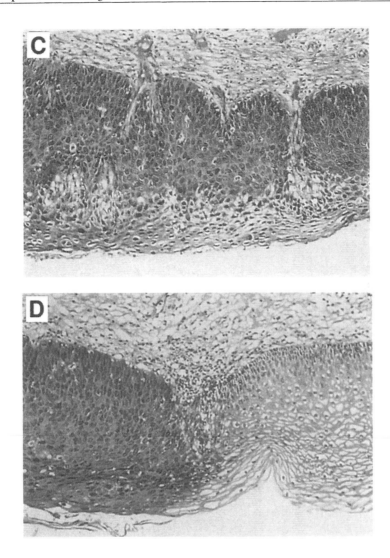

Fig. 2. (C) Moderate dysplasia (CIN 2); **(D)** carcinoma *in situ* (CIN 3/CIS).

Colposcopy

The colposcope is an instrument used to magnify and examine the transformation zone of the cervix to identify abnormal areas warranting biopsy. A patient with an abnormal Pap smear should undergo colposcopy using acetic acid and colposcopically directed biopsies of lesions and endocervical sampling to evaluate the endocervical canal. The goals of any clinician dealing with an abnormal Pap smear are twofold: (1) to identify any occult, invasive cancer and (2) to determine the extent of

Table 1

The 1991 Bethesda System

Adequacy of the specimen
 Satisfactory for evaluation
 Satisfactory for evaluation but limited by (specify reason)
 Unsatisfactory for evaluation (specify reason)
General categorization (optional)
 Within normal limits
 Benign cellular changes: *see* descriptive diagnosis
 Epithelial cell abnormality: *see* descriptive diagnosis
Descriptive diagnoses
 Benign cellular changes
  Infection
   Trichomonas vaginalis
    Fungal organisms morphologically consistent with *Candida* spp
   Predominance of *Coccobacilli* consistent with shift in vaginal flora
   Bacteria morphologically consistent with *Actinomyces* spp
   Cellular changes associated with herpes simplex virus
   Other
    Reactive changes
     Reactive cellular changes associated with:
      Inflammation (includes typical repair)
      Atrophy with inflammation (atrophic vaginitis)
      Radiation
      Intrauterine contraceptive device (IUD)
      Other
Epithelial cell abnormalities
 Squamous cell
  Atypical squamous cells of undetermined significance: qualify[a]
  Low-grade squamous intraepithelial lesion encompassing HPV[b], mild
   dysplasia
  High-grade squamous intraepithelial lesion encompassing moderate and
   severe dysplasia, CIS/CIN II, and CIN III
  Squamous-cell carcinoma
 Glandular cell
  Endometrial cells, cytologically benign, in a postmenopausal woman
  Atypical glandular cells of undetermined significance: qualify[a]
  Endocervical adenocarcinoma
  Endometrial adenocarcinoma
  Extrauterine adenocarcinoma
  Adenocarcinoma, NOS
Other malignant neoplasms: specify hormonal evaluation (applies to
 vaginal smears only)
  Hormonal pattern compatible with age and history
  Hormonal pattern incompatible with age and history: specify
  Hormonal evaluation not possible because of (specify)

Chapter 3 / Screening for Cervical Cancer

Table 1 *(continued)*

HPV, human papillomavirus; CIN, cervical intraepithelial neoplasia; NOS, not otherwise specified.

[a] Atypical squamous or glandular cells of undetermined significance should be further qualified as to whether a reactive or a premalignant/malignant process is favored.

[b] Cellular changes of HPV (previously termed koliocytosis, koliocytotic atypia, or condylomatous atypia) are included in the category of low-grade squamous intraepithelial lesion.

Source: ref. *15*.

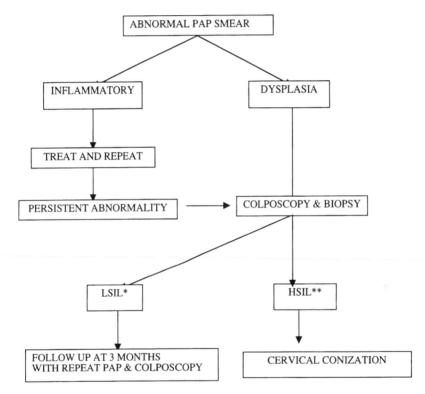

Algorithm 1. Screening algorithm. *, Low-grade squamous intraepithelial lesion; **, high-grade squamous intraepithelial lesion.

the abnormality and to treat, if treatment is likely to decrease the chance of developing cervical cancer in the future.

The acetic acid serves to dehydrate cells and reveals "aceto-white epithelium" that results from piling up of cells with an increased nuclear–cytoplasm ratio. The main criteria to establish the degree of atypia and identify sites for biopsy are (1) vascular patterns, (2) intensity of aceto-white areas, and (3) sharpness of borders of suspicious areas.

Table 2
Natural History of Squamous Intraepithelial Lesions at 24-mo Follow-up

Cytology	Regression	Progression	Cancer
ASCUS[a]	68%	7%	0.25%
LGSIL[b]	47%	21%	0.15%
HGSIL[c]	35%	23%	1.4%

[a]Atypical squamous cells of undetermined significance.
[b]Low-grade squamous intraepithelial lesion.
[c]High-grade squamous intraepithelial lesion.
Source: ref. 27.

Further evaluation by staining with iodine using Lugol's or Schiller's solution can be performed. Abnormal areas show mustard yellow staining or a mottled appearance compared to the deep mahogany of normal epithelium. Colposcopy of the cervix is a careful inspection under magnification and careful evaluation of the cervical squamo-columnar transformation zone, where most abnormalities are likely to be found.

TREATMENT OPTIONS

All methods of treatment for cervical neoplasia are nearly equivalent, and 90–95% of patients are successfully cured by these methods. Biopsy is successful and curative in patients with small, low-grade lesions that are entirely visualized by colposcopy. An inadequate colposcopic examination, however, is an indication for further evaluation. Colposcopy is considered inadequate if the following criteria exist:

1. The transformation zone is not fully visualized.
2. A visible lesion extends into the endocervical canal.
3. An endocervical lesion is suspected based on abnormal endocervical sampling.
4. There is discordance of more than one grade in other diagnostic evaluations.

If colposcopy is considered inadequate, cervical conization is generally indicated. Cervical conization can be performed by a number of methods, including loop electro-excision procedures, laser conization, and cold-knife conization. The choice of method depends on the size of the lesion, the size of the transformation zone, the extent of the abnormality suspected, and physician preference. Cryotherapy is an ablative therapy used to treat cervical dysplasia. Since the advent of loop electro-

Chapter 3 / Screening for Cervical Cancer 39

excision, its role has decreased, but cryotherapy remains an option for the treatment of patients with a satisfactory colposcopic examination, a negative endocervical margin, and persistent low-grade dysplasia.

Micro-invasive and early-stage cervical cancers are highly curable, and such patients should be referred to a trained gynecologic oncologist for surgical treatment or conservative management when appropriate.

CERVICAL NEOPLASIA AND HIV

Human immunodeficiency virus (HIV) and acquired immunodeficiency syndrome (AIDS) in women are becoming a worldwide public health issue, and the occurrence of cervical neoplasia in this group of women presents a particular challenge to the clinician. In 1993, the Centers for Disease Control classified cervical cancer as an AIDS-defining illness. Immunodeficiency predisposes women to the development of neoplasia, and immunosuppressed patients such as renal transplant patients are known to be at high risk for cervical dysplasia. Women who are HIV-positive have as much as a 10-fold increased rate of abnormal cytology *(16)* and this rate appears to increase with decreasing CD4 counts *(17)*.

Screening strategies in HIV-positive women must take into account the high prevalence of cervical dysplasia, the higher grade of dysplasia encountered, and the rapid progression of the disease in this group of women. Several studies have highlighted a higher discordance rate between cytology and histology in the HIV-positive women, and many authors recommend baseline colposcopy and frequent evaluation of cervical cytology in these women *(18)*. Furthermore, a more aggressive and a "see-and-treat" approach may be warranted in this group of women *(27)*.

The treatment of preinvasive cervical disease in HIV-infected women is often challenging to the practitioner. There is an increased incidence of treatment failures and standard therapies such as cryotherapy, laser therapy, cone biopsy, and loop excision have been shown to have a recurrence rate of 40–60%. The following treatment guidelines have been developed for treating HIV-infected women with cervical neoplasia:

1. Baseline colposcopy.
2. Pap smear every 6 mo.
3. Excision is preferred over ablative therapy.
4. Indications for conization are similar in HIV-positive and HIV-negative women.
5. Aggressive follow-up and liberal use of colposcopy.
6. Aggressive retreatment for persistent or recurrent disease.

GENETIC TESTING

Cervical cancer is etiologically associated with HPV and multiple environmental host factors. No genetically determined cause for cervical cancer has been identified to date and only a few anecdotal reports of familial clusters of cervical cancer have been described.

FUTURE DIRECTIONS

In order to improve the sensitivity of cervical cytologic screening, several new technologies have evolved. These address the false-negative rate by automatic rescreening of negative Pap smears and by optimizing the collection and preparation of cells.

Automated Cytologic Screening

Automated cytologic screening involves computerized instrumentation for the analysis of conventionally prepared cervical smears. Currently, there are two Food and Drug Administration (FDA) approved tests: PAPNET7 (Neuromedical Systems, Suffern, NY) and AutoPap 300 QC7 (NeoPath, Redmond, WA). They have been approved for rescreening of previous manually screened Pap smears. AutoPap and PAPNET have been found to be sevenfold more sensitive in detecting missed abnormalities, as compared to manual rescreening. Neither of these systems, however, has been currently approved for primary screening.

Fluid-Based Technology

Fluid-based technology (monolayers) changes the method by which cells are collected and processed. Two systems are currently available for monolayer cervical cytologic screening, but only ThinPrep7 (Cytyc Corporation, Boxborough, MA) has been FDA approved. The other system, CytoRich7 (AutoCyte, Burlington, NC), is being studied currently. In collecting specimens with ThinPrep, the cells are rinsed from a collection brush into a vial solution. After processing, the cells are touch-transferred onto a glass slide and stained. The clinical trials of monolayers as compared to the conventional smear have shown that they have a concordance rate of over 90%. ThinPrep has been found to increase detection of premalignant lesions while improving specimen adequacy *(28,29)*.

SUMMARY

The incidence of cervical cancer has declined in the developed countries of the world because of easy access to health care and widespread

Chapter 3 / Screening for Cervical Cancer 41

implementation of screening programs. There remain, however, large segments of the population who do not undergo regular screening. Future directions in cervical cancer screening should include efforts to include of the entire population at risk.

REFERENCES

1. Devesa SS, Silverman DT, Young JJ, et al. (1987) Cancer incidence and trends among whites in the United States, 1947–1984. *J Natl Cancer Inst* 79(4):701–770.
2. Christopherson WM, Parker JE, Mendez WM, et al. (1970) Cervix cancer death rates and mass cytologic screening. *Cancer* 26:808.
3. Brinton LA, Hoover RN. (1997) In: Hoskins WJ, Perez CA, Young RC, eds., *Epidemiology of Gynecologic Cancers, in Principles and Practice of Gynecologic Oncology*, 2nd edition. Philadelphia: Lippincott-Raven.
4. Bosch FX, Manos MM, Munoz N, et al. (1995) Human papillomavirus in cervical cancer: a worldwide perspective. *J Natl Cancer Inst* 87:796.
5. Herrero R, Brinton LA, Reeves WC, et al. (1990) Sexual behavior, venereal diseases, hygiene practices and invasive cervical cancer in a high-risk population. *Cancer* 65(2):380–386.
6. Brinton LA, Hamman RF, Huggins GR, et al. (1987) Sexual reproductive risk factors for invasive squamous-cell cervical cancer. *J Natl Cancer Inst* 79(1):23–30.
7. Peters RK, Thomas D, Hagan DG, et al. (1986) Risk factors for invasive cervical cancer among Latinos and non-Latinos in Los Angeles County. *J Natl Cancer Inst* 77(5):1063–1077.
8. Winkelstein WJ. (1990) Smoking and cervical cancer-current status: a review. *Am J Epidemiol* 131(6):945–950.
9. Bosch FX, Munoz M, de Sanjose S, et al. (1992) Risk factors for cervical cancer in Colombia and Spain. *Int J Cancer* 52(5):750–758.
10. Sawaya GF, Berlin M. (1996) Epidemiology of Cervical Neoplasia In: Rubin SE, Hoskins WJ, eds. *Cervical Cancer and Preinvasive Neoplasia*. Philadelphia: Lippincott-Raven.
11. Pater A, Bayatpour M, Pater MM. (1990) Oncogenic transformation by human papillomavirus type 16 deoxyribonucleic acid in the presence of progesterone or progestins from oral contraceptives. *Am J Obstet Gynecol* 162:1099.
12. Munger K, Werness BA, Dyson N, et al. (1989) Complex formation of human papillomavirus E7 proteins with the retinoblastoma tumor suppressor gene product. *EMBO J* 8:4099.
13. Werness BA, Levine AJ, Howley PM. (1990) Association of human papillomavirus types 16 and 18 E6 proteins with p53. *Science* 248:76.
14. Parker M, Sausville E, Birrer M. (1997) Basic biology and biochemistry of gynecological cancer. In: Hoskins WJ, Perez CA, Young RC, eds. *Principles and Practice of Gynecologic Oncology*. 2nd edition. Philadelphia: Lippincott-Raven, pp. 61–86.
15. Broders S. (1992) Report of the 1991 Bethesda Workshop. *JAMA* 267:1892.
16. Chilvers C, Mant D, Pike MC. (1987) Cervical adenocarcinoma and oral contraceptives. *Br Med J* 295:1446.
17. Eide TJ. (1987) Cancer of the uterine cervix in Norway by histologic type, 1970–1984. *J Natl Cancer Inst* 79:199.
18. Parazzini F, LaVecchia C. (1990) Epidemiology of adenocarcinoma of the cervix. *Gynecol Oncol* 39:40.

42 **Part II** / Screening for Breast and Gynecological Cancers

19. Schwartz SM, Weiss NS. (1986) Increased incidence of adenocarcinoma of the cervix in young women in the United States. *Am J Epidemiol* 124:1045.
20. Guzick DS. (1978) Efficacy of screening for cervical cancer: A review. *Am J Public Health* 68:125.
21. Clarke EA, Anderson TW. (1979) Does screening by "Pap" smears help prevent cervical cancer? A case-control study. *Lancet* 2:1.
22. La Vecchia C, Franceschi S, Decarli A, et al. (1984) Pap smear and the risk of cervical neoplasia. Quantitative estimates from a case-control study. *Lancet* 2:779.
23. Olesen F. (1988) A case-control study of cervical cytology before diagnosis of cervical cancer in Denmark. *Int J Epidemiol* 17:501.
24. American College of Obstetrics and Gynecology. (1995) Committee opinion: recommendations on frequency of Pap test screening. *Int J Gynaecol Obstet* 49:210.
25. Wingo, PA, Tong T, Bolden S. (1995) Cancer statistics, 1995. *CA Cancer J Clin* 45(1):8–30.
26. Maiman M, Fruchter RG. (1996) Cervical neoplasia and the human immunodeficiency virus. In: Rubin SC, Hoskins WJ, eds. *Cervical Cancer and Preinvasive Neoplasia.* Philadelphia: Lippincott-Raven.
27. Diaz-Rosario LA, Kabawat SE. (1999) Performance of a fluid-based thin-layer Papiancolaou smear method in the clinical setting of an independent laboratory and an outpatient screening population in New England. *Arch Pathol Lab Med* 123:817–821.
28. Lee KR, Ashfaq R, Birdsong GG, et al. (1997) Comparison of conventional papanicolau smears and a fluid-based, thin-layer system for cervical cancer screening. *Obstet Gynecol* 90:278–284.
29. Melnikow J, Nuovo J, Willan AR, et al. (1998) Natural history of cervical squamous intraepithelial lesions: a meta-analysis. *Obstet Gynecol* 92:727–735.

4 Screening for Ovarian Cancer

Beth E. Nelson, MD
and Allan R. Mayer, DO

KEY PRINCIPLES

- Ovarian cancer is the most common cause of death from gynecological cancer in women.
- The majority of the patients are diagnosed at an advanced stage, with significant mortality and morbidity.
- Several risk factors have been identified and include old age, personal history of other cancers, reproductive risk factors, and family history.
- Recently, several genetic abnormalities are found that are linked to breast and ovarian cancer.
- Screening for ovarian cancer is controversial and, at present, screening is not recommended for the general population.
- Screening should be offered to women who are at high risk of developing ovarian cancer.

INTRODUCTION

Epithelial ovarian cancer is the fifth most common malignancy in women and is the most common cause of death from gynecologic cancer. Every year in the United States 25,200 women are diagnosed with ovarian cancer and 14,500 succumb to this illness *(1)*. Because approx 60% of women are diagnosed at advanced Stage (III or IV), improved methods of early detection or screening should result in improved survival statistics *(2)*. Successful screening depends on the appropriate identification of a high-risk group, the ability to detect an early or

From: *Cancer Screening: A Practical Guide for Physicians*
Edited by: K. Aziz and G. Y. Wu © Humana Press Inc., Totowa, NJ

44 Part II / Screening for Breast and Gynecological Cancers

preclinical stage of the disease for which effective treatment is available as well as the existence of an appropriate test that is accurate, inexpensive, safe and acceptable to the patients. This chapter will investigate whether ovarian cancer as a disease entity meets these criteria and the manner in which the available screening tests may be applied.

EPIDEMIOLOGY

Risk factors for ovarian cancer include Caucasian race, older age, residence in an industrialized country, Jewish heritage, family history of ovarian cancer, personal or family history of breast, endometrial, or colon cancer, nulliparity, and other reproductive risk factors. Additional possible risk factors include the use of fertility drugs, the use of talcum powder, and a high-fat diet. Reproductive risk factors can be summarized by assessing the ovulatory years—the time period from menarche to menopause during which a woman is experiencing regular ovulation *(3)*. Thus, the duration of all pregnancies, breast-feeding, and the use of oral contraceptive pills would be subtracted from the total time period of ovulation. The greater the duration of ovulation, the greater the risk for ovarian cancer. Oral contraceptives exert a protective effect, reducing the risk of ovarian cancer by 40–50%, presumably by reducing the number of ovulatory cycles *(4,5)*. Tubal ligation and hysterectomy are associated with decreased risks, possibly because the ovaries of these women have been "screened" through visual inspection at the time of surgery *(6)*. Others have used these data in support of the theory of ascending pathogens. Bilateral oophorectomy at the time of hysterectomy also reduces the likelihood of developing ovarian cancer *(7–9)*, although primary peritoneal cancer is well documented following oophorectomy and cancer may also occur in residual ovary syndrome in which the ovary is inadvertently incompletely resected *(10–12)*.

Risk for ovarian cancer clearly increases with age. At age 40, the risk is 15.7 per 100,000 and increases to 54 per 100,000 by age 75 *(13)*. Approximately one-third of affected women are over age 65 at the time of diagnosis. In the group of women with a hereditary syndrome, the disease occurs approx 10 yr earlier than the average age of 59–62, developing between the ages of 45 and 50 *(14)*.

Family history appears to be among the most important risk factors. The lifetime risk of ovarian cancer for the 'average' American woman with no family history of breast or ovarian cancer is about 1 in 70 or 1.5%. For a woman with one first-degree relative with ovarian cancer, the lifetime risk increases to approx 4%. If two first-degree relatives are

Chapter 4 / Screening for Ovarian Cancer

affected, this risk is about 8%. For a family with a true genetic syndrome, which is inherited in an autosomal dominant fashion, the lifetime risk for a female family member is approx 40–50% because of incomplete penetrance. Mutations in BRCA1 and 2 genes have been identified, which confirm a genetic basis for increased risk for ovarian and breast cancer. It is important to recognize that the genetic abnormality may be inherited from either mother or father. The three major recognized syndromes are the Breast–Ovarian Cancer syndrome, conferred by mutations in the BRCA 1 gene on chromosome 17q12-21, which may result in familial breast and/or ovarian cancers, the site-specific Ovarian syndrome, probably also resulting from BRCA1, and Hereditary Nonpolyposis Colorectal Cancer syndrome (HNPCC). The BRCA2 gene, on chromosome 13q12-13, has now been linked to breast and ovarian cancer and particularly to male breast cancer. Women with mutations in BRCA1 have a lifetime incidence of ovarian cancer of approx 45%, and those with BRCA2 mutations, about 25% *(15)*. Families with HNPCC, formerly termed Lynch Syndrome II, show an overabundance of ovarian, colon, breast, and endometrial cancers as well as some less frequent malignancies. HNPCC is related to inherited mutations in the MLH1, PMS2, MSH2, MSH3, and MSH6 genes *(16)*. Despite recent advances in molecular diagnosis, inherited causes of ovarian cancer appear to account for only 5–10% of cases. Of these women with inherited ovarian cancer, it has been estimated that mutations in BRCA1 account for 76–100% of cases, whereas those in BRCA2 account for 10–35%, and those in HNPCC genes, 10–15% *(17)*. It has recently been reported that the reduction in risk conferred by the use of oral contraceptives also applies to women with an inherited genetic risk *(15,18)*.

The risk of developing ovarian cancer is elevated for a woman with a personal history of certain cancers, in some cases because of shared risk factors. Women with a past history of breast or colon cancer are at increased risk. Most women with endometrial cancer undergo bilateral oophorectomy as part of their primary therapy, but if not, these women also face heightened risk of ovarian cancer.

Fertility drugs, particularly clomiphene, have been associated with a possible increased risk of both invasive ovarian cancer and ovarian tumors of low malignant potential *(19,20)*. Early studies had some methodological problems, including lack of information about specific drugs. Current studies suggest that the primary at-risk group may be those women who are unable to conceive even with drug therapy *(21)*.

The data regarding postmenopausal use of estrogen replacement are conflicting, with a relative risk of developing ovarian cancer ranging from 0.6 to 2.5, but it is generally held that the risk of ovarian cancer is not increased by postmenopausal estrogen. A recent meta-analysis including nine studies concluded that prolonged use of hormone replacement therapy (HRT) for greater than 10 yr may be associated with a slight increased risk of ovarian cancer (odds ratio 1.27) *(22)*.

PATHOPHYSIOLOGY

The primary theory of ovarian cancer pathogenesis is termed *incessant ovulation*—essentially, the monthly ovulation occurring in the nonpregnant reproductive-age woman. Epithelial ovarian cancer, the most common ovarian malignancy, derives from the surface epithelium of the ovary. It is this epithelium that ovulation disrupts each month. The presence of invaginations in the ovarian surface and inclusion cysts has been well documented and they are believed to result from ovulation *(23)*. Researchers hypothesize that healing following this disruption results in both angiogenesis and metaplasia on the ovarian surface, both of which may be fertile sites for carcinogenesis.

A second and possibly interrelated theory holds that ascending carcinogens may enter the peritoneal cavity via the vagina. The female pelvis is essentially open to the outside environment by way of the vagina, the uterine cavity, and then the fallopian tubes. Talc exposure has been variably related to ovarian cancer risk *(24,25)*. Particles of talc and asbestos have been demonstrated in the ovarian epithelium and within cancers *(26)*. Although this is not proof of etiology, it certainly lends support to this theory, as does the finding of reduction in ovarian cancer cases among women with tubal ligation or hysterectomy with preservation of ovaries.

Because epithelial ovarian cancer arises on the ovarian surface, the most common route of spread is via direct extension to the peritoneal cavity. Because the ovarian surface epithelium shares a common embryologic origin with the peritoneum, it is possible that peritoneal involvement occurs simultaneously with ovarian tumor development, rather than as a metastatic site. Although the data are not yet conclusive, genetic studies have suggested that primary peritoneal carcinoma may be multifocal, whereas ovarian carcinoma is unifocal in origin *(27–29)*. Once malignant cells are present within the peritoneal fluid, they are spread by the normal, clockwise circulation of peritoneal fluid, with the highest concentration of tumor deposits along the right pericolic gutter and diaphragm. Very commonly, the omentum, bowel surface, liver or splenic surface, and pelvic peritoneum are involved. Ascites frequently develops, probably as a result of secretions by cancer cells but also

Chapter 4 / Screening for Ovarian Cancer

because of decreased absorption of fluid by the tumor-coated right diaphragm. Development of a pleural effusion frequently occurs as well, although solid metastasis to the lung, liver parenchyma, bone, or brain is less common.

Symptoms at presentation typically relate to digestive disturbances caused by ascites or tumor spread to the omentum or bowel surface. Patients frequently have vague gastrointestinal symptoms and are often falsely reassured or may begin a gastrointestinal (GI) workup entailing weeks or months of testing before a pelvic exam is performed. A rectovaginal pelvic exam by an experienced clinician should be among the first evaluations in any woman with vague digestive symptoms. Early-stage disease, when the tumor is confined to the ovary, often produces no symptoms unless the patient is able to appreciate a mass or it is discovered serendipitously on routine pelvic exam. If ascites or a pelvic mass are appreciated on examination, imaging studies such as ultrasound and/or computed tomography can aid in further diagnosis. CA 125, a glycoprotein serum tumor marker, is elevated in 83% of advanced-stage cases, but only 25–50% of stage I and II cancers (30).

Primary treatment includes surgery and usually chemotherapy (31). Ovarian cancer is arguably the only malignancy in which cytoreduction (the surgical attempt to remove a maximum amount of tumor) is beneficial even with widespread disease. It is well substantiated that the more tumor that is removed, at both the primary and metastatic sites, the better the prognosis (32). In all but the earliest cases, chemotherapy with platinum and a taxane is recommended. Carcinomas of the fallopian tube and peritoneum are histologically identical to ovarian cancer and are delineated from ovarian cancer by anatomical factors, including the presence, degree, and type of ovarian involvement as well as exact findings within the fallopian tube. Tubal and peritoneal carcinomas in women share the same treatment and natural history as ovarian carcinoma. A description of stages and survival by stage is noted in Table 1.

RATIONALE FOR SCREENING

Approximately 25,000 American women are diagnosed with ovarian cancer annually. Of these, 60%, or about 15,000, are found to have Stage III or IV disease. Only 30% of these, or approx 4500, will survive 5 yr. If a screening test were available that could shift the stage at diagnosis to Stage I in 70%, with a 5-yr survival rate of 90%, nearly four times as many, or 15,750 women, would live to 5 yr. Clearly, detection of a premalignant precursor is optimal. This is best illustrated by one of the most successful cancer screening programs, the Papanicolau smear, in

Table 1

Incidence and Survival by Stage

Stage		Incidence	Survival
I	Confined to the ovaries	24%	90%
II	Extension to pelvic organs	9%	70%
III	Extension to abdomen or nodes	61%	28%
IV	Extension to liver parenchyma, lungs		

Source: ref. *1*.

which detection and treatment of cervical dysplasia has reduced the incidence and mortality of cervical cancer. Unfortunately, it is unclear that such a precursor exists in ovarian cancer. At present, borderline ovarian tumors (tumors of low malignant potential) are commonly believed to have a distinct pathogenesis from invasive epithelial cancers, although one study of mutations of the K-ras proto-oncogene reveals a similar pattern in both borderline and invasive ovarian cancers, suggesting a relationship *(33)*. However, several authors have documented what has been termed *ovarian dysplasia* with architectural abnormalities and cytologic atypia in twin sisters of women with ovarian cancer, in women undergoing prophylactic oophorectomy because of a strong family history, and in the opposite ovary or adjacent to the malignant epithelium of early ovarian cancers *(23,34–37)*.

SCREENING METHODS

The most important step in screening may be to obtain an accurate, detailed family history encompassing both maternal and paternal relatives and extending back at least three generations. It is important to get a sense of the number of female relatives, because in small families, a genetic inheritance pattern may not be as obvious as in large families. Patients should be specifically queried about ovarian, breast, uterine, and colon cancers, including breast and colon cancers in both male and female relatives. Cases of abdominal cancer, female cancer, and stomach cancer, may or may not refer to ovarian cancer. Pathology reports should be sought for family members seemingly afflicted, for confirmatory purposes prior to embarking on what may be a long, expensive, and invasive series of tests. However, in a study of 116 ovarian cancer patients who underwent genetic testing, the 12 patients with germline mutations in BRCA1 or 2, MSH2, or MLH1 did not have highly suggestive family histories *(38)*. Although family history may guide us in selecting candidates for screening, family history is frequently inaccurate and may require research on the part of the patient.

Chapter 4 / Screening for Ovarian Cancer

Pelvic Examination

Yearly, bimanual, and rectovaginal pelvic exams in reproductive-age women are important for many reasons such as assessment of contraceptive needs, cytologic screening for cervical cancer, sexually transmitted disease screening, and ovarian/adnexal assessment. However, pelvic exam alone is a poor screening test for ovarian cancer because of the inability to detect a cancer prior to extraovarian spread in most cases. Because of the epithelial surface site at which ovarian cancer develops, spread to the peritoneal cavity is likely to be an early event in many cases, probably before an abnormality is detected even by an experienced gynecologist.

CA 125

In a recent ovarian cancer screening study utilizing pelvic exam and CA 125 for the initial screening technique, with ultrasound of women with abnormal results, in 2623 healthy, asymptomatic women (57% were perimenopausal or postmenopausal), 1.5% were found to have abnormal adnexae on the bimanual exam *(39)*. Among these 40 women, ultrasound revealed normal findings in 45%, uterine fibroids in 33%, and abnormal ovaries in 22%. All of the ovarian abnormalities were benign, with no cases of ovarian cancer detected. Seventy-nine women had elevated CA 125 levels at the initial screening. One woman with a CA 125 elevation but normal pelvic exam and ultrasound developed ovarian cancer during the first year of follow-up, detected by a further rise in CA 125.

CA 125 is a glycoprotein serum tumor marker originally described in 1983 by Bast et al. *(30)*. Although elevated in 83% of advanced ovarian cancers, it is only elevated in 23–50% of Stage I and II cancers. Frequently, other benign and malignant conditions are associated with elevated values, as outlined in Table 2. One of the initial screening studies utilizing CA 125 was a case control study involving the JANUS serum bank *(40)*. Between 1974 and 1986, 39,300 women were registered in the bank, of which 105 developed ovarian cancer and were matched with 323 controls. Among controls, 4.6% had CA 125 values over 35 U/mL. In comparison, at 60 mo prior to diagnosis, 15% of cases had elevations, which increased to 33% by 18 mo prior to diagnosis. Subsequently, the same investigator prospectively screened 1082 women, of whom 36 had abnormal CA 125 results *(41)*. The CA 125 doubled in two women, and this elevation was sustained in the only patient who was found to have ovarian cancer. Another study of 1010 asymptomatic postmenopausal women reported a specificity of 97% for CA 125 screening, however, 75 false-positive elevations were noted for

Table 2
Frequency of CA 125 Elevation and Causation

Disease state	% >35 U/mL
Benign	
Healthy	1
First-trimester pregnancy	16
Pelvic inflammatory disease	10
Leiomyoma	4
Cirrhosis	70
Pericarditis	70
Endometriosis	54
Malignancies	
Ovarian Stage I/II	23–50
Stage III/IV	83
Pancreatic	59
Lung	32
Colorectal	23
Other GI	27
Other non-GI	25
Breast	12

every case of ovarian cancer detected *(42)*. In a prospective cohort study of 22,000 women, subjects with a CA 125 level over 30 U/mL were 35.9 times more likely to develop ovarian cancer within 1 yr as compared to women with CA 125 values under 30 U/mL *(43)*. It has been suggested that the rate of rise of CA 125, in addition to the absolute value, may be indicative of cancer development. Incorporation of this parameter into the screening algorithm may reduce the false-positives and improve the sensitivity *(44)*. Many other tumor markers have been studied with the intent to identify a complementary marker, which would decrease the false-positive rate of screening with CA 125 alone or offer a more cost-effective test than ultrasound. Unfortunately, none has yet been confirmed *(45)*. Because of the low percentage of early-stage cancers with elevated CA 125, this test alone is insufficient for screening, as the goal is detection of early-stage disease.

Ultrasonography

At the present time, ultrasound is the optimal imaging technique for visualization of the ovaries and has been extensively studied as a screening modality since the late 1980s *(42,46)*. Transvaginal scans are superior to transabdominal scans for ovarian assessment and are quite

Chapter 4 / Screening for Ovarian Cancer　　　　　　　　**51**

tolerable for most women *(47,48)*. Both excessive ovarian volume and abnormal morphology have been utilized as criteria for an abnormal screening test *(46,49)*. The important morphologic abnormalities are complexity (multiloculation) of cysts, particularly when solid components or papillary projections are noted. More recently, color Doppler flow has been added to the armamentarium, although larger studies have not provided confirmation of its accuracy in differentiating benign from malignant ovarian lesions *(50–52)*. In premenopausal women, ultrasound should be performed between cycle d 3 and 8 to prevent false-positive scans related to physiologic cysts.

The seminal American work, and one of the largest ultrasound screening studies to date, has been performed at the University of Kentucky *(53)*. Between 1987 and 1999, these investigators performed annual transvaginal sonography on 14,469 asymptomatic women who were either over age 50, or over age 30 with a family history of ovarian cancer. Ultrasound was considered abnormal if the volume exceeded established values dependent on menopausal status or if morphology was abnormal. An abnormal scan was repeated in 4–6 wk. Twenty-three percent had a family history of ovarian cancer and underwent an average of four scans over the course of the study. One hundred eighty women had persistently abnormal scans and underwent laparotomy or laparoscopy. Seventeen cancers were detected, of which 11 were invasive epithelial malignancies and the remainder low malignant potential or granulosa-cell tumors. There were four false-negative scans in women who developed cancer within 12 mo of ultrasound. The sensitivity of ultrasound in this large study was 81%, the specificity was 98.9%, and the positive predictive value was 9.4%. The positive predictive value would rise to 20% by excluding women with unilocular cysts under 5 cm. These patients could be followed with ultrasound instead of immediate surgical intervention. There did appear to be a shift to earlier stage at diagnosis in these women with 45% detected in Stage I and 27% detected in Stage II.

Limitations of ultrasound screening include the cost, the relatively high false-positive rate, and the fact that up to 50% of postmenopausal ovaries cannot be visualized *(54)*. Another important potential limitation of ultrasound screening directed at the ovaries is that it is unlikely to detect primary peritoneal carcinoma, which, by definition, affects the ovarian surface in a minimal fashion or not at all *(55)*.

The use of several companion tests, termed *multimodal screening*, has been reported in several studies. One small European pilot study of 180 women with a strong family history of ovarian cancer, many of whom had a personal history of breast cancer, reported a 5% prevalence of ovarian cancer *(56)*. The group underwent transvaginal ultrasound, CA 125, and breast exam. Of nine ovarian cancers detected, seven were identified by ultrasound. Four of the nine had elevated CA 125 determinations. Thirteen women underwent oophorectomy for treatment of breast cancer, with two ovarian cancers detected. Another study of 2000 women over age 45 utilized pelvic examination and CA 125 as the initial screen, with 174 and 18 abnormal studies, respectively *(57)*. Ultrasound was performed in this second tier of women, with 15 abnormal scans resulting in surgery. One Stage IA ovarian cancer, one borderline tumor, and one cancer metastatic to the ovary were detected. The sensitivity was 100%, specificity 99.7%, and positive predictive value 22%. However, this screening intervention was unlikely to improve the prognosis for the woman with a metastatic cancer, and for the woman with a borderline tumor who would have been likely to have a good prognosis had diagnosis been delayed until symptoms developed.

In an analysis of 25 studies of ovarian cancer screening, for every ovarian cancer detected, between 2.5 and 60 women undergo surgical evaluation *(58)*. Clearly, in an accounting of the risk–benefit ratio and a cost analysis, the morbidity and mortality of surgery must be assessed, as well as direct and indirect costs such as days lost from work. Proponents of screening argue that most of the adnexal masses discovered on ultrasound require surgical intervention even if they are ultimately found to be benign disease.

The underlying question for screening trials is whether prognosis will be improved for women with cancers diagnosed. Many of the early-screening trials detected women with late-stage disease or nonepithelial tumors for whom diagnosis was unlikely to impact prognosis. In a prospective randomized British trial of screening involving nearly 22,000 women, half of whom were randomized to screening with CA 125, followed by ultrasound for women with values over 30 U/mL, 20 cancers were diagnosed *(59)*. Women with abnormal ovarian morphology on ultrasound were significantly more likely to be diagnosed with cancer than women with normal morphology. In a companion article, the 16 women in the screening arm who were diagnosed with cancer demonstrated a median survival of 72.9 mo compared with 41.8 mo for the 20 women diagnosed with ovarian cancer in the control group of nonscreened women ($p = 0.0112$) *(60)*.

Recommendations regarding ovarian cancer screening have been issued by several national groups. The National Institutes of Health held a Consensus Development Conference on Ovarian Cancer in April 1994 *(61,62)*. The conclusion regarding screening was that an effective test did not exist for general population screening. The recommendation continued that high-risk women, based on family history, should be referred to a specialist in gynecologic oncology for consideration of screening with a combination of pelvic exam, transvaginal ultrasound and CA 125 testing, or prophylactic surgery. Participation in clinical trials is an important option and should be encouraged for eligible women when available. The American College of Obstetricians and Gynecologists guidelines for screening state that no techniques that have proven to be effective in reducing the disease-specific mortality of ovarian cancer are currently available *(63)*.

Genetic Testing

Experts generally recommend genetic testing for women with an estimated 10–20% chance of finding a genetic mutation *(17)*. This risk is realized in a woman with two first- or second-degree relatives with either ovarian cancer at any age or breast cancer under age 50. In contrast, the risk of a mutation in a family with a single relative over age 50 diagnosed with ovarian cancer is under 3%. At the opposite end of the spectrum, a family with two cases of ovarian cancer and two cases of breast cancer faces an 80–90% risk of a mutation in BRCA1 or 2. The frequency of mutations in BRCA1 in the general US population is approx 1 in 800. Several specific mutations, called founder mutations, have been described with enhanced prevalence in the Ashkenazi Jewish population with a frequency of about 2% for BRCA1 and BRCA2 *(64)*. The U.S. Preventive Services Task Force issued consensus guidelines for follow-up care of individuals with known mutations of BRCA1 and 2 in 1997, concluding that cancer screening tests should be performed *(65)*.

Genetic testing is commercially available to the practitioner, but haphazard use of such tests, even by the well-intentioned and well-informed physician, is fraught with harmful consequences. There are significant ethical, psychological, and legal risks to the patient, including possible discrimination in her job and insurance, as well as the major potential for depression or suicide with either negative or positive results. Additionally, because of the large number of known mutations and the fact that many potential mutations are as yet undiscovered, initial identification of a potential mutation in a family may be difficult and false-negative results are possible. This is particularly true if the affected individuals are not available for testing. Virtually all experts strongly recommend the use of genetic testing only by expert practitioners in concert with genetic counselors and psychological support. It is wise to learn of your own local resources and to refer patients for participation in clinical trials whenever available.

COST OF SCREENING

The cost of a single screen ranges from $30 to perhaps $500. The lower figure is the actual cost for a single ultrasound scan in the dedicated screening program at the University of Kentucky *(66)*. The latter is an estimated cost for a screening visit, which includes transvaginal ultrasound, CA 125, and physician fee for pelvic exam on an established patient in a typical American health care setting. Not included in either estimate is the "excess" cost for medical care, including surgery for women with false-positive screening tests. The cost of screening must be multiplied by the number of women to be screened and the frequency of screening. Total cost would depend on whether all women over a certain age were to be screened or if the focus were further narrowed to include only women with a family history. Finally, these costs must be balanced against costs to treat a woman with advanced ovarian cancer, which were estimated at $32,900 in 1994, including surgical, hospital, laboratory, and chemotherapy charges for initial treatment *(67)*. This estimate excludes costs for treatment of recurrent disease, complications, or terminal care.

The cost for screening could be reduced by the use of dedicated screening programs, limitation of tests used (initial screening with one test, with further testing only for abnormal results), and selection of a high-risk group. Additionally, costs for cancer care would be lower if screening shifted stage at diagnosis to a lower stage. However, a public health prevention program to widen the use of oral contraceptives, with the anticipated 40–50% reduction in risk of ovarian cancer, may be the most cost-effective alternative.

Several mathematical models assessing the risk–benefit ratios have been published *(68,69)*. In one, annual CA 125 screening between ages 50 and 75 was estimated to save 3.4 yr of life per case of ovarian cancer at a cost of $36,000 to $95,000 per year of life saved *(68)*. The second model was based on a one-time screen at either age 40 or age 65 with serum CA 125 and transvaginal sonography, resulting in an increase in average life expectancy by less than 1 d at either age *(69)*.

PREVENTIVE STRATEGIES

Even if generally applicable screening strategies for ovarian cancer do not exist at present, other preventive measures should be more widely publicized and applied. Women are often well informed about the risks of oral contraceptives, yet few realize that even relatively short-term use can significantly reduce their risk of both ovarian and endometrial cancers. Oral contraceptive use is also a good strategy throughout the childbearing years in women with a strong family cancer history who may

Chapter 4 / Screening for Ovarian Cancer 55

ultimately opt for prophylactic oophorectomy once their families are complete *(15,18)*. Additionally, routine use of bilateral oophorectomy in women undergoing hysterectomy after the age of 40 or 45 will prevent ovarian cancer in approx 1000 women each year, and both the female public and gynecologists need to be educated about this rationale for oophorectomy *(7,8)*. Obviously, women should receive appropriate preoperative counseling regarding the risks and benefits of this approach, as well as guidance concerning the decision about hormone replacement therapy.

The prophylactic removal of ovaries may be warranted in certain women at extremely high risk of developing ovarian cancer, particularly those with a true family cancer syndrome *(70)*. This is generally performed at completion of childbearing, with an attempt to perform the procedure 10 yr earlier than the age of diagnosis of the youngest affected family member. Hereditary cancers tend to occur at earlier ages than the same cancer in the general population and may occur at a younger age in each succeeding generation. Because endometrial cancer occurrence is high in families with HNPCC, hysterectomy should also be performed if the patient chooses a prophylactic surgical approach. These young women then face the difficult decision regarding initiation of hormone replacement therapy and the increased risk of breast cancer, which appears to be dose and duration related. Additionally, for women with an intact uterus, the need to use combination estrogen and progesterone therapy may further increase risk over estrogen use alone *(71)*. If oophorectomy is selected, the surgeon must be certain to remove the entire ovary, as cancers may occur in a fragment of retained ovarian tissue. This procedure may be performed laparoscopically in many women, provided that the ureter can be visualized in such a manner to allow complete ovarian resection. Visualization of the peritoneal surfaces should also be performed, as the peritoneum appears to be an at-risk organ as well.

Many gynecologic oncologists will perform peritoneal washings for cytology and some have advocated peritoneal biopsies in these high-risk women as well. When an ovary is removed from a woman with a family history of cancer, the pathologist must be alerted to carefully section the entire ovary. Cases of "peritoneal" cancer have been reported following prophylactic oophorectomy in which small foci of cancer were detected in the previously removed ovary when retrospective sectioning was performed.

RECOMMENDATIONS

A simple, cost-effective screening test for ovarian cancer, which can be widely applied to the US population, does not exist, so the screening

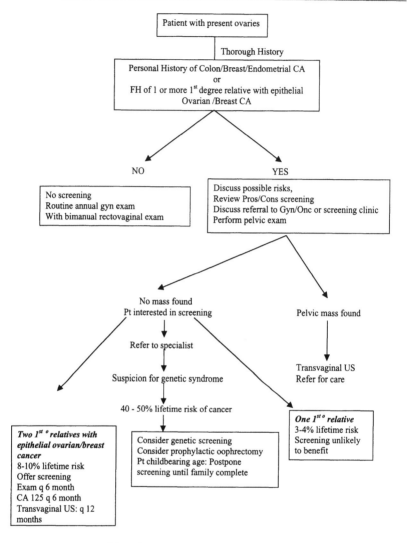

Algorithm 1. Screening algorithm.

focus must be narrowed. The women at highest risk for ovarian cancer are those with a significant family history of ovarian cancer or ovarian and breast cancer, and current screening modalities should target these individuals. However, this group represents less than 10% of women with ovarian cancer, so current screening efforts are being applied to a small minority of women at risk. Guidelines for screening are summarized in Algorithm 1.

First, a careful family history should be obtained from all patients. In women with no family history of cancer and no personal history of breast, colon, or endometrial cancer, routine annual bimanual and

Chapter 4 / Screening for Ovarian Cancer

rectovaginal pelvic exams should be performed. In women with a personal history of the index cancers or a family history of ovarian cancer or breast and ovarian cancer in two or more first-degree relatives, a discussion of the possible increased risk of ovarian cancer should be conducted. If a pelvic mass is appreciated on the exam, imaging studies should be carried out and the patient referred for surgery.

High-risk patients with no mass on the exam should be referred to a specialist, generally a gynecologic oncologist, for possible screening. Those with one first-degree relative face a minimal increased risk and screening will not be encouraged. Women with two first-degree relatives will generally be offered screening. Women with a pedigree suspicious for a genetic cancer syndrome will be offered genetic testing after careful counseling by a trained genetic counselor and then may undergo prophylactic surgery. In the absence of a clinical trial, screening commonly includes a pelvic exam, tumor marker determinations, and transvaginal ultrasound screening based on the risk assessment performed by the gynecologic oncologist and/or geneticist. Participation in clinical trials of screening should be encouraged, so that answers to the dilemma of screening may be answered most expeditiously.

SUMMARY

Epithelial ovarian cancer is one of the most common malignancies in women. The majority of the patients have advanced disease at the time of presentation. Currently available screening techniques are not cost-effective for the general population and have not proven to be effective in reducing the disease-specific mortality. Screening is highly recommended in the high-risk patients who have personal or family history of ovarian, breast, and certain other genetic cancers.

REFERENCE

1. Landis SH, Murray T, Bolden S, Wingo PA. (1999) Cancer statistics 1999. *CA Cancer J Clin* 49:8–31.
2. Menck HR, Garfinkel L, Dodd, GD. (1991) Preliminary report of the National Cancer Data Base. *CA Cancer J Clin* 41:7.
3. Wu ML, Whittemore AS, Paffenbarger RS, et al. (1988) Personal and environmental characteristics related to epithelial ovarian cancer, Part I. Reproductive and menstrual events and oral contraceptive use. *Am J Epidemiol* 216:1227.
4. The Cancer and Steroid Hormone Study of the Centers for Disease Control and the National Institute of Child Health and Human Development. (1987) The reduction in risk of ovarian cancer associated with oral-contraceptive use. *N Engl J Med* 16:650–656.
5. Hankinson SE, Colditz GA, Hunter DJ, et al. (1992) A quantitative assessment of oral contraceptive use and risk of ovarian cancer. *Obstet Gynecol* 80:708–714.

58   Part II / Screening for Breast and Gynecological Cancers

6. Weiss NS, Harlow BL. (1986) Why does hysterectomy without bilateral oophorectomy influence the subsequent incidence of ovarian cancer? *Am J Epidem* 124:856–858.
7. Sightler S, Boike G, Estape R, Averette H. (1991) Ovarian cancer in women with prior hysterectomy: a 14-year experience at the University of Miami. *Obstet. Gynecol* 78(4):681–684.
8. Nguyen HN, Averette HE, Janicek M. (1994) A review of the significance of familial risk factors and the role of prophylactic oophorectomy in cancer prevention. *Cancer* 74:545–555.
9. Prophylactic Oophorectomy. (1999) *ACOG Practice Bulletin 7.* Washington, DC, ACOG, pp. 998–1003.
10. Tobacman J, Tucker M, Kase R, et al. (1982) Intra-abdominal carcinomatosis after prophylactic oophorectomy in ovarian-cancer-prone families. *Lancet* Oct:795–797.
11. Weber AM, Hewett WJ, Gajewski WH, Curry SL. (1992) Serous carcinoma of the peritoneum after oophorectomy. *Obstet Gynecol* 80:558–560.
12. Piver M, Jishi M, Tsukada Y, Navas G. (1993) Primary peritoneal carcinoma after prophylactic oophorectomy in women with a family history of ovarian cancer: a report of the Gilda Radner familial ovarian cancer registry. *Cancer* 71(9):2751–2755.
13. Yancik R, Gloeckler RL, Yates JW. (1986) Ovarian cancer in the elderly: an analysis of the surveillance, epidemiology and end results program data. *Am J Obstet Gynecol* 154:639–647.
14. Lynch HT, Watson P, Lynch JF, Conway TA, Fili M. (1993) Hereditary ovarian cancer: heterogeneity in age at onset. *Cancer* 71:573–581.
15. Narod SA, Risch H, Moslehi R, et al. (1998) Oral contraceptives and the risk of hereditary ovarian cancer. *N Engl J Med* 339:424–428.
16. Lynch HT, Casey MJ, Shawn TG, Lynch, JF. (1998) Hereditary factors in gynecologic cancer. *Oncologist* 3:319–338.
17. Boyd J, Rubin SC. (1997) Hereditary ovarian cancer: molecular genetics and clinical implications. *Gynecol Oncol* 64:196–206.
18. Gross TP, Schlesselman JJ. (1994) The estimated effect of oral contraceptive use on the cumulative risk of epithelial ovarian cancer. *Obstet Gynecol* 83:419–424.
19. Whittemore AS, Harris R, Intyre J. (1992) Collaborative ovarian cancer group. Characteristics relating to ovarian cancer risk: collaborative analysis of 12 US case-control studies. II. Invasive epithelial ovarian cancers in white women. *Am J Epidemiol* 136:1184–1203.
20. Rossing MA, Daling JR, Weiss NS, Moore DE, Self SG. (1994) Ovarian tumors in a cohort of infertile women. *N Engl J Med* 331:771–776.
21. Venn A, Watson L, Lumley J, et al. (1995) Breast and ovarian cancer incidence after infertility and in vitro fertilization. *Lancet* 346:995–1000.
22. Garg PP, Kerlikowsk K, Subak L, Grady D. (1998) Hormone replacement and the risk of epithelial ovarian carcinoma: a meta-analysis. *Obstet Gynecol* 92:472–479.
23. Resta L, Russo S, Colucci GA, Prat J. (1993) Morphologic precursors of ovarian epithelial tumors. *Obstet Gynecol* 82(2):181–186.
24. Chang S, Risch HA. (1996) Perineal talc exposure and risk of ovarian carcinoma. *Cancer* 79:2396–2401.
25. Wong C, Hempling RE, Piver S, Natarajan N, Mettlin CJ. (1999) Perineal talc exposure and subsequent epithelial ovarian cancer: a case-control study. *Obstet Gynecol* 93:372–376.
26. Heller DS, Westhoff C, Gordon RE, Katz N. (1996) The relationship between perineal cosmetic talc usage and ovarian talc particle burden. *Am J Obstet Gynecol* 174:1507–1510.

Chapter 4 / Screening for Ovarian Cancer

27. Gallion H, Guarino A, DePriest P, et al. (1996) Evidence for a unifocal origin in familial ovarian cancer. *Am J Obstet Gynecol* 174(4):1102–1108.
28. Tsao SW, Mok CH, Knapp RC, et al. (1993) Molecular genetic evidence of a unifocal origin for human serous ovarian carcinomas. *Gynecol Oncol* 48(1):5–10.
29. Muto MG, Welch WR, Mok SC, et al. (1995) Evidence for a multifocal origin of papillary serous carcinoma of the peritoneum. *Cancer Res* 55(3):490–492.
30. Bast RC, Klug TL, St. John E, et al. (1983) A radioimmunoassay using a monoclonal antibody to monitor the course of epithelial ovarian cancer. *N Engl J Med* 309:883–887.
31. McGuire WP, Hoskins WJ, Brady MF, et al. (1996) Cyclophosphamide and cisplatincompared with paclitaxel and cisplatin in patients with stage III and stage IV ovarian cancer. *N Engl J Med* 334:1–52.
32. Ozols RF, Rubin SC, Thomas G, Robboy S. (1997) Epithelial ovarian cancer. In: Hoskins WJ, Perez CA, Young RC, eds., *Principles and Practice of Gynecologic Oncology*, 2nd ed, Philadelphia: Lippincott-Raven, p. 941.
33. Mok SC, Bell DA, Knapp RC, et al. (1993) Mutation of K-ras protooncogene in human ovarian epithelial tumors of borderline malignancy. *Cancer Res* 53(7):1489–1492.
34. Gusberg SB, Deligdisch L. (1984) Ovarian dysplasia. A study of identical twins. *Cancer* 54:1–4.
35. Salazar H, Godwin AK, Daly MB. (1996) Microscopic benign and invasive malignant neoplasms and a cancer-prone phenotype in prophylactic oophorectomies. *J Natl Cancer Inst* 88:1810–1820.
36. Plaxe SC, Deligdisch L, Dottin, PR, Cohe, CJ. (1990) Ovarian intraepithelial neoplasia demonstrated in patients with stage I ovarian carcinoma. *Gynecol Oncol* 38:367–372.
37. Deligdisch L, Gil J, Kerner K, et al. (1999) Ovarian dysplasia in prophylactic oophorectomy specimens: cytogenetic and morphometric correlations. *Cancer* 86:1544–1550.
38. Rubi, SC, Blackwood MA, Bandera C, et al. (1998) BRCA1, BRCA2 and hereditary nonpolyposis colorectal cancer gene mutations in an unselected ovarian cancer population: relationship to family history and implications for genetic testing. *Am J Obstet Gynecol* 178:670–677.
39. Grover S, Quinn M. (1995) Is there any value in bimanual pelvic examination as a screening test? *Med J Aust* 162:408–410.
40. Zurawski V, Orjaseter H, Andersen A, Jellum E. (1988) Elevated serum CA 125 levels prior to diagnosis of ovarian neoplasia: relevance for early detection of ovarian cancer. *Int J Cancer* 42:677–680.
41. Zurawski VR, Sjovall K, Schoenfeld DA, et al. (1990) Prospective evaluation of serum CA 125 levels in a normal population, phase I: the specificities of single and serial determinations in testing for ovarian cancer. *Gynecol Oncol* 36:299–305.
42. Jacobs I, Bridges J, Reynolds C, et al. (1988) Multimodal approach to screening for ovarian cancer. *Lancet* Feb:268–271.
43. Jacobs IJ, Skates S, Davies AP, et al. (1996) Risk of diagnosis of ovarian cancer after raised serum CA 125 concentration: a prospective cohort study. *BMJ* 313(7069): 1355–1358.
44. Skates SJ, Singer DE. (1991) Quantifying the potential benefit of CA 125. Screening for ovarian cancer. *J Clin Epidemiol* 4:365–380.
45. Berek J, Bast R. (1995) Ovarian cancer screening: the use of serial complementary tumor markers to improve sensitivity and specificity for early detention. *Cancer* Suppl 76(10):2092–2096.
46. Higgins R, Van Nagell J, Donaldson E, et al. (1988) Transvaginal sonography as screening method for ovarian cancer. *Gynecol Oncol* 34:402–406.

60   Part II / Screening for Breast and Gynecological Cancers

47. Crvenkovic G, Karlan B, Platt L. (1996) Current role of ultrasound in ovarian cancer screening. *Clin Obstet Gynecol* 39(1):59–67 .

48. Gynecologic Ultrasonography (1995) ACOG Technical Bulletin 215. Washington, DC: ACOG, pp. 461–470.

49. Campbell S, Royston P, Bhan V, Whitehead M, Collins W. (1990) Novel screening strategies for early ovarian cancer by transabdominal ultrasonography. *Brit J Obstet Gynecol* 97:304–311.

50. Vuento M, Pirhonen J, Mäkinen J, et al. (1995) Evaluation of ovarian findings in asymptomatic postmenopausal women with color doppler ultrasound. Ovarian cancer screening. *Cancer* 76(7):1214–1218.

51. Van Nagell JR, Ueland FR. (1999) Ultrasound evaluation of pelvic masses: predictors of malignancy for the general gynecologist. *Curr Opin Obstet Gynecol* 11(1):45–49.

52. Tekay A, Jouppila P. (1996) Controversies in assessment of ovarian tumors with transvaginal color doppler ultrasound. *Acta Obstet Gynecol Scand* 75(4):316–329.

53. VanNagell JR, DePriest PD, Reedy M, et al. (2000) The efficacy of transvaginal sonographic screening in asymptomatic women at risk for ovarian cancer. Society of Gynecologic Oncologists, Annual Meeting, San Diego, CA, p. 84.

54. Wolf SI, Gosink BB, Feldesman MR, et al. (1991) Prevalence of simple adnexal cysts in postmenopausal women. *Radiology* 180:65–71.

55. Karlan BY, Baldwin RL, Lopez-Luevanos E, et al. (1999) Peritoneal serous papillary carcinoma, a phenotypic variant of familial ovarian cancer: implications for ovarian cancer screening. *N Engl J Med* 180:917–928.

56. Dorum A, Kristensen GB, Abeler VM, Trope CG, Moller P. (1996) Early detection of familial ovarian cancer. *Eur J Cancer* 32A(10):1645–1651.

57. Adonakis GL, Paraskevaidis E, Tsiga S, Seferiadis K, Lolis DE. (1996) A combined approach for the early detection of ovarian cancer in asymptomatic women. *Eur J Obstet Gynecol Repro Biol* 65:221–225.

58. Bell R, Petticrew M, Sheldon T. (1998) The performance of screening tests for ovarian cancer: results of a systematic review. *Br J Obstet Gynecol* 105:1136–1147.

59. Menon U, Talaat A, Jeyarajah AR, et al. (1999) Ultrasound assessment of ovarian cancer risk in postmenopausal women with CA 125 elevation. *Br J Cancer* 80(10):1644–1647.

60. Jacobs IJ, Skates SJ, MacDonald N, et al. (1999) Screening for ovarian cancer: a pilot randomized controlled trial. *Lancet* 353(9160):1207–1210.

61. Ovarian Cancer: Screening, Treatment and Follow-up. (1994) NIH Consensus Statement. April 5–7; 12(3):1–30.

62. National Institutes of Health Consensus Development. (1994) Conference Statement Ovarian Cancer: screening, treatment, and follow-up. *Gynecol Oncol* 55:S4–S14.

63. Routine Cancer Screening (1997) *ACOG Committee Opinion 185.* Washington, DC: ACOG, pp. 225–229.

64. Struewin JP, Hartge P, Wacholder S, et al. (1997) The risk of cancer associated with specific mutations of BRCA1 and BRCA2 among Ashkenazi Jews. *N Engl J Med* 336:1401–1408.

65. Burke W, Daly M, Garber J. (1997) Recommendations for follow-up care of individuals with an inherited predisposition to cancer. *JAMA* 227:997–1003.

66. VanNagell JR, Gallion HH, Pavlik EJ, DePriest PD. (1995) Ovarian cancer screening. *Cancer* 6:2086–2091.

67. Cohen CJ, Jennings TS. (1994) Screening for ovarian cancer: the role of noninvasive imaging techniques. *Am J Obstet Gynecol* 170:1088–1094.

68. Carlson KJ, Skates SJ, Singer DE. (1994) Screening for ovarian cancer. *Ann Intern Med* 121:124–132.

69. Schapira MM, Matchar DB, Young MJ. (1993) The effectiveness of ovarian cancer screening. *Ann Intern Med* 118:838–843.
70. Berchuck A, Schildkraut JM, Marks JR, Futreal PA. (1999) Managing hereditary ovarian cancer risk. American Cancer Society National Conference on Cancer Genetics. *Cancer* 1697–1704.
71. Schairer C, Lubin J, Troisi R, et al. (2000) Menopausal estrogen and estrogen-progestin replacement therapy and breast cancer risk. *JAMA* 283:485–491.

5 Screening for Endometrial Cancer

Allan R. Mayer, DO
and Beth E. Nelson, MD

KEY PRINCIPLES

- Endometrial carcinoma is a relatively common cancer in the United States, mostly affecting postmenopausal women.
- Most of the patients are diagnosed early and prognosis is generally favorable.
- Several risk factors have been identified, which include older age group, states of unopposed hyperestrogenemia, Tamoxifen therapy, and personal history of breast, colon, or ovarian carcinoma.
- Routine screening for general population is not recommended.
- Patients on tamoxifen therapy should be educated regarding the risk of endometrial carcinoma and need to seek immediate medical advice in case of abnormal vaginal bleeding.

INTRODUCTION

Endometrial carcinoma is the eighth most common cancer in women worldwide and the fourth most commonly diagnosed cancer in US women, with 36,100 new cases annually *(1–3)*. An estimated 1–3% of postmenopausal females will be diagnosed before age 75 *(4)*. Because of identifiable symptoms, the diagnosis is frequently made in early stage (I and II) disease with excellent (83%) overall survival statistics *(5)*. This is a disease of the sixth and seventh decades, with the mean age at diagnosis of 62 yr. Twenty-five percent of cases occur perimenopausally, with 5% of women under age 40. Traditional thinking

From: *Cancer Screening: A Practical Guide for Physicians*
Edited by: K. Aziz and G. Y. Wu © Humana Press Inc., Totowa, NJ

64 Part II / Screening for Breast and Gynecological Cancers

associates prolonged, unopposed estrogen with the diagnosis *(5–7)*. Patients may demonstrate chronic anovulation resulting from polycystic ovarian disease, nulliparity/infertility, or perimenopausal anovulatory menstrual cycles.

Postmenopausally, unopposed exogenous estrogen or hyperestrogenism as a result of peripheral conversion of adrenal androstenedione to estrone may predispose women to this cancer. Other associated risk factors include obesity, early menarche, and late menopause, estrogen-secreting tumors, and personal or family history of breast, ovarian, or colonic malignancies *(6,7)*. Recent medical literature identifies tamoxifen, an antiestrogenic breast cancer therapy, as another risk factor for endometrial carcinoma *(8–12)*. This is related to the drug's paradoxical secondary agonist effect on the reproductive tract. Conversely, associated risk factors of diabetes mellitus and hypertension appear to be related but not causal *(5,6)*.

This chapter will review the disease process, including epidemiology and pathophysiology, with an emphasis on screening techniques and mechanisms of prevention. Finally, recommendations for referral and therapy are suggested.

DEFINITION

The endometrial lining of the uterine cavity is hormonally mediated tissue *(13)*. It is comprised of endometrial glands (epithelium) supported by stromal cells. These glands are stimulated by both estrogen and progesterone and carry cytoplasmic receptors for both. Exposure to estrogen causes the glands to proliferate. Progesterone, either endogenously from the ovarian corpus luteum or exogenously, will convert the endometrial glands and stroma to a luteal phase.

Postovuluation, if conception does not occur or if exogenous progesterone is interrupted, the endometrial lining of the uterus will shed as menstrual flow and then regenerate with subsequent estrogenic stimulation. Postmenopausally, without estrogen, the endometrial lining atrophies and flattens. Chronic estrogenic stimulation of the endometrium may lead to a pathologic finding of hyperplastic epithelium (glands). Many pathologists believe that hyperplastic glands without nuclear atypia are a benign process. If cellular nuclei become cytologically atypical, the endometrium is at risk for developing an adenocarcinoma *(13,14)*.

EPIDEMIOLOGY

As stated earlier, endometrial adenocarcinoma appears related to states of unopposed hyperestrogenism. Additionally, age, race, obesity,

Chapter 5 / Screening for Endometrial Cancer 65

and family history also impact on the disease. Endometrial adenocarcinoma occurs more frequently in the United States, Canada, and Western European countries (15 per 100,000 women), with lower incidence rates in Asia, Africa, and Latin America (<8 per 100,000 women) *(15)*. Endometrial cancer is most commonly a condition of the postmenopausal woman. Frequently the perimenopausal ovary becomes anovulatory (i.e., progesterone deficient) while estrogen production continues. Age impacts on disease survival with a poorer prognosis in women over age 72. Race also appears to affect disease *(16,17)*. It is found more frequently in Caucasian women than in African-American or non-Caucasians. Caucasian females have a 2.4 lifetime risk compared to 1.3 in African-American women. However, when occurring in non-Caucasians, the diagnosis is often at a higher stage or grade, yielding a (30%) lower survival *(16)*.

Obesity plays a powerful role in this diagnosis *(15,18)*. The adrenal hormone androstenedione is converted to estrone in peripheral adipose tissue. Additionally, sex-hormone-binding globulin levels are decreased, compounded by differences in estrogen metabolism in obese women *(18)*. This can create a milieu of unopposed estrogenic stimulation of the postmenopausal uterus. In premenopausal women, obesity is associated with a higher frequency of anovulation, suggesting that progesterone deficiency may be an important factor. The risk of cancer increases with the degree of obesity, ranging from a 2- to 20-fold rise *(15)*. In societies with a low prevalence both of obesity and endometrial cancer, increased body weight becomes a major risk factor for endometrial cancer *(19)*. Frequently, excessive estrogen stimulation creates endometrial proliferation, shedding, and bleeding. Unfortunately, obesity complicates the surgical staging and anesthesia required for disease treatment.

Often, patients with endometrial cancer are nulliparous or of low parity *(20–23)*. Again, this feature reflects ovarian anovulation. When ovulation does not occur, a corpus luteum is not formed and the endometrium escapes progestational opposition and withdrawal, again leading to a state of unopposed estrogen. Elective infertility with contraception does not have a similar impact. In fact, women who use combination oral contraception have a 50% risk reduction *(21)*. This is attributed to the progestational component of oral contraceptive pills (OCP's), with regular endometrial withdrawal bleeding.

Postmenopausal hormone replacement therapy especially when used without progesterone opposition has been related to a higher risk of endometrial adenocarcinoma *(24–26)*. Several studies in the mid-1970s linked increased estrogen sales with a four- to sevenfold elevated risk of endometrial cancer *(4,24–26)*. In 1995, Grady published a meta-analysis revealing a 2.3 (95% confidence interval [CI] 2.1–2.5) relative risk for ever users of estrogen replacement therapy (ERT) over nonusers. The cancer risk is dose and duration (5–10 yr) dependent. A 10-fold-higher risk has been reported for use >10 yr *(25)*. The risk also declines with time following discontinuation but remains elevated even 5–10 yr later *(24,26)*. Grady revealed a relative risk of 3.9 (95% CI 1.6–9.5.) for 0.3 mg, 3.4 (95% CI 0–5.6) for 0.625 mg, and a 5.8 RR (95% CI 4.5–7.5) for >1.25-mg doses *(25)*.

Current evidence suggests the addition of cyclic or continuous progesterone reduces or eliminates the cancer risk by interruption of endometrial proliferation *(27)*. An odds ratio of 1.9 (95% CI 0.9–3.8) is reported for use of combination therapy *(24,26)*. Most current gynecologists recognize that keeping the ERT doses as low as possible (≤0.625 mg daily and providing Provera 10 mg daily × 10 d as cyclic therapy or 2.5 mg daily continuously) minimizes the malignant transformation risk. It should be stated that the cardiovascular and skeletal benefits derived from postmenopausal ERT far outweight any reported cancer risk in carefully managed patients. Of note, there are 467,613 cardiovascular and cerebral vascular deaths reported annually in US women compared to 6500 endometrial and 40,800 breast cancer mortalities *(3)*.

Women with a personal history of breast cancer are at increased risk for second adenocarcinoma primaries and especially colon, ovarian, and endometrial disease *(5,27)*. These women should undergo regular screening with their gynecologist, including a careful history for symptoms, a comprehensive physical with pelvic examination, and rectovaginal and stool hemoccult evaluation. This becomes particularly important past the age of 50, when routine asymptomatic colon screening is recommended at 5-yr intervals by the American College of Gastroenterology *(28)*. In addition, with increasing frequency, breast cancer patients are receiving the antitumor drug tamoxifen *(29)*. This medication replicates the endometrial agonist effect of estrogen. In postmenopausal or anovulatory women, this may result in a two- to threefold increased risk of endometrial adenocarcinoma *(8,9,11,12)*. The surveillance recommendations in this clinical scenario are more completely discussed in the section Patients on Tamoxifen Therapy.

Family cancer history may also impact on the disease *(5,27)*. An important aspect of well-woman care includes a thorough family history and pedigree, focusing on cases of adenocarcinoma. The affected organ sites may be breast, colon, ovary, endometrium, or even pancreas or prostate. Five to seven percent of adenocarcinomas have a genetic link. Pedigrees with three or more cases should prompt further investigations and possibly genetic counseling and screening by a comprehensive genetic laboratory service.

Chapter 5 / Screening for Endometrial Cancer 67

Finally, several diagnoses have been postulated to be risk factors that may, in fact, be cofactors. Hypertension and diabetes mellitus are two diseases that commonly occur in women of advancing age. These disease complexes may all be associated with underlying obesity. No literature to date has found them to be causal *(22,30)*.

PATHOPHYSIOLOGY

Pathologists are not in complete agreement concerning the effects of estrogen on the endometrium *(13,14)*. Estrogen stimulates endometrial tissue to proliferate. It will promote tissue thickening by increasing gland proliferation. In the progesterone-deficient scenario, the endometrial lining may become hyperplastic; that is, the endometrial gland-to-stroma ratio will increase with intraglandular cribriforming or bridging and formation of solid areas without intervening stroma. However, the hallmark of malignancy is nuclear atypia, hyperchromatism, and mitoses. Pathologists disagree on the potential for unopposed estrogen to convert a normal endometrial lining into complex hyperplasia with atypia, which is now widely accepted as the preinvasive stage of endometrial adenocarcinoma. Kurman demonstrated that in the presence of atypia, there is a 29% lifetime risk of developing cancer and a 19% incidence of a coexistent endometrial adenocarcinoma *(14)*.

Therefore, when an office biopsy returns complex hyperplasia with atypia, a dilation and curettage (D&C) is required to exclude coexistent adenocarcinoma. Post-D&C therapy includes progestational hormonal treatment or total hysterectomy, depending on the clinical scenario.

CLINICAL ASPECTS OF SCREENING

The 1999 US cancer statistics revealed 36,100 new endometrial cancer cases. Paradoxically, there were only 6500 deaths attributed to this diagnosis that year *(3)*. This is primarily the result of rapid diagnosis at early stages of the disease (Stages I and II) because women with abnormal uterine or postmenopausal bleeding frequently present to their physician and receive diagnosis by endometrial sampling. Eighty percent of cases are found prior to metastasis outside the uterus and cervix. Stage I disease confined to the uterus occurs in 60% of cases and Stage II disease with cervical extension in 20% *(5)*. More advanced disease, Stage III (extrauterine pelvic disease) and Stage IV (extrapelvic spread) occur least commonly, in less than 20% of women. The physician's index of suspicion should be raised in any patient greater than 35 yr of age with persistent, irregular vaginal bleeding or sporadic brown, watery, or mucoid discharge which should prompt an endometrial

68 Part II / Screening for Breast and Gynecological Cancers

biopsy. Rarely do other symptoms of pelvic pain, gastrointestinal (GI) or GU complaints, fatigue, or weight loss coexist. General gynecologists are confronted with the management of abnormal uterine bleeding in up to 20% of ambulatory visits *(31)*. As the life expectancy of American women increases and more women use postmenopausal hormone replacement, screening becomes a more common clinical consideration.

Any vaginal bleeding determined by physical examination to be of uterine origin requires an endometrial biopsy in women over age 40. The dilemma comes with the asymptomatic patient. The other group of patients without symptoms is the high-risk cohort. Women taking tamoxifen or those who come from high-risk cancer families have in the past undergone aggressive screening, even in the absence of symptomatology *(30,32)*. Although not well supported by the literature, this screening may have been with semiannual pelvic examination and cervical cytology, or even endometrial surveillance via transvaginal ultrasonography and random, outpatient endometrial biopsy *(32)*. Any woman using prolonged unopposed estrogen should have consideration of endometrial sampling prior to adding a progestin. Biopsy is mandatory if she has symptoms of abnormal or postmenopausal bleeding.

Acceptable screening tests have specific criteria regarding technique and reliability. Screening is used primarily in malignant conditions where there is a detectable preinvasive phase. A screening test should be reproducible, minimally invasive, and cost-effective. It should be sufficiently sensitive and specific to remain valuable. Commonly acceptable medical screening tests are the Papanicolaou smear and mammogram.

Unfortunately, there is no clear consensus regarding who, when, and how to screen for endometrial cancer *(31,33)*. Many gynecologists will submit all asymptomatic patients to endometrial sampling prior to the initiation of postmenopausal estrogen replacement therapy. Others will follow high-risk cancer women with frequent clinical and pelvic ultrasound evaluations with or without endometrial biopsy. However, the 1997 screening recommendations of the American College of Obstetricians and Gynecologists clearly state that endometrial assessment in the asymptomatic female is unwarranted and not cost-effective *(32)*. Most current practices reserve ultrasound, hysteroscopy, and biopsy for women with symptoms.

ENDOMETRIAL SCREENING METHODS

Pap Smear

Traditionally, cervical cytologic screening has demonstrated low sensitivity (40%) in diagnosing endometrial cancer *(34–36)*. There are several retrospective reports of postmenopausal women with endome-

Chapter 5 / Screening for Endometrial Cancer

trial cells identified on Pap smear. In 1 series of 74 postmenopausal patients with benign endometrial cells on cervical cytology, 63 (85%) had benign disease, 9 (12%) hyperplasia, and 1 carcinoma *(35)*. When atypia is identified, the risk of hyperplasia (5/22, 22.7%) increases. With a suspicious smear, (25/31, 74.5%), the diagnosis of carcinoma predominates. Interestingly, many articles have shown that 23–82% of endometrial cancer patients may present with a normal smear *(34,36–39)*. However, most articles concede that this finding predicts a higher stage or grade in the presence of a malignant diagnosis *(34,36–40)*. In 1992, the Bethesda system of Pap smear reporting developed a specific category called atypical glandular cells of uncertain significance (AGUS), directed at the diagnosis of glandular lesions of the endocervix and endometrium. This category of reporting is further subdivided into the following: favor reactive, favor premalignant or malignant, or unable to further classify.

Eddy reviewed 112 endometrial cancer patients, looking for AGUS Pap smears *(40)*. This article found that up to 29% of endometrial cancer patients have AGUS and 15% had a malignant diagnosis at presentation. In a second publication, Eddy also retrospectively reviewed endocervical and endometrial biopsy results of 531 patients with AGUS Paps *(41)*. These histologic specimens revealed 17% invasive carcinomas (29/531), with 88% (28/29) of these malignancies originating in the endometrial cavity. However, even with a near 50% diagnostic rate, Pap smear is not considered a particularly reliable screen for endometrial cancer. The Endopap (Monoject Division, Sherwood Medical, St. Louis, MO) is a new technique to cytologically evaluate the endometrial cavity *(42)*. The 2-mm-diameter, 9-cm-long, soft plastic microcuret is inserted into the endometrial cavity and 5–10 strokes are taken from the anterior and posterior endometrium.

In studies comparing this technique to the Pipelle (Uniman, Wilton, CT), a 3-mm, piston-action suction biopsy instrument, the sensitivity for endometrial disease was 56 and 51%, respectively, with a specificity of 94 and 100%. The sensitivity in diagnosing endometrial cancer was 80% vs 100% for the Pipelle *(42)*.

Endometrial Sampling

An endometrial sampling or biopsy should be the initial evaluation for women with suspected endometrial carcinoma *(43)*. The cytologic sampling requires identical endometrial manipulation with less diagnostic accuracy compared to histologic specimens. In other literature, the Pipelle histologic aspiration has been shown to yield a 98 and 99% sensitivity and specificity when compared to D&C or hysterectomy

70 Part II / Screening for Breast and Gynecological Cancers

specimens *(44)*. The use of these techniques may be limited in postmenopausal women with cervical stenosis or who have flattened, atrophic endometrial tissue *(31)*.

Transvaginal Ultrasonography

Transvaginal ultrasonography (TVS) is a useful technique for visualizing the entire pelvis, uterus, endometrium, ovaries, and cul-de-sac *(45,46)*. Some ultrasonographers report one-sided (single-layer) endometrial thickness *(47)*. The endometrial stripe usually measures the distance between basement membranes on each side of the cavity *(48,49)*. This gives an estimate of the diameter of the endometrial cavity. This is referred to as the double-layer thickness or endometrial stripe. The premenopausal endometrial stripe varies in width based on the phase of menstrual cycle and on hormonal stimulation *(50)*. The double-layer thickness range may be greater than 1 cm. Postmenopausally, without the use of estrogen replacement, the endometrial stripe should measure no more than 4 mm across *(51,52)*. Transvaginal ultrasonography will also outline uterine or endometrial abnormalities such as leiomyoma, endometrial polyps, stromal edema, or endometrial-cavity fluid collections *(53–57)*. Often these findings require clinical coordination and may be pathologic or artifactual, based on hormonal or tamoxifen use *(50,53)*. Additional consideration of patient symptomatology and medical history will factor into the need for further evaluation *(50,53)*.

There is voluminous recent literature reviewing TVS and its sensitivity, specificity, and positive and negative predictive values in the diagnosis of endometrial hyperplasia and adenocarcinoma *(48–56)*. Authors tend to stratify premenopausal from postmenopausal women and often exclude tamoxifen users and even women on estrogen *(50–53)*. Most articles tend to use a 5-mm double-layer endometrial stripe thickness as the critical value *(50,53,54–56)*. Asymptomatic menopausal screening will show significantly wider values if patients are within 5 yr of menopause or using steroid hormones that affect the endometrial lining *(58)*. When assessing TVS for endometrial pathology there is 90% sensitivity, 48% specificity, and 99% negative predictive value but only a 9–23% positive predictive value for diagnosing cancer *(59,60)*. It remains more sensitive and specific than endometrial cytology (97.4 vs 78.9% sensitive and 99.7 vs 88.5% negative predictive value, respectively) *(60)*. In the most stringent articles, TVS is compared to the D&C gold standard *(51,52,58)*. Even adding color Doppler to traditional sonography does not appear to improve the detection of malignant lesions over measurement of endometrial stripe thickness *(61,62)*.

Chapter 5 / Screening for Endometrial Cancer 71

When confronted with potential endometrial pathology, the practitioner has several options for tissue sampling *(31)*. As stated earlier, the Papanicolaou smear has the unacceptably low (<40%) sensitivity for the detection of endometrial cancer. However, when either endometrial cells or atypical glandular cells (AGUS) are recovered in a Pap smear screen, particularly in a postmenopausal female, endometrial histologic evaluation is indicated *(38,43)*. The outpatient clinic technique of Vabra (electrical suction instrument) or Pipelle (manual internal Piston) biopsy offers effective and comprehensive sampling. These techniques have a 91% correlative accuracy with the gold standard, fractional dilatation and curettage (D&C) *(31,33,43)*.

The critical feature is to obtain tissue for pathologic evaluation to rule out neoplasia. Once the pathologist identifies the status of the endometrium, particularly if there is endometrial hyperplasia with atypia, the clinician should complete a fractional D&C, which is considered to be the most thorough endometrial evaluation without hysterectomy *(28)*.

Sonohysterogram

Additional endometrial evaluation may be accomplished using a sonohysterogram *(63–67)*. This technique, originally described by Beyth in 1982, employs sterile placement of a 5F intrauterine catheter into the endometrial cavity, followed by insertion of a transvaginal ultrasound probe *(63)*. The cavity is then filled with saline and visualized in the transverse and longitudinal planes to recreate three-dimensional anatomy. Fifty to sixty-five percent of patients with wide (>5 mm) endometrial stripes will demonstrate endometrial polypoid masses, submucous leiomyomata, or other endometrial pathology *(63,65)*. Unfortunately, this technique offers no improvement over Pipelle biopsy in the diagnosis of endometrial cancer *(66)*. Finally, direct visualization with/without biopsy may be accomplished by a flexible office or an operative hysteroscopy *(67)*. The 8-mm hysteroscope allows a more focused and directed sampling or excision of pathologic tissues. Although hysteroscopic inspection of the endometrial cavity does yield 16% more histologic information over findings from blind uterine curettage, the majority of these additional findings are benign *(67,68)*. Usually, the hysteroscope is reserved for cases in which random endometrial sampling is noninformative or nondiagnostic *(31,33)*. The 1991 and 1997 American College of Obstetricians and Gynecologists ACOG Technical Bulletins acknowledge that there is no effective screening test for endometrial adenocarcinoma and specifically state that routine endometrial biopsy in asymptomatic women is not cost-effective *(6,69)*.

GENETIC TESTING

Several genetic syndromes link multiple organ sites to uterine carcinomas *(70–75)*. Commonly associated are breast, ovarian, colon, and endometrial adenocarcinomas. Some are by site-specific syndromes, associated with gene mutations on chromosome 17q21, the BRCA1 gene locus *(71)*. Others are clusters identified by Lynch as familial disease *(72)*. Lynch described two specific groups, one previously recognized as a Lynch II syndrome and now termed Hereditary Nonpolyposis Colon Cancer (HNPCC) *(72–75)*. This autosomal dominant inheritance is also associated with DNA mismatch repair genes HMSH2 (chromosome 2P), HMLH1 (chromosome 3P), HPMS 1 (chromosome 2q31-33), and PMS2 (chromosome 7p22). These family syndromes have at least three or more cancer cases including nonpolyposis colon cancer, or two family cases diagnosed at an early age (<50 yr) *(73,74)*. These patients are also at increased risk of developing an endometrial adenocarcinoma *(73–75)*.

The serum of affected patients may be screened for linkage mutations, which have been identified as markers for the disorder. Patients and their families may strongly consider genetic screening. Genetically affected individuals would merit earlier and more stringent cancer screening because these cancers occur at a younger age (10–15 yr younger) than expected. At-risk individuals might consider early colonoscopy (younger than age 50) looking for right-sided lesions *(74)*. Also, there should be consideration of prophylactic hysterectomy and oophorectomy upon completion of childbearing *(74)*. Identification of high-risk families allows heightened awareness of cancer potential. Fortunately, only 5–7% of all adenocarcinoma patients come from genetically predisposed families *(73–75)*. In these instances, the endometrial cancer cases appear to be in slightly younger women but with early-stage and low-grade disease. Options for heightened gynecologic surveillance are presented in the following section.

SCREENING ALGORITHM

The approach to abnormal uterine bleeding (premenopausal diagnosis) and postmenopausal bleeding is based on the clinical presentation. The clinician must consider patient age and other risk factors when deciding on screening and endometrial biopsy *(see* Algorithm 1). One end of the spectrum at low risk is a young woman (<35 yr age) with no abnormal uterine bleeding. She requires annual gynecological evaluation and comprehensive patient counseling. Similarly, the postmenopausal woman, posthysterectomy, experiencing no bleeding symptoms,

Chapter 5 / Screening for Endometrial Cancer

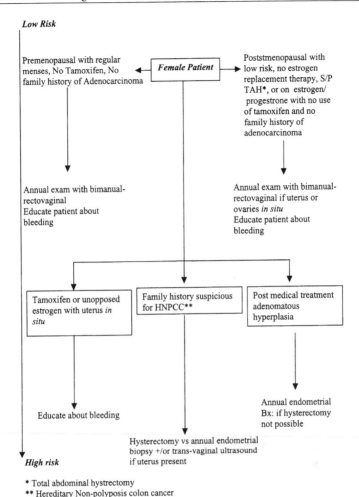

Algorithm 1. Endometrial cancer risk.

or at low cancer risk may undergo annual evaluation, again with patient education concerning the symptoms of cancer. Less straightforward are patients who are experiencing bleeding symptoms or are at risk because of personal and family cancer history or who use medications such as tamoxifen. This latter, common situation merits a discussion unto itself. The surveillance of patients on tamoxifen therapy remains contentious and a diagnostic dilemma for the practitioner. Historically, options range from patient education to semiannual clinical examinations, transvaginal ultrasound, periodic endometrial sampling, and progesterone-withdrawal testing.

As outlined earlier, at-risk HNCPP family members require consideration of prophylactic hysterectomy/oophorectomy or at least height-

74   Part II / Screening for Breast and Gynecological Cancers

ened clinical observation. Finally, women with a personal history of atypical endometrial tissue on biopsy deserve similar intensive surveillance.

COST-EFFECTIVENESS

This is a particularly important consideration in today's medical economy *(31,43)*. There is clearly no cost-effective screening technique for a high-risk asymptomatic patient *(6,69)*. Thorough counseling regarding personal risk factors and symptoms provides a woman with a good comprehension of her cancer status. The ultimate diagnosis is by outpatient endometrial sampling, however, this falls short of a true screening procedure. Biopsy may be painful and not particularly well tolerated. Also, office histology will cost $200 to 300 and is usually reserved for symptomatic cases. Other options include transvaginal sonography ($350) and office sonohysterography or hysteroscopy, both more invasive and cost prohibitive for consideration as screening techniques. The ACOG recommends reserving these modalities for symptomatic cases only *(6,69)*.

PATIENTS ON TAMOXIFEN THERAPY

One area of controversy surrounds the evaluation and surveillance of patients using tamoxifen. A nonsteroidal antiestrogenic breast cancer drug, it was originally used in ER-positive, postmenopausal breast cancer patients *(11,12,32)*. More recently, the indications have been extended to premenopausal women with node-negative, breast disease and even as chemoprophylaxis in high-risk breast cancer families *(12,29)*. Although generally estrogen antagonistic, tamoxifen has a paradoxical effect on the female reproductive tract. Studies have shown a 35–39% prevalence of endometrial polyps or stromal edema, an 11–16% prevalence of endometrial hyperplasia, and a 2–3% prevalence of endometrial cancer associated with its use *(9,75–77)*. Other gynecologic changes found secondary to tamoxifen include vaginal tissue proliferation and maturation, as well as an increase in sex-hormone-binding globulin levels and an effect on trabecular bone density and serum cholesterol *(9,32,77)*. These changes have been reported with as little as 14 mo of medication and are dose (>20 mg daily) and duration dependent *(9,32)*. The majority of literature documents that the stage, grade, histology, and tumor biology of tamoxifen-associated endometrial cancers are no different than in the general population *(9,12,32)*.

Two large National Cancer Institute (NCI) sponsored trials demonstrated the cancer survival benefits of tamoxifen use. The National Surgical Adjuvant Breast and Bowel Project (NSABP) trial recently

Chapter 5 / Screening for Endometrial Cancer

showed a 38% increase in disease-free survival rates in breast cancer tamoxifen users over nonusers *(11)*. Also, recent data from the Breast Cancer Prevention Trial (BCPT) reveal a decrease in the prevalence of breast cancer in unaffected patients who come from high-risk families *(78)*. Unfortunately, these clinical trials also confirm a 39% incidence of abnormal endometrial tissue associated with tamoxifen use, in addition to a 2–3/1000 annualized risk of endometrial cancer. Over the past 10 yr, researchers have attempted to identify the most effective technique for assessment of endometrial pathology during tamoxifen use. The surveillance process is confounded by the fact that endometrial cancers are frequently diagnosed at low grades and early stages. Most current authors promote patient education of symptoms and a low threshold for endometrial biopsy in the face of abnormal bleeding as the most sensitive and cost-effective mechanism of diagnosis. Other clinicians recommend a careful medical history for symptoms followed by semi-annual clinical examinations (for uterine enlargement).

There is copious literature evaluating the value of transvaginal (+/– Doppler) ultrasonography *(79–87)*, sonohysterography *(88–90)*, and even magnetic resonance imaging (MRI) *(91,92)* as radiologic screening modalities. Pelvic ultrasound demonstrated a thickened endometrial stripe (>8 mm) in 45–52% of tamoxifen users, particularly if use is greater than 5 yr *(79)*. Fourty-four to fifty-eight percent of these women had abnormal biopsies *(79,85)*. The leading pathologic finding is endometrial polyps in 33% of biopsies performed for increased endometrial thickness *(79,85,93,94)*. Most other studies cite up to a 58% incidence of endometrial thickening, but all conclude that the histological risk of cancer is extremely low (1–2%) *(75,93,94)*. Also, the high prevalence of false positive abnormal endometrial findings makes ultrasound a poor screening test for endometrial cancer. Recent articles couple color Doppler flow to ultrasonography but concede that little improvement in diagnostic sensitivity or specificity is derived from calculating mean pulsatility or resistance indices *(82,86,87)*.

Finally, in women with thickened endometrial stripes, a sonohysterogram may allow better clarification of the endometrial cavity *(88,89)*. In one recent study of 68 asymptomatic postmenopausal women on tamoxifen with an endometrial thickness of >8 mm, 33% demonstrated abnormal findings *(89)*. Sonohysterography correctly identified endometrial pathology in 95% of cases with no false-negative diagnoses *(89)*. However, none of this literature reported a marked improvement in early diagnosis at preinvasive stages or in disease prevention. Frequently, false-positive findings result in excessive patient concern and medical expense for noninvasive, asymptomatic pathology *(93)*. There is no literature that supports random, invasive endometrial sampling in asymptomatic women. That merely results in increased expense and patient discomfort. Biopsy reports in that clinical scenario show a 35–39% incidence of insufficient or atrophic tissue *(80,84)*.

Recent presentations at the American Society of Clinical Oncologists (ASCO) and in the ACOG Technical Practice Bulletins recommend frequent detailed clinical history and physical examination, with radiographic or pathologic intervention only when uterine abnormalities are detected.

Future investigations will evaluate the impact of raloxifen on asymptomatic but high-risk cancer patients. Investigational consideration might be directed to intermittent or continuous oral progesterone therapy during tamoxifen use *(95,96)*. Women with sufficient endometrial proliferation from any source to generate a progesterone-withdrawal bleeding/menses may be at greater risk for neoplastic endometrial pathology. These women might merit annual sampling *(96)*.

Finally, endometrial genetic testing may someday hold the key to which breast cancer patients on tamoxifen are at greatest risk for developing endometrial pathology. Naturally, posthysterectomy women have no risk of disease and to date, only benign cysts and no ovarian malignancies have been reported from tamoxifen use *(97)*.

INDICATIONS FOR REFERRAL

One issue that confronts primary care providers is the indication for referral to a subspecialist practitioner. Breast cancer patients with reproductive tract organs who use tamoxifen must have an annual gynecologic evaluation. This may be accomplished by any physician trained in current gynecology. Frequently, routine gynecologic care, cervical cytologic screening, and even postmenopausal counseling and hormone replacement therapy are all provided by primary care physicians. When any female over the age of 40 develops abnormal bleeding, she requires endometrial sampling *(15,31)*. This may trigger consultation with a gynecologic specialist. Women with more complicated gynecologic histories, chronic anovulation, polycystic ovarian disease, or unexplained abnormal bleeding require gynecologic evaluation and intervention. Patients who have unopposed endogenous estrogen or who take exogenous estrogen in an unopposed (without progesterone) fashion are also at risk for endometrial cancer and probably merit specialist care. These women need a thorough examination and comprehensive risk–benefit counseling concerning hormone replacement and progesterone-withdrawal therapy. Certainly any patient diagnosed with

Chapter 5 / Screening for Endometrial Cancer

endometrial hyperplasia with or without atypia should be referred to a gynecologic specialist. Often, these women at increased risk for endometrial cancer will be evaluated and counseled by a gynecologic oncologist.

Finally, there are several circumstances that might generate consultation with a gynecologic oncologist. Patients with a breast cancer history on tamoxifen who retain their reproductive tract organs will often meet the subspecialist. Certainly, women with a personal cancer history or who are part of high-risk families, where uterine cancer is a potential diagnosis, deserve the expertise of a gynecologic oncologist. This includes families with site-specific cancer symptoms or Lynch HNPCC-type genetic syndromes.

PREVENTION

Probably the most important section of the chapter centers on disease prevention. Although not entirely preventable, endometrial cancer may be avoided in many instances *(96)*. This begins primarily with education of both patient and health care providers. Knowledge of the disease pathophysiology, risk factors, and symptoms helps raise the clinical consciousness and prompts early biopsy diagnosis. Even earlier, hormonal adjustments with intermittent progestin withdrawals may prevent low-grade disease in anovulatory women *(15)*.

Gynecologists agree that postmenopausal estrogen replacement when the uterus is retained requires some method of progestional opposition. This may be with continuous (medroxy progesterone acetate, 2.5 mg daily) low-dose therapy or cyclic (intermittent) progesterone (10 mg daily × 10–14 d), which results in a withdrawal bleed. Women with uterine hyperplasia may require long-term, higher-dose progestin therapy or even hysterectomy *(95,96)*. In 1997, Gambrell published a meta-analysis evaluating methods for diagnosing and treating endometrial cancer patients *(95)*. His focus was to better define the role of progestin therapy in postmenopausal estrogen replacement therapy. He concluded that endometrial cancer can occur in cases of combination estrogen–progesterone therapy when the progestin dose is less than optimal: medroxy progesterone acetate 2.5 mg daily. He stressed that the latter continuous therapy may not be fully protective, citing 67 published cases, which occurred on that daily therapy. He also promoted the progesteone challenge test as a mechanism to identify at-risk postmenopausal women. The progesterone challenge test involves oral medroxy progesterone acetate 10 mg daily for 13 d. When this is stopped or withdrawn, an estrogen-primed endometrium will shed or menstruate.

78 Part II / Screening for Breast and Gynecological Cancers

Table 1
Guidelines for Reducing Endometrial Cancer

1. Encourage oral contraceptive use in premenopausal women needing family planning.
2. Identify postmenopausal women at risk for endometrial cancer.
   a. Use progestogen challenge test as part of initial evaluation and repeat annually in untreated asymptomatic women.
   b. Perform endometrial biopsy for positive bleeding responses to progestogen challenge test.
   c. Pretreatment endometrial biopsies need not be done with negative responses to progestogen challenge test; however, any abnormal bleeding with hormone replacement therapy should be promptly sampled.
   d. Treat precancerous lesions with progestogens.
3. Use adequate durations and dosages of progestogens.
   a. Duration: 12–14 d each cycle or month
   b. Dosage: 10 mg medroxy-progesterone acetate 2.5 mg norethindrone acetate.
4. Continuous combined hormone replacement therapy may not be fully endometrial protective.
5. Cyclic combined hormone replacement therapy is clinically superior and may be more endometrial protective.
6. There are no adverse effects of progestogens on lipids and lipoproteins, especially when adequate dosages of estrogen are used.
7. Manage hormone replacement therapy side effects by adding diuretic, or changing the type, dosage, or route of administration of progestogens.

Reproduced from Gambrell, Jr RD. (1997) Strategies to reduce the incidence of endometrial cancer in postmenopausal women. *Am J Obset Gynecol* 177(5):1196–1204, with permission.

The test attempts to identify the patient who theoretically requires a more invasive evaluation with ultrasound or biopsy.

Gambrell reviewed progestin therapy, including progesterone-induced premenstrual symptoms and its therapy. He emphasized the estrogen-dependent lipid profile benefit with no diminution by the addition of progesterone *(97)*. He also presented guidelines for reduction or prevention of endometrial cancer (*see* Table 1). These include patient education, aggressive use of combination hormone therapy, and judicious use of diagnostic testing when indicated. Careful consideration must be given to the risks and benefits of both alternatives. Long-term (especially high-dose) progestin therapy may negatively impact the cardiac/lipid profile benefit of estrogen *(98)*. According to recent literature, it may also impact on the risk of subsequent breast cancers

Chapter 5 / Screening for Endometrial Cancer

(99). Clearly, this complicated scenario must be addressed in an individualized fashion with each patient.

SUMMARY

Endometrial carcinoma is the fourth most commonly diagnosed cancer in women in the United States. The majority of the cases occur in elderly women. Prognosis is excellent. Only a minority of the patients has Stage III or VI disease at the time of presentation. Certain hereditary factors, estrogen therapy without progesterone, and tamoxifen use are associated with increased risk of endometrial carcinoma. Routine screening for endometrial carcinoma is not recommended. However, it is highly recommended in high-risk patients.

REFERENCES

1. Parkin DM, Pisani P, Ferlay J. (1993) Estimates of the worldwide incidence of eighteen major cancers in 1985. *Int J Cancer* 54(4):594–606.
2. Parkin DM, Muir CS, Whelan SL, et al. (1992) Cancer incidence in five continents VI. *IARC Sci Publ* 120:45–173.
3. *American Cancer Society Facts and Figures.* (1999) Atlanta, GA: American Cancer Society.
4. Miller BA, Riles LAG, Hankey BF. (1993) *SEER Cancer Statistics Review: 1973–1990.* Bethesda, MD: National Cancer Institute, p. 2789.
5. Brinton LA, Hoover RN. (1992) Epidemiology of gynecologic cancers. In: Hoskins WJ, Perez, CA, Young RC, eds., *Principles and Practice of Gynecologic Oncology.* Philadelphia: JB Lippincott, pp. 3–26.
6. ACOG Technical Bulletin. (1991) *Carcinoma of the Endometrium.* Washington, DC: ACOG.
7. Zweizig SL. (1999) Office screening for gynecologic cancer. *Obstet Gynecol* 42(2):267–275.
8. Suh-Burgmann EJ, Goodman A. (1999) Surveillance for endometrial cancer in women receiving Tamoxifen. *Ann Intern Med* 131:127–135.
9. Barakat RR. (1998) Tamoxifen and the endometrium. In: Foon, KA, Muss, HB, eds., *Biological and Hormonal Therapies of Cancer.* Kluwer Academic, Boston, MA, pp. 195–207.
10. Cohen I, Altaras MM, Shapira J. (1997) Different coexisting endometrial histological features in asymptomatic postmenopausal breast cancer patients treated with tamoxifen. *Gynecol Obstet Invest* 43:60–63.
11. Fisher B, Costantino JP, Redmond CK, et al. (1994) Endometrial cancer in tamoxifen treated breast cancer patients: findings from the National Surgical Adjuvant Breast and Bowel Project (NSABP) B-14. *J Natl CA Inst* 86:527–537.
12. Fishe B, Costantino JP, Wickerham DL. (1998) Tamoxifen for prevention of breast cancer: report of the National Surgical Adjuvant Breast and Bowel Project, P-1 Study. *J Natl Cancer Inst* 90(18):1371–1388.
13. Skully RE, Bonfiglio TA, Kurman RJ, Silverburg SG, Wickinson EJ. (1994) *Uterine Corpuy in Histological Typing of Female Genital Tract Tumors.* New York: Springer-Verlag. p. 13.

80   Part II / Screening for Breast and Gynecological Cancers

14. Kurman R, Kaminski P, Norris H. (1985) The behavior of endometrial hyperplasia: a long term study of "untreated hyperplasia in 170 patients." *Cancer* 56:403–412.
15. Burke TW, Tortolero-Luna G, Malpica A, et al. (1996) Endometrial hyperplasia and endometrial cancer. *Obstet Gynecol* 3:411–456.
16. Brooks SE. (1997) A review of screening and early detention of endometrial cancer and use of risk assessment. *J Assoc Acad Minority Physicians* 8:24–37.
17. Hill HA, Coutes RJ, Austin H, et al. (1995) Racial differences in tumor grade among women with endometrial cancer. *Gynecol Oncol* 56:154–163.
18. Pike MC. (1990) Reducing cancer risk in women through life style-mediated changes in hormone levels. *Cancer Detect Prev* 14:595–607.
19. Shuxo XO, Brinton LA, Zheng W, et al. (1992) Relation of obesity and body fat distribution to endometrial cancer in Shanghai, China. *Cancer Res* 52(14):3865–3870.
20. Brinton LA, Barret RJ, Berman ML, et al. (1993) Cigarette smoking and the risk of endometrial cancer. *Am J Epidemio* 137(3):281–291.
21. Jick SS, Walhen AM, Jick H. (1993) Oral contraceptives and endometrial cancer. *Obstet Gynecol* 82(6):931–935.
22. Parazzini F, LaVecchia C, Bocciolone L, Franceschi S. (1991) The epidemiology of endometrial cancer. *Gynecol Oncol* 41(1):1–16.
23. Parazzini F, LaVecchia C, Negri E, Fedele L, Balotta F. (1991) Reproductive factors and risk of endometrial cancer. *Am J Obstet Gynecol* 164(2):522–527.
24. Brinton LA, Hoover RN. (1993) Estrogen replacement therapy and endometrial cancer risk: unresolved issues. The endometrial cancer collaborative group. *Obstet Gynecol* 81(2):265–271.
25. Grady D, Gemetsadik T, Kerlikowske K, Ernster V, Petitti D. (1995) Hormone replacement therapy and endometrial cancer risk: a meta-analysis. *Obstet Gynecol* 85(2):304–313.
26. Jick SS, Walker AM, Jick H. (1993) Estrogens, progesterone and endometrial cancer. *Epidemiology* 4(1):20–24.
27. Woodruff JD, Pickar JH. (1994) Incidence of endometrial hyperplasia in post-menopausal women taking conjugated estrogens (Premarin) with medroxy-progesterone acetate or conjugated estrogen alone. The Menopause Study Group. *Am J Obstet Gynecol* 170(5 pt 1):1213–1223.
28. American Cancer Society. (1993) *Guidelines for Cancer Related Check Up: An Update.* Atlanta, GA: American Cancer Society.
29. Early Breast Cancer Trialists Collaborative Group. (1988) Effects of adjuvant tamoxifen and of cytotoxic therapy on mortality. *N Engl J Med* 319:1681–1685.
30. Brinton LA, Berman ML, Mortel, R, et al. (1993) Reproductive, menstrual and medical risk factor for endometrial cancer: results from a case-control study. *Am J Obstet Gynecol* 167(5):1317–1325.
31. Chambers JT, Chambers SK. (1992) Endometrial sampling: When? Where? Why? With what? *Obstet Gynecol* 5:28–39.
32. ACOG Committee Opinion. (1996) Tamoxifen and endometrial cancer. *Int J Gynecol Obstet* 53:197–199.
33. Kim YB, Ghosh K, Ainbinder S, Berek JS. (1998) Diagnostic and therapeutic advances in gynecologic oncology: screening for gynecologic cancer. In: Ozeols, RF, eds., *Gynecology Oncology.* Kluwer Academic, Boston, MA, pp. 253–276.
34. DuBeshter B, Warshal DP, Angel C, et al. (1991) Endometrial carcinoma: the relevance of cervical cytology. *Obstet Gynecol* 77:458–462.
35. Yancey M, Magelssen D, Demaurez A, Lee RB. (1990) Classification of endometrial cell on cervical cytology. *Obstet Gynecol* 76:1000–1005.

Chapter 5 / Screening for Endometrial Cancer

36. Demirkiron F, Arvas M, Erkum E, et al. (1995) The prognostic significance of cervico-vaginal cytology in endometrial cancer. *Eur J Gynecol Oncol* 16:403–409.
37. Mitchell H, Giles G, Medley G. (1994) Accuracy and survival benefits of cytologic prediction of endometrial carcinoma on routine cervical smears. *Int J Gynecol Pathol* 12:34–40.
38. Larson DM, Johnson K, Reyes CN, Brosk SK. (1994) Prognostic significance of malignant cervical cytology in patients with endometrial cancer. *Obstet Gynecol* 84:399–403.
39. Burk JR, Lehman HF, Wolf FS. (1984) Inadequacy of papanicolaou smears in the detection of endometrial cancers. *N Eng J Med* 291:191,192.
40. Eddy GL, Wojtowycz MA, Piraino PS, Mazur M. (1997) Papanicolaou smears by the Bethesda system in endometrial malignancy: utility and prognostic importance. *Obstet Gynecol* 90:999–1003.
41. Eddy GL, Strumpf KB, Wojtowycz MA, Piraino PS, Mazur MT. (1997) Biopsy findings in five hundred thirty-one patients with atypical glandular cells of uncertain significance as defined by the Bethesda system. *Am J Obstet Gynecol* 177(5):1188–1195.
42. Van Den Bosch T, Vandendael A, Wranz P, Lombard CJ. (1996) Endopap-versus Pipelle-sampling in the diagnosis of postmenopausal endometrial disease. *Eur J Obstet Gynecol* 64:91–94.
43. Schirch-Shelly M. (1997) Endometrial biopsy. *Am Fam Physician* 55(5):1731–1736.
44. Shapley M, Redman CWE. (1997) Endometrial sampling and general practice. *Br J Gen Prac* 47:387–392.
45. Bourne T, Hamberger L, Hahlin M, Granberg S. (1997) Ultrasound in gynecology: endometrium. *Int J Gynecol Obstet* 56:115–127.
46. Bree RL. (1997) Ultrasound of the endometrium: facts, controversies and future trends. *Abdom Imaging* 22:557–568.
47. Tesoro MR, Borgida AF, MacLaurin NA, Asuncion CM. (1999) Transvaginal endometrial sonography in postmenopausal women taking tamoxifen. *Obstet Gynecol* 93(3):363–366.
48. Gruboeck K, Jurkovic D, Lawton F, et al. (1996) The diagnostic value of endometrial thickness and volume measurements by three-dimensional ultrasound in patients with postmenopausal bleeding. *Ultrasound Obstet Gynecol* 8:272–276.
49. Fleischer AC. (1997) Optimizing the accuracy of transvaginal ultrasonograpy of the endometrium. *N Eng J Med* 337(25):1839,1840.
50. Goldstein SR, Zeltser I, Horan CK, Snyder JR, Schwartz LB. (1997) Ultrasonography-based triage for perimenopausal patients with abnormal uterine bleeding. *Am J Obstet Gynecol* 177(1);102–108.
51. Güner H, Tiras BM, Karabacak O, et al. (1996) Endometrial assessment by vaginal ultrasonography might reduce endometrial sampling in patients with postmenopausal bleeding: a prospective study. *Aust NZ J Obstet Gynecol* 36(2):175–178.
52. Büyük E, Durmusolu F, Erenus M, Karakoç B. (1999) Endometrial disease diagnosed by transvaginal ultrasound and dilatation and curettage. *Acta Obstet Gynecol Scand* 78:419–422.
53. Smith-Bindman R, Kerlikowke K, Feldstein VA, et al. (1998) Endovaginal ultrasound to exclude endometrial cancer and other endometrial abnormalities. *JAMA* 280(17):1510–1530.
54. Briley M, Lindsell, DRM. (1998) The role of transvaginal ultrasound in the investigation of women with post-menopausal bleeding. *Clin Radiol* 53:502–505.

82 Part II / Screening for Breast and Gynecological Cancers

55. Bakour SH, Dwarakanath LS, Khan KS, Newton JR, Gupta JK. (1999) The diagnostic accuracy of ultrasound scan in prediction endometrial hyperplasia and cancer in postmenopausal bleeding. *Acta Obstet Gynecol Scand* 78:447–451.

56. Langer RD, Pierce JJ, O'Hanlan KA. (1997) Transvaginal ultrasonography compared with endometrial biopsy for the detention of endometrial disease. *N Engl J Med* 337:1792–1798.

57. Vuento MH, Pirhonen JP, Mäkinen JI, et al. (1996) Endometrial fluid accumulation in asymptomatic postmenopausal women. *Ultrasound Obstet Gynecol* 8:37–41.

58. Tsuda H, Kawabata M, Kawabata K, Yamamoto K, Umesaki N. (1997) Improvement of diagnostic accuracy of transvaginal ultrasound for identification of endometrial malignancies by using cutoff level of endometrial thickness based on length of time since menopause. *Gynecol Oncol* 64:35–37.

59. Tsuda H, Kawabata M, Yamamoto K, Inoue T, Umesaki N. (1997) Prospective study to compare endometrial cytology and transvagina ultrasonography for identification of endometrial malignancies. *Gynecol Oncol* 65:383–386.

60. Kufahl J, Pedersen I, Eriksen PS. (1997) Transvaginal ultrasound, endometrial cytology sampled by Gynoscann and histology obtained by UterineExplora Curette compared to the histology of the uterine specimen. *Acta Obstet Gynecol Scand* 76:790–796.

61. Bonilla-Musoles F, Raga F, Osborne N, Blanes J, Coelho F. (1996) Three-dimensional hysterosonography for the study of endometrial tumors:Comparison with conventional trasnvaginal sonography, hysterosalpingography and hysteroscopy. *Gynecol Oncol* 65:245–252.

62. Vuento MH, Pirhonen J, Mäkinen JI. (1999) Screening for endometrial cancer in asymptomatic postmenopausal women with conventional and colour dopler sonography. *Br J Obstet Gynecol* 106:14–20.

63. Aviram R, Michaeli G, Lew S. (1999) The value of sonohysterography combined with cytological analysis of the fluid retrieved from the endometrial cavity in prediction histological diagnosis. *Ultasound Obstet Gynecol* 14:58–63.

64. Sohaey R, Woodward P. (1999) Sonohysterography: technique, endometrial finding and clinical applications. *Sem Ultrasound, CT MRI* 20(4):250–258.

65. Goldstein SR. (1996) Saline infusion sonohysterography. *Obstet Gynecol* 39(1):248–258.

66. O'Connell LP, Fries MH, Zeringue E, Brehm W. (1998) Triage of abnormal postmenopausal bleeding: a comparison of endometrial biopsy and transvaginal sonohysterography versus fractional curettage with hysteroscopy. *Am J Obstet Gynecol* 178:956–961.

67. Wildrich T, Bradley LD, Mitchinson AR, Collins RL. (1996) Comparison of saline infusion sonography with office hysteroscopy for the evaluation of the endometrium. *Am J Obstet Gynecol* 74:1327–1334.

68. Maia H, Barbosa IC, Marques D, et al. (1996) Hysteroscopy and transvaginal sonography in menopausal women receiving hormone replacement. *J Am Assoc Gynecol Lapar* 4(1):13–18.

69. Routine Cancer Screening. (1997) *ACOG Committee Opinion.* Washington, DC: ACOG.

70. ACOG Educational Bulletin. (1998) *Ovarian Cancer.* Washington, DC: ACOG.

71. Toribara NW, Sieisenger MH. (1995) Screening for colorectal cancer. *N Engl J Med* 332:861–867.

72. Winawer SJ, Schottenfeld D, Flehinger BJ. (1991) Colorectal cancer screening. *J Natl Cancer Inst* 83:243–253.

Chapter 5 / Screening for Endometrial Cancer 83

73. Boyd J. (1998) Molecular genetics of hereditary ovarian cancer. *Oncology* 12(3):399–413.
74. Boyd J, Rubic SC. (1997) Hereditary ovarian cancer: molecular genetics and clinical implications. *Gynecol Oncol* 64:196–206.
75. Lynch HT, Casey MJ, Lynch J, White T, Goodwin, AK. (1998) Genetics and ovarian carcinoma. *Semin Oncol* 25(3):265–280.
76. Assikis VJ, Jorda, VC. (1995) Gynecologic effects of Tamoxifen and the association with endometrial carcinoma. *Int J Gynecol Obstet* 49:241–257.
77. Neven P, Vergote I. (1998) Should Tamoxifen users be screened for endometrial lesions? *Lancet* 351:155,156.
78. Friedrich M, Villena-Heinsen C, Mink D, et al. (1998) Ultrasonography of the endometrium and endometrial pathology under tamoxifen treatment. *Eur J Gynecol Oncol* 6:536–540.
79. Keda, RP, Bourne TH, Powles TJ, et al. (1994) Effects of tamoxifen on uterus and ovaries of postmenopausal women in a randomized breast cancer prevention trial. *Lancet* 343:1318–1321.
80. Hann LE, Giess CS, Bach AM, et al. (1997) Endometrial thickness in Tamoxifen-treated patients: correclation with clinical and pathologic findings. *Am J Roentgenol* 168:657–661.
81. Cecchini S, Ciatto S, Bonardi R, et al. (1996) Screening by ultrasonography for endometrial carcinoma in postmenopausal breast cancer patients under adjuvant tamoxifen. *Gynecol Oncol* 60:409–411.
82. Nahari C, Tepper R, Beyth Y, et al. (1999) Long-term transvaginal ultrasonographic endometrial follow-up in postmenopausal breast cancer patients with tamoxifen treatment. *Gynecol Oncol* 74:222–226.
83. Cohen I, Beyth Y, Tepper R. (1998) The role of ultrasound in the detection of endometrial pathologies in asymptomatic postemenopausal breast cancer patients with tamoxifen treatment. *Obstet Gynecol* 53(7):429–438.
84. Franchi M, Ghezzi F, Donadello N, et al. (1999) Endometrial thickness in Tamoxifen-treated patients: an independent predictor of endometrial disease. *Obstet Gynecol* 93:1004–1008.
85. Anteby EY, Yagel S, Weissman A. (1996) Sonographic evaluation of the uterus in postmenopausal women receiving Tamoxifen: characterization of mid-uterine abnormalities. *Eur J Obstet Gynecol* 69:115–119.
86. McGonigle KF, Shaw SL, Vasilev SA, et al. (1998) Abnormalities detected on transvaginal ultrasonography in tamoxifen-treated postmenopausal breast cancer patients may represent endometrial cystic atrophy. *Am J Obstet Gynecol* 178:1145–1150.
87. Spencer C. (1999) Screening for endometrial cancer in asymptomatic postmenopausal women with conventional and colour dopler sonography. *Br J Obstet Gynecol* 106:612–613.
88. Marconi D, Exacoustos C, Cangi B. (1997) Transvaginal sonographic and hysteroscopic findings in postmenopausal women receiving Tamoxifen. *J Am Assoc Gynecol Laparosc* 4(3):331–339.
89. Scwartz LB, Snyder J, Horan C, et al. (1998) The use of transvaginal ultrasound and saline infusion sonohysterography for the evaluation of asymptomatic postmenopausal breast cancer patients on Tamoxifen. *Obstet Gynecol* 1:48–53.
90. Tepper R, Beyth Y, Altaras MM, et al. (1997) Value of sonohysterography in asymptomatic postmenopausal tamoxifen-treated patients. *Gynecol Oncol* 64:386–397.
91. Dubisnky TJ, Stroenhlein K, Abu-Chazzeh Y, Parvey HR, Maklad N. (1999) Prediction of benign and malignant endometrial disease: hysterosonographic-pathologic correlation. *Radiology* 210:393–397.

84 Part II / Screening for Breast and Gynecological Cancers

92. Gordon AN, Fleischer AC, Dudley BS, et al. (1989) Preoperative assessment of myometrial invasion of endometrial adenocarcinoma by sonography (US) and magnetic resonance imaging (MRI). *Gynecol Oncol* 34:175–179.
93. Chen SS, Rumancik WM, Spiegel G. (1990) Magnetic resonance imaging in stage I endometrial carcinoma. *Obstet Gynecol* 5:274–277.
94. Mourits MJ, Van Der Zee GJ, Willemse P, et al. (1999) Discrepancy between ultrasono-graphy and hysteroscopy and histology of endometrium in postmenopausal breast cancer patients using tamoxifen. *Gynecol Oncol* 73:21–26.
95. Timmerman D, Deprest J, Bourne T, et al. (1998) A randomized trial on the use of ultrasonography or office hysteroscopy for endometrial assessment in postmenopausal patients with breast cancer who were treated with tamoxifen. *Am J Obstet Gynecol* 179:62–70.
96. Cohen I, Figer A, Altaras MM, et al. (1996) Common endometrial decidual reaction in postmenopausal breast cancer patients treated with Tamoxifen and progestogens. *Int J Gynecol Pathol* 15(1):17–22.
97. Gambrell RD. (1997) Strategies to reduce the incidence of endometrial cancer in post-menopausal women. *Am J Obstet Gynecol* 177:1196–1207.
98. Schwartz LB, Rutkowski N, Horan C, et al. (1998) Use of transvagianal ultrasonography to monitor the effects of Tamoxifen on uterine leiomyoma size and ovarian cyst formation. *J Ultrasound Med* 17:699–703.
99. Gambrell RD, Teran AZ. (1991) Changes in lipids and lipoproteins with long-term estrogen deficiency and hormone replacement therapy. *Am J Obstet Gynecol* 165:307–317.

III SCREENING FOR GASTROINTESTINAL CANCERS

6 Screening for Colorectal Cancer

Kittichai Promrat, MD, Khalid Aziz, MD, and George Y. Wu, MD, PhD

KEY PRINCIPLES

- Colorectal carcinoma is the second leading cause of cancer-related deaths in the United States.
- Most deaths from colorectal cancer are preventable through screening.
- Natural history of colorectal cancer is ideal for screening.
- Precursor lesion (adenomatous polyp) is readily identifiable by various screening techniques.
- Removal of adenomatous polyps prevents progression to cancer.
- Several options for colorectal cancer screening are widely available and cost-effective.
- Persons age 50 and older should have screening test for colorectal cancer, depending on their risk.

EPIDEMIOLOGY

Adenocarcinoma of the colon and rectum is the second leading cause of cancer-related deaths in the United States. During 1999, approx 129,400 new cases of colorectal cancer were diagnosed and approx 56,600 persons died from the disease *(1)*. Worldwide, an estimated 875,000 cases of colorectal cancer occurred in 1996, accounting for 8.5% of all new cases of cancer *(2)*. The cumulative lifetime risk is approx 5%. The incidence of colorectal cancer increases with age and occurs with about equal frequency in women and men.

From: *Cancer Screening: A Practical Guide for Physicians*
Edited by: K. Aziz and G. Y. Wu © Humana Press Inc., Totowa, NJ

Colorectal cancer is uncommon among those younger than age 40. Rates of disease begin to rise sharply after age 50, which has implications for screening. Recent data have continued to show a decrease in incidence rates of colorectal carcinoma in whites since the mid-1980s, particularly for the distal colon and rectum *(3)*. Mortality rates of colorectal cancer also have decreased. These trends could be explained by the current strategy of polyp removal, early stage of detection, more accurate diagnosis, lower incidence, or more effective treatment; it is uncertain in what proportions each of these contribute. Incidence rates of colorectal cancer vary approx 20-fold around the world, with the highest rates seen in the developed world. This may be explained, in large part, by dietary and other environmental differences *(4)*. The incidence rates of colorectal cancer in Hawaiian Japanese are among the highest rates in the world, whereas the incidence rates in Japan have been quite low *(4)*. Among US populations, the incidence rate of colorectal carcinoma in whites peaked in the 1980s and subsequently declined. In contrast, incidence rates among African-Americans continue to rise, especially in males *(3)*. Overall, the majority of tumors arise in the proximal colon (from splenic flexure to cecum) (38.8%) and approximately equal numbers arise in the distal colon (descending colon and sigmoid colon) (29.6%) and rectum (28.5%) *(3)*. Proximal carcinoma incidence rates among African-American are considerably higher than in whites and continue to increase, whereas rates in whites show signs of decline *(3)*. Factors that contribute to this observed discrepancy remain unclear.

BIOLOGY OF ADENOMA AND COLORECTAL CARCINOMA

It is generally accepted that most cancers of the colon and rectum develop from adenomatous polyps. The progression from normal mucosa to adenomatous polyp to cancer appears to be associated with an accumulation of genetic alterations that are acquired after birth, resulting in genes that promote the development of cancer (oncogenes) as well as loss of genes that suppress tumor development. Several specific genetic abnormalities have been identified. Adenomatous polyps are found in about a quarter of people by age 50 yr, and the prevalence increases with age. Few adenomatous polyps progress to cancer; the rate is estimated at about 2.5 polyps per 1000 per year *(5,6)*. In those that do, the transformation from small adenoma to cancer seems to occur slowly over many years. The average time taken for this transformation (polyp dwell time) is estimated to be about 10 yr, particularly for ones less than

1 cm in diameter. The probability that an adenomatous polyp will progress to cancer and the probability that the patient will develop other adenomatous polyps or cancer elsewhere in the colon and rectum can be estimated from characteristics of the polyp at the time it is first examined. In the National Polyp Study, 1.1% of adenomatous polyps <5 mm in diameter, 4.6% of those 5–9 mm in diameter, and 20.6% of those >1 cm had high-grade dysplasia, an early sign of preinvasive cancer *(7)* (Table 1). A British study *(8)* followed 1618 patients in whom adenomas were removed from the rectum and sigmoid colon and received no additional testing for about 14 yr/patient. Those whose original polyps had been tubulovillous, villous, or large (more than 1 cm in diameter) were more than three times more likely to develop colon cancer than people in the general population (odds ratio 3.6; 95% confidence interval [CI] 2.4–5.0) (Table 2). If, in addition, there were multiple rectosigmoid polyps with advanced pathology, affected people were more than six times more likely to develop colon cancer (odds ratio 6.6; 95% CI 3.3–11.8). On the other hand, in patients with small tubular adenoma (whether single or multiple), the risk of subsequent cancer was found to be no more than in the general population *(8)*.

RATIONALE FOR SCREENING

Most colorectal cancers develop from benign adenomatous polyps and develop slowly over many years. This provides a window of opportunity for detecting and removing precancerous lesions and early-stage cancers. Survival from colorectal cancer is closely related to the clinical and pathological stage of the disease at detection. Up to 90% of patients with cancer limited to the bowel wall will be alive 5 yr after diagnosis *(9)* compared with 35–60% of those with involvement of the lymph nodes, and less than 10% of patients with metastatic disease *(10)*. These features make colorectal cancer an ideal target for screening and early detection. Screening tests, such as fecal occult blood test (FOBT) and/ or flexible sigmoidoscopy, are sufficiently accurate in detecting early-stage disease. They are acceptable to patients and are feasible in general clinical practice. Several controlled trials and case-control studies suggest that removing adenomatous polyps reduces incidence of colorectal cancer and detecting early-stage cancers reduces mortality from the disease. Screening for colorectal cancer in average risk-people has been shown in several models to be cost-effective. All strategies (FOBT, flexible sigmoidoscopy, barium enema, colonoscopy) cost less than $20,000 per year of life saved and are within an acceptable range of cost-effectiveness by US health standards *(11,12)*.

Part III / Screening for Gastrointestinal Cancers

Table 1

Polyp Size and Risk of High-Grade Dysplasia/Cancer

Polyp size (mm)	High-grade dysplasia/cancer
Less than 5	1.1%
5–9	4.6%
Greater than 10	20.6%

Table 2

Characteristic of Rectosigmoid Polyps and Risk of Subsequent Colon Cancer

Characteristics	Odds ratio (95% CI)
Single tubulovillous, villous, >1 cm	3.6 (2.4–5.0)
Tubulovillous, villous, >1 cm	6.6 (3.3–11.8)
Single or multiple tubular adenoma, <1 cm	0.5 (0.1–1.3)

METHODS OF SCREENING

Fecal Occult Blood Testing

The concept of detecting colorectal cancers by testing for blood in the stool is based on the observation that cancers bleed more than normal mucosa. About two-thirds of cancers bleed in the course of a week *(13)* and a higher proportion, perhaps more than 90%, will be detected with repeated testing over several years. Bleeding tends to be intermittent and blood is distributed unevenly in the stool. The amount of bleeding increases with the size of the polyp and the stage of cancer. People with small polyps bleed scarcely more than those without polyps, whereas those with very large polyps (>2 cm) often bleed *(14)*. Testing for fecal occult blood will, therefore, lead to detection of cancers; however, it also will lead to the detection of polyps because they are much more common.

The test most widely used for detecting blood in the stool is the guaiac-based test for peroxidase activity. The version of the test most commonly used is the Hemoccult II test (SmithKline Diagnostics Inc., San Jose, CA). Several limitations of the test have to be kept in mind. It detects blood from any source in the gastrointestinal tract from nose, gum diseases, gastritis, peptic ulcer disease, and hemorrhoids. The test is also not specific for blood. It can detect other substances that contain peroxidase or pseudoperoxidase activity. Certain foods and vegetables (red meat, turnips, horseradish) with peroxidase activity can cause false-

Table 3

Factors Affecting FOBT (Guaiac Based)

False-positive
  Rare red meat (nonhuman hemoglobin)
  Turnips, horseradish (dietary peroxidase)
  Aspirin, NSAID (gastric irritants)
False-negative
  Vitamin C (antioxidant)
  Storage

positive reaction (*see* Table 3). The person being tested, therefore, should avoid rare red meat, turnips, horseradish, aspirin, and NSAID for 2 d before the test and during the test period. The number of samples per stool and the number of stools sampled increase the sensitivity of the FOBT. The person undergoing the test should take samples of stool from different sites, smear them onto the FOBT card, and then repeat the procedure for the next two bowel movements. The cards should then be returned to a screening center, either by mail or in person within 4 d. Patients with positive results should undergo complete colonic evaluation, preferable with colonoscopy. Complications of FOBT result mainly from the diagnostic evaluation of people with positive tests. Data from the UK trial showed 0.5% complication rate (perforation and bleeding) as a result of colonoscopy and polypectomy without observed mortality *(15)*.

EFFECTIVENESS OF FOBT

The evidence to support the effectiveness of population-based screening by FOBT continues to mount. Three large prospective randomized controlled trials, involving more than 250,000 participants, showed statistically significant reduction of colorectal mortality from 15% to 33% *(9,16,17)* (Table 4). The first published randomized trial was conducted in Minnesota *(9)* on 46,551 people, age 50–80, who were randomized into three groups. One was screened annually, the second screened every 2 yr, and the third received usual care. After 13 yr of follow-up, annual fecal occult blood testing reduced colorectal cancer mortality by at least 33%, and after 18 yr of follow up, a 21% reduction in colorectal cancer mortality was observed in the biennial group (every other year) *(18)*. The major differences of the Minnesota colon cancer study from other studies were the technique of testing guaiac slides. In this trial *(9)*, they mainly used a rehydration method, by adding few drops of water before adding hydrogen peroxide reagent. This increased sensitivity resulted in a high positivity rate, and more patients underwent colonoscopy. In

92 Part III / Screening for Gastrointestinal Cancers

this trial, 38% of the group offered annual screening had at least one colonoscopy. Because the number of colonoscopies performed was large, the mortality reduction in the Minnesota study could be predominantly the result of chance detection, as suggested by Ahlquist et al. *(19)* and Lang and Ransohoff *(20)*. In 1997, the Minnesota investigators used a mathematical model developed by Lang and Ransohoff and found that only up to 25% of the reduction in colorectal cancer deaths was the result of chance detection. The remainder resulted from sensitive detection *(21)*. They concluded that chance played a minor role in the detection of colorectal cancer by FOBT in the Minnesota study. Two other large randomized trials from Europe (England and Denmark) showed colorectal cancer mortality reduction of 15 and 18% from biennial (every 2 yr) FOBT with the nonrehydration method *(16,17)*. These three randomized controlled trials achieved a high quality of study design and follow-up. Recent meta-analysis of six trials (four randomized *[9,16,17,22]*, two nonrandomized *[23,24]*) showed a reduction in mortality from colorectal cancer of 16% (relative risk [RR] 0.84, 95% CI 0.77–0.93) in those allocated to FOBT screening *(25)*. When adjusted for attendance for screening, this reduction was 23% (RR 0.77, 95% CI 0.57–0.89).

Sensitivity and Specificity of FOBT

Sensitivity is defined as the proportion of all colorectal cancers that are detected by screening, with all colorectal cancers being the sum of screen-detected cancers (true-positive) and interval cancers within 1 or 2 yr of screening (false-negative). Specificity is defined as the proportion of all people without cancers that are correctly classified by a screening test. The sensitivity and specificity of FOBT for colorectal cancer reported in different studies vary considerably. The sensitivity reported in these studies usually reflects the performance of a program of repeated screening rather than a single test. The highest sensitivity was achieved with rehydration of slides as was performed in the Minnesota trial *(9)*. In that study, the sensitivity was 88–92%, but with loss of specificity to 90–92% and positive predictive value for cancer (from 10–17% to 2–6%). In its nonrehydrated form, the sensitivity of hemoccult test for detecting cancer range from 46–78% with 98% specificity *(16,17,25)*.

Sigmoidoscopy

Three different types of sigmoidoscope have been used for colorectal cancer screening: the rigid 25-cm scope and the 35- and 60-cm flexible scopes. Flexible sigmoidoscopes have largely replaced rigid scopes because of better visualization of bowel, longer depth of insertion, and more comfort for the patients. The 60-cm flexible sigmoidoscope is the type that is most commonly used currently. There is good evidence that primary care physicians and nonphysician health professionals can be trained to perform sigmoidoscopy with equal polyp detection rates and complication rates as those achieved by gastroenterologists *(26–29)*. The advantages of sigmoidoscopy are direct visualization of the large bowel, with high sensitivity and specificity for polyps and cancers. The polyps and cancers also can be biopsied as part of the procedure. The major limitation of sigmoidoscopy is disparity in the length of the instrument and target organ (colon). The 60-cm flexible sigmoidoscope can usually visualize up to splenic flexure. Several studies showed significant variability in depth of insertion, depending on bowel preparation, patient tolerance, and distal colonic anatomy. In a recent study *(30)*, the descending colon was not visualized in 61% of patients and splenic flexure was not reached in majority of patients. In general, the sigmoid colon can be reached in 80% of the examinations and should, therefore, detect 40–60% of adenomatous polyps and colorectal cancers *(31)*.

When adenomatous polyps were found in the rectosigmoid colon, patients had about a one in three chance of having adenomas in proximal colon *(6)*. Abnormal screening sigmoidoscopy should be followed by colonoscopy to identify additional lesions and excise them. In current algorithms for average-risk screening *(6)*, flexible sigmoidoscopy serves as a gatekeeper, because colonoscopic inspection of the proximal colon is pursued only if rectosigmoid adenomas are found. It is clear that polyps that are shown on biopsy to be hyperplastic or to consist of normal mucosa are not premalignant and need not be followed up by colonoscopic examination. If cancer or polyps with high-grade features (>1 cm in diameter, villous component, high-grade dysplasia on histology) are found, a full colonoscopy should be performed. The risk of subsequent colon cancer in patients with polyps with high-grade feature increases 3.6-fold and up to 6.6-fold if multiple polyps are found *(8)*.

More controversial is the question of rectosigmoid polyps that are less than 1 cm with no villous component or high-grade dysplasia. Small tubular adenomas are uncommonly associated with more advanced lesions proximally *(32)* and are associated with a risk of colorectal cancer no greater than of the general population *(8)*. Some investigators advocate no follow-up colonoscopy in this group of patients to enhance the economy of sigmoidoscopic screening. Others prefer to follow up such lesions with colonoscopy because it offers greater certainty that proximal adenomas will be identified and excised. The AHCPR/AGA recommendations *(6)* leave this issue up to patients and physician to decide whether to undergo colonoscopy. Data from subsequent studies,

94 Part III / Screening for Gastrointestinal Cancers

however, indicate a much higher prevalence of proximal advanced adenoma (more than 1 cm in size, villous component, and high-grade dysplasia) in those with only a small distal tubular adenoma *(33–36)*. The prevalence of advanced proximal adenomas ranged from 3.1 to 6.9% in these studies *(33–36)*, as compared to 0.8% in the original study *(32)*. These findings support performing full colonoscopic inspection for any adenomatous polyp found at flexible sigmoidoscopy.

EFFECTIVENESS OF SIGMOIDOSCOPY

In contrast to FOBT, there have been no randomized controlled trials addressing the effectiveness of screening sigmoidoscopy. An ongoing National Cancer Institute sponsored trial (Prostate, Lung, Colon, and Ovary Trial) is not expected to yield result until 2008. Data supporting screening sigmoidoscopy come from three case-control studies *(37–39)*. A significant reduction in mortality from rectosigmoid cancers (part of the colon screened by sigmoidoscopy) was observed consistently from these studies and ranges from 59–80% reduction.

SENSITIVITY AND SPECIFICITY OF SIGMOIDOSCOPY

The sensitivity of flexible sigmoidoscopy is 96.7% for cancer and large polyps and 73.3% for small polyps within the reach of the 60-cm flexible instrument. Specificity is 94% for cancers and large polyps and 92% for small polyps *(6)*. Generally, the 60-cm flexible scope can reach the proximal end of the sigmoid colon in 80% of cases and should, therefore, detect 40–60% of adenomatous polyps and colorectal cancer.

Combined FOBT and Flexible Sigmoidoscopy

Annual FOBT plus flexible sigmoidoscopy every 5 yr is currently recommended by American Cancer Society as screening tests for people age 50 or older with average risk *(40)*. There are theoretical reasons for combining FOBT with sigmoidoscopy. Two-thirds of the interval cancers being diagnosed between screening rounds were within the reach of the 60-cm flexible sigmoidoscopy in Danish and English fecal occult blood trials *(16,17)*. Winawer et al. compared annual screening either with rigid sigmoidoscopy combined with FOBT or with rigid sigmoidoscopy alone *(23)*. After 5–11 yr of follow-up, mortality from colorectal cancer was lower in those receiving FOBT and sigmoidoscopy (0.36 vs 0.63) with borderline significance. FOBT and sigmoidoscopy as compared to sigmoidoscopy alone detected a substantial number of early-stage cancers. Several studies have shown much higher diagnostic yield with combined screening than FOBT alone in detecting colorectal neoplasia *(41,42)*. In addition, sigmoidoscopy is more accurate than FOBT for detecting adenomatous polyps. Therefore, sigmoidoscopy offers the possibility of reducing the incidence of colorectal cancer as well as detecting cancers at an earlier stage. The additional effectiveness of combined testing is unknown at present because of the lack of studies. It is estimated that 21% more colorectal cancer deaths would be prevented if sigmoidoscopy were added to an FOBT program *(43)*.

Colonoscopy

Colonoscopy is the only technique that can detect cancers and polyps throughout the colon and rectum and remove them in a single sitting. There are no published studies that directly examine the effectiveness of colonoscopy as a screening test for colorectal cancers. It has been shown that detecting and removing polyps reduces the incidence of colorectal cancer. Data from the National Polyp Study showed a 76–90% reduction in the incidence of colorectal cancer as compared to reference groups after colonoscopic polypectomy *(44)*. In a recent multicenter, prospective study, only 34.5% of patients with cancer proximal to the splenic flexure had adenomas distal to the splenic flexure *(45)*. This indicates that the majority of patients with cancer proximal to the splenic flexure will have a normal screening flexible sigmoidoscopy. Levin et al. have shown that the prevalence of advanced proximal adenomas (>1 cm, villous feature, and severe dysplasia) are as common in people without distal adenomas as with them *(35)*. Based on this indirect evidence, total colonic examination should, therefore, be used as a goal for colorectal cancer screening.

The performance of colonoscopy has been verified in several studies. The cecum is reached in 80–95% of procedures. The miss rate of colonoscopy for large polyps (more than 1 cm) as determined by back-to-back colonoscopy was found to be low (6%) *(46)*. Colonoscopy is less accurate for small adenomas, however. The miss rate for adenomas less than 5 mm was 27%, and 13% for adenomas 6–9 mm in size *(46)*.

Colonoscopy, unlike other screening tests, can cause morbidity and mortality on its own. It can be complicated by perforation, hemorrhage, respiratory distress resulting from sedation, arrhythmia, transient abdominal pain, and ileus and nosocomial infection. Based on data from several studies, the perforation rate is approx 0.1%, major bleeding is 0.3%, and the mortality rate is 1–3 in 10,000 *(6)*. Complications usually occur as a result of intervention and polypectomy. Recently, the American College of Gastroenterology (ACG) has adopted colonoscopy every 10 yr for average-risk individuals as the preferred screening strategy *(47)*.

Barium Enema

Barium enema is another screening method that examines the entire colon. A double-contrast barium enema, in which air is instilled after most of the barium has been removed from the colon, is substantially more sensitive and specific than a single-contrast study at detecting mucosal lesions, including small polyps. The examination takes 20–30 min and is generally well tolerated. Results from several studies suggest a reasonably high sensitivity for large polyps (>1 cm). Sensitivity for small polyps drops significantly, however. Average sensitivity and specificity for large polyps are 70% and 90%, respectively *(48)*. False-positive findings are mainly caused by adherent stools or non-neoplastic mucosal irregularities. In a recent study by Rex et al. *(49)*, the sensitivity of colonoscopy for colorectal cancer (95%) was greater than that for barium enema (82.9%), with an odds ratio of 3.93 for a missed cancer by barium enema compared with colonoscopy *(49)*.

Cancers detected by colonoscopy were more likely to be Dukes' class A (24.9% vs 9.8%) *(49)*. Overall performance of double-contrast barium enema, although less sensitive than colonoscopy, is felt to be sufficient in detecting clinically important lesions *(6)*. Barium enema is relatively safer compare to colonoscopy. The most serious complication is bowel perforation, which occurs approx 1 in 25,000 cases *(50)*. The mortality rate was 1 in 56,786 in a recent study from the United Kingdom *(50)*. The causes of death were cardiac arrhythmia, followed by bowel perforation. Expert panels for Agency for Health Care Policy and Research (AHCPR) included double-contrast barium enema every 5–10 yr in their screening options for average-risk asymptomatic individual *(6)*. Barium enema has been shown to be cost-effective as a screening tool if sensitivity for polyps 5 mm and larger is more than 70% *(48)*.

NEW TECHNIQUES FOR COLORECTAL CANCER SCREENING

Computed Tomographic Colonography (Virtual Colonoscopy)

Computed tomographic (CT) colonography is a new imaging technique for detection of colonic polyps and cancers. The colonic mucosa is evaluated by acquisition of planar helical CT images, with interactive display using a variety of two-dimensional (2D) and 3D visualization techniques *(51)*. Virtual colonoscopy refers to computer-simulated 3D endoscopic visualization of the colonic mucosal surface. This rapidly growing field has gained multidisciplinary attention as a potential noninvasive test for colorectal cancer screening. Patient preparation is similar to that of colonoscopy and barium enema. Just before image acquisition, air or carbon dioxide is insufflated through the rectum to distend the entire colon. Cross-sectional computerized tomographic scans are taken at multiple levels in both prone and supine positions *(52–54)*. The procedure takes less than 1 min, although manipulation and interpretation of virtual colonoscopic examination remains time-consuming, requiring on average of 20–30 min per patient *(52)*. Radiation exposure to patients with this technique is small, less than that of standard abdominal pelvic CT. The total effective dose is 1.1 REM, which is approx 22% of the annual limit to a radiation worker *(51)*. Data from early experience with CT colonography showed variable sensitivity and specificity. The sensitivity and specificity for polyps 10 mm or larger were 57–75% and 90%, respectively. For polyps less than 10 mm, the sensitivity and specificity were significantly lower *(53,54)*.

The technology in CT colonography continues to evolve rapidly, however. Later experience showed much better results *(52)*. In a more recent study, the sensitivity of virtual colonoscopy for the detection of polyps was 91% for large polyps (more than 10 mm in diameter), 82% for medium-sized polyps (6–9 mm), and 55% for small polyps (1–5 mm) as compared to conventional colonoscopy as the gold standard *(55)*. This technique is a promising approach to become an important tool for colorectal cancer screening. Several issues remain to be resolved. A cost-effective analysis *(56)* suggested that in order for CT colonography to be cost-effective, it would need to be offered at a very low price (54% less than colonoscopy) or associated with a better compliance rate (15–20% better than colonoscopy).

Fecal Occult Blood Tests: Newer Techniques

An immunochemical test (HemeSelect, FlexSure OBT) reacts specifically with hemoglobin *(57)*. It detects colonic blood with great sensitivity and does not detect small quantities of blood from the upper gastrointestinal tract *(58)*. It is not, at present, an office-based test. The study in average-risk individuals showed that immunochemical testing had higher sensitivity without a loss of specificity *(59)*. When the combination of an immunochemical-based test with Hemoccult II Sensa was evaluated, this approach yielded the highest positive predictive value, with sensitivity and specificity of 66 and 97%, respectively *(59)*. Therefore, it is likely that an immunochemical test or a combination with a guaiac-based test may become a component of FOBT screening program.

GENETIC TESTING

Approximately 5% of colorectal cancers are accounted for by two well-defined genetic syndromes: familial adenomatous polyposis (FAP)

98 Part III / Screening for Gastrointestinal Cancers

and hereditary nonpolyposis colorectal cancer (HNPCC). Recently, a variant of APC (I1307K APC allele), the gene responsible for FAP, has been described *(60)*, which may account for some cases of familial colon cancer in Ashkenazi Jews. At present, genetic tests are commercially available for FAP, HNPCC, and the I1307K APC allele. Testing for FAP mutation is part of the standard care for affected individuals and families; however, the role of genetic testing for HNPCC and I1307K APC is not fully established. Genetic counseling should always be performed before and after genetic test by qualified consultants. Detrimental consequences of genetic testing, such as genetic discrimination, psychological harm, and confidentiality need to be addressed.

Familial Adenomatous Polyposis

Familial adenomatous polyposis is an autosomal dominant disorder that accounts for approx 1% of colorectal cancer. FAP is caused by a germline mutation of *APC* gene located on chromosome 5q21. Affected individuals develop hundreds to thousands of colonic adenomas by their mid to late teens with variable extracolonic manifestations. Colorectal cancer is inevitable in the untreated, usually by age 45. Different specific mutations have been described, which may correlate with phenotypic expression. The majority of APC mutations result in truncated gene product, which can be detected by a protein truncation test (PTT) or in vitro synthesized protein assay (IVSP), the test that is currently used in FAP genetic testing *(61)*. The sensitivity of the test is approx 80% *(61)*. Genetic testing of a FAP family should start with an affected family member. Detection of a mutation among one of the affected members of the family permits genetic testing of at-risk relatives. Those free of mutation need no longer participate in the screening program, whereas those with the mutation must continue screening. If the mutation is not found in an affected individual, it does not mean that FAP is not present; an individual may still harbor a mutation that cannot be detected by the current test. It is important to keep in mind that a negative test result rules out FAP only if an affected family member has an identified mutation. Recently, Laken et al. used monoallelic mutation analysis (MAMA) to determine the status of the APC gene in FAP patients with a negative protein truncation test *(62)*. With a combination of MAMA and a standard genetic test, 95% of patients with FAP were shown to have inactivated mutations in APC. The results suggest that there may be another gene, besides APC, that can give rise to FAP *(62)*.

Hereditary Nonpolyposis Colorectal Cancer

Hereditary nonpolyposis colorectal cancer is an autosomal dominantly inherited disorder of cancer susceptibility with high penetrance (80–85%). The cause is an inherited mutation in one of the following mismatch repair (MMR) genes: *hMSH2, hMLH1, PMS1, PMS2,* and *hMSH6 (63)*. The disorder is characterized by development of colorectal cancer at an early age (mean age 45 yr). The cancer is usually located in the proximal colon with a high degree of microsatellite instability (MSI) (>90%). HNPCC accounts for approx 5% of all colorectal cancer cases. HNPCC is diagnosed based on Amsterdam criteria, which were recently revised to include other associated cancers in their diagnostic requirements *(63)*. The criteria are as follows: three or more relatives with an HNPCC-associated cancers (colorectal cancer, cancer of the endometrium, small bowel, ureter, or renal pelvis); one patient a first-degree relative of the other two; at least two successive generations affected, at least one diagnosed before age 50.

Current available genetic tests for HNPCC are limited to *hMSH2* and *hMLH1*, which account for 90% of identified mutations. Detection of MSI in tumor tissue is also commercially available. The so-called "Bethesda guidelines" have been developed to identify the patient's characteristics in whom tumors should be tested for MSI *(64)*. A logistic model for estimating the likelihood of a mutation of *hMSH2* and *hMLH1* has been developed *(65)*. A younger age of diagnosis of colorectal cancer (CRC), fulfillment of the Amsterdam criteria, and the presence of endometrial cancer in the family are independent predictors of a MMR mutation. Individuals with a more than 20% likelihood of having a mutation based on the logistic model should have HNPCC genetic testing, whereas those with less than 20% probability should have their tumors assessed for MSI first, then genetic testing only if tumors are positive for MSI *(65)*. The value of genetic testing and subsequent medical intervention for HNPCC, at present, are unproved, however.

I1307K Mutation of APC Gene

This mutation was recently described and the genetic testing is commercially available. This mutation may account for some cases of familial colon cancer in Ashkenazi Jews *(66,67)*. The risk of colorectal cancer in an individual with this mutation appears to be low to modest. Testing for this mutation, outside the research setting, is not recommended at this point.

COST-EFFECTIVENESS ANALYSIS

Screening for CRC has been shown to be cost-effective by several studies *(11,12)*. Lieberman compared five screening strategies: FOBT, flexible sigmoidoscopy, FOBT and sigmoidoscopy combined, one-time colonoscopy, and air-contrast barium enema *(11)*. The analysis was based on various assumptions regarding the sensitivity and specificity of the screening tests, the complication rates, the cost of screening programs and of treating detected cancers, and so forth. All strategies were found to be cost-effective. FOBT alone was the most cost-effective of the programs, but the cost was sensitive to several key variables. The most important variable is compliance to the screening program, which remains a significant issue in the US population screening. The cost-effectiveness analysis by the Office of Technology Assessment (OTA) of the US Congress showed that all strategies cost less than $20,000 per year of life saved *(12)*. This is well within an acceptable range of cost-effectiveness by US health standards.

CRC SCREENING: PROBLEMS AND CONTROVERSIES

What Is the Best Screening Strategy?

The fecal occult blood test and flexible sigmoidoscopy are currently recommended as screening tools for colorectal cancer in an average-risk individual *(6,40,68)*. The recommendation is based on strong scientific data that screening can reduce CRC-related mortality and is cost-effective. It is also clear that better screening strategy is needed. Newer screening techniques are now being developed and studied to better assess the whole colon. Preliminary data from the VA Cooperative Colonoscopy Screening for Colorectal Cancer showed promising results *(69)*. More than 3000 subjects underwent screening colonoscopy, there was no perforation or morbidity directly attributed to colonoscopy. The cecum was successfully reached in 95%. These data suggest that screening colonoscopy is feasible and safe. CT colonography is another promising approach. Recent experience showed much improved sensitivity and specificity in detecting polyps larger than 10 mm *(52)*. This technique may be more acceptable to the general population because of the noninvasive nature of the test.

Low Participation Rate in CRC Screening

Data from the 1997 Behavioral Risk Factor Surveillance System (BRFSS) analyzed by the Centers for Disease Control (CDC) showed low rates of use of colorectal cancer screening tests *(70)*. Approximately 40% of respondents reported ever having had a FOBT or sigmoidoscopy/proctoscopy. Only 20% of respondents reported having had a FOBT during the preceding year, and 30% reported having had a sigmoidoscopy during the preceding 5 yr, durations recommended by several guidelines *(70)*. It has been shown that local educational programs and on-site sigmoidoscopy services can enhance primary care provider utilization of screening sigmoidoscopy *(71)*. The issue of scope disinfection, which may not be possible in an office setting, can be overcome by using disposable endoscope sheaths *(71)*. Public health officials, health care providers, and health plans need to intensify efforts to increase awareness of the effectiveness of screening and to promote the widespread use of colorectal cancer screening tests.

In order for FOBT to be effective, proper follow-up testing and treatment need to be performed. It has been shown that only a minority of patients has an appropriate diagnostic workup after a positive screening FOBT. Data from Medicare's National Claims History System showed that only 34% of Medicare beneficiaries with positive FOBT had the recommended evaluation of their colons *(72)*. Obviously, this will further reduce the effectiveness of screening program. Efforts need to be made to ensure proper follow-up after a positive screening test.

People with Small (Less Than 1 cm) Distal Tubular Adenoma: Do They Need Colonoscopy?

Current practice guidelines do not recommend routine colonoscopy in an individual with a single small tubular adenoma discovered at screening sigmoidoscopy, but encourage individuals to decide with their physicians whether to undergo colonoscopy *(6)*. It has been shown that the risk of colorectal cancer in such an individual is apparently no more than in the general population *(8)*. The practice on this issue has varied quite significantly. Recent data, however, suggest that the finding at screening sigmoidoscopy may not be a good predictor of proximal colonic findings. The prevalence of advanced proximal neoplasia has been shown to be similar among patients with no tubular adenoma at sigmoidoscopy, those with tubular adenoma less 1 cm, and those with tubular adenoma 1 cm or larger *(35)*. The majority of patients with proximal colon cancer did not have adenomas distal to splenic flexure in a large prospective study *(45)*. These data support the importance of total colonic evaluation as a goal for screening. Based on the current recommended algorithm (*see* Algorithm 1), individuals with adenomas of any size detected during screening sigmoidoscopy and their physicians may prefer to follow up such lesions with colonoscopy to ensure that proximal adenomas have been identified and excised.

Screening Strategies Are Not Well Defined for Certain High-Risk Groups

Approximately 25% of sporadic colorectal cancers occur in individuals with a family history of colorectal cancer that do not belong to well-

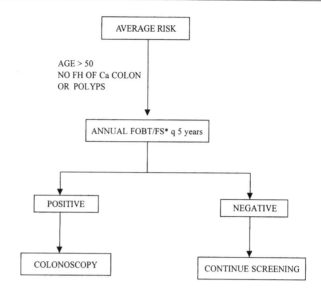

Algorithm 1. CRC screening in average-risk patients.

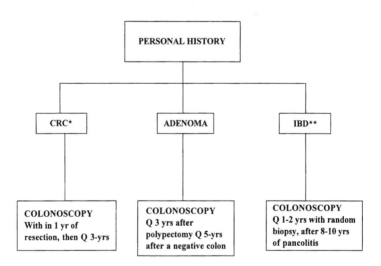

Algorithm 2. CRC screening in high-risk patients: 1.

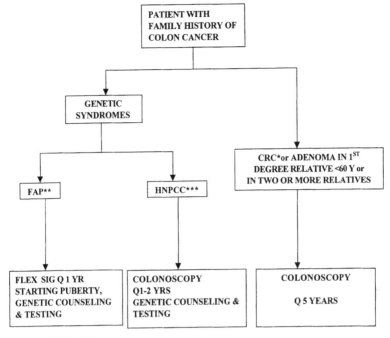

Algorithm 3. CRC screening in high-risk patients: 2.

defined genetic syndromes (FAP and HNPCC). First-degree relatives of persons with colorectal carcinoma or adenomatous polyps have an approximately twofold risk of developing colorectal carcinoma *(73–76)*. The risk increases with the number of relatives affected and younger age at diagnosis. Current practice guidelines *(see* Algorithms 2 and 3) recommend colonoscopy every 5 yr as a screening tool for a person with a family history of colorectal cancer or adenomas in a first-degree relative younger than 60 yr or in two or more first-degree relatives of any age *(40)*. For individuals with a family history of CRC or adenomas, not included above, the screening strategy is similar to average-risk individual, but begins at earlier age *(6,40)*. Additional studies are needed to better characterize this group of patients who may be most benefit from more intense screening program.

The risk of colorectal cancer after gynecologic cancer has been shown to be higher than the general population. Among women with a history of ovarian cancer or endometrial cancer diagnosed before age of 50, the risk of colorectal cancer is substantially elevated with standardized incidence ratios of 3.67 (95% CI, 2.74–4.80) and 3.39 (95% CI, 2.73–4.17), respectively *(77)*.

The risk remains elevated even among women with previous ovarian cancer between 50 and 64 yr of age *(77)*. So far, there has been no established guidelines for colorectal cancer screening for this particular group.

CONCLUSIONS

Significant numbers of the US population die each year of invasive colorectal carcinoma. Screening for colorectal cancer has been shown by several randomized controlled trials to be effective in decreasing CRC-related deaths and cost saving. At present, all asymptomatic, average-risk individuals over 50 yr of age should undergo screening for colorectal cancer with annual FOBT and flexible sigmoidoscopy every 5 yr. Those at higher risk should be offered more intensive screening and follow-up surveillance according to guidelines. In the future, screening colonoscopy or CT colonography (virtual colonoscopy) may prove effective and feasible.

SUMMARY OF RECOMMENDATIONS FOR CRC SCREENING *(6,40,68)*

1. People with average risk, age 50 yr or older
   - FOBT every year plus flexible sigmoidoscopy every 5 yr.
   - Other options; FOBT every year alone, flexible sigmoidoscopy every 5 yr alone, colonoscopy every 10 yr or double-contrast barium enema every 5–10 yr.
   - Positive test should be followed by colonoscopy.
2. People with high-risk family history: colorectal cancer or adenomatous polyps in first-degree relative younger than 60 yr or in two or more first-degree relatives at any ages
   - Colonoscopy every 5 yr, start age 40 or 10 yr before the youngest case in the family, whichever is earlier.
3. People with low-risk family history: CRC in other relatives, not included in Recommendations 1 and 2
   - As per average risk; start at age 40.
4. People with a family history of familial adenomatous polyposis
   - Flexible sigmoidoscopy every 12 mo, beginning at puberty.
   - Consideration of colectomy when polyps are detected.
   - Genetic counseling and genetic testing.
   - Consider colonoscopy for attenuated FAP, start at later age.
5. People with a family of hereditary nonpolyposis colorectal cancer
   - Colonoscopy every 1–2 yr, start age 20, until age 40, then every year.
   - Genetic counseling and consideration of genetic testing.
6. People with a personal history of adenomatous polyps
   - Colonoscopy within 3 yr after initial polyp removal; if normal, then colonoscopy every 5 yr.

7. People with a personal history of CRC
   - Colonoscopy within 1 yr after curative resection; if normal, colonoscopy in 3 yr; if still normal, then every 5 yr.
8. People with inflammatory bowel disease
   - Colonoscopy with biopsies for dysplasia, every 1–2 yr, beginning 8 yr of disease in pancolitis and after 15 yr in left-sided colitis.
   - Consideration of colectomy if dysplasia is detected.

REFERENCES

1. Landis SH, Murray T, Bolden S, Wingo PA. (1999) Cancer statistics, 1999. *CA Cancer J Clin* 49:8–31.
2. *World Health Organization. (1997)* The World Health Report. Geneva: WHO.
3. Troisi RJ, Freedman AN, Devesa SS. (1999) Incidence of colorectal carcinoma in the U.S.: an update of trends by gender, race, age, subsite, and stage, 1975–1994. *Cancer* 85:1670–1676.
4. Potter JD. (1999) Colorectal cancer: molecules and populations. *Rev J Natl Cancer Inst* 91:916–932.
5. Eide TJ. (1986) Risk of colorectal cancer in adenoma-bearing individuals within a defined population. *Int J Cancer* 38:173–176.
6. Winawer SJ, Fletcher RH, Miller L, et al. (1997) Colorectal cancer screening: clinical guidelines and rationale [see comments]. *Gastroenterology* 112:594–642 [errata: 1997;112(3):1060 and 1998;114(3):625].
7. O'Brien MJ, Winawer SJ, Zauber AG, et al. (1990) The National Polyp Study. Patient and polyp characteristics associated with high-grade dysplasia in colorectal adenomas. *Gastroenterology* 98:371–379.
8. Atkin WS, Morson BC, Cuzick J. (1992) Long-term risk of colorectal cancer after excision of rectosigmoid adenomas [see comments]. *N Engl J Med* 326:658–662.
9. Mandel JS, Bond JH, Church TR, et al. (1993) Reducing mortality from colorectal cancer by screening for fecal occult blood. Minnesota Colon Cancer Control Study. *N Engl J Med* 328:1365–1371 [erratum: 1993;329(9);672].
10. Wingo PA, Tong T, Bolden S. (1995) Cancer statistics, 1995. *CA Cancer J Clin* 45:8–30 [erratum: 1995;45(2):127,128].
11. Lieberman DA. (1995) Cost-effectiveness model for colon cancer screening. *Gastroenterology* 109:1781–1790.
12. Wagner J L, Tuni, S, Brown M, et al. (1996) Cost-effectiveness of colorectal cancer screening in average-risk adults. In: Young G, Levin B, eds. *Prevention and Early Detection of Colorectal Cancer.* London: Saunders, pp. 321–356.
13. Young GP, St John DJ. (1991) Selecting an occult blood test for use as a screening tool for large bowel cancer. *Front Gastrointest Res* 18:135–156.
14. Macrae FA, St. John DJ. (1982) Relationship between patterns of bleeding and hemoccult sensitivity in patients with colorectal cancers or adenomas. *Gastroenterology* 82:891–898.
15. Robinson MH, Hardcastle JD, Moss SM, et al. (1999) The risk of screening: data from the Nottingham randomised controlled trial of faecal occult blood screening for colorectal cancer. *Gut* 45:588–592.
16. Hardcastle JD, Chamberlain JO, Robinson MH, et al. (1996) Randomized controlled trial of fecal-occult-blood screening for colorectal cancer [see comments]. *Lancet* 348:1472–1477.

106   **Part III** / Screening for Gastrointestinal Cancers

17. Kronborg O, Fenger C, Olsen J, Jorgensen OD, Sondergaard O. (1996) Randomized study of screening for colorectal cancer with fecal-occult-blood test [see comments]. *Lancet* 348:1467–1471.
18. Mandel JS, Church TR, Ederer F, Bond JH. (1999) Colorectal cancer mortality: effectiveness of biennial screening for fecal occult blood [see comments]. *J Natl Cancer Inst* 91:434–437.
19. Ahlquist DA, Moertel CG, McGill DB. (1993) Screening for colorectal cancer [letter; comment]. *N Engl J Med* 329:1351–1354.
20. Lang CA, Ransohoff DF. (1994) Fecal occult blood screening for colorectal cancer. Is mortality reduced by chance selection for screening colonoscopy? [see comments]. *JAMA* 271:1011–1013.
21. Ederer F, Church TR, Mandel JS. (1997) Fecal occult blood screening in the Minnesota study: role of chance detection of lesions [see comments]. *J Natl Cancer Inst* 89:1423–1428.
22. Kewenter J, Brevinge H, Engaras B, Haglind E, Ahren C. (1994) Results of screening, rescreening, and follow-up in a prospective randomized study for detection of colorectal cancer by fecal occult blood testing. Results for 68,308 subjects. *Scan J Gastroenterol* 29:468–473.
23. Winawer SJ, Flehinger BJ, Schottenfeld D, Miller DG. (1993) Screening for colorectal cancer with fecal occult blood testing and sigmoidoscopy [see comments]. *J Natl Cancer Inst* 85:1311–1318.
24. Faivre J, Arveux P, Milan C, et al. (1991) Participation in mass screening for colorectal cancer:Results of screening and rescreening from the Burgundy study [see comments]. *Eur J Cancer Prev* 1:49–55.
25. Towler B, Irwig L, Glasziou P, et al. (1998) A systematic review of the effects of screening for colorectal cancer using the fecal occult blood test, hemoccult [see comments]. *Br Med J* 317:559–565.
26. Maule WF. (1994) Screening for colorectal cancer by nurse endoscopists [see comments]. *N Engl J Med* 330:183–187.
27. Schoenfeld PS, Lipscomb S, Crook J, et al. (1999) Accuracy of polyp detection by gastroenterologists and nurse endoscopists during flexible sigmoidoscopy: a randomized Trial. *Gastroenterology* 11:312–318.
28. Schoenfeld PS, Cash B, Kita J, et al. (1999) Effectiveness and patient satisfaction with screening flexible sigmoidoscopy performed by registered nurses [see comments]. *Gastrointest Endosc* 49:158–162.
29. Wallace MB, Kemp JA, Meyer F, et al. (1999) Screening for colorectal cancer with flexible sigmoidoscopy by nonphysician endoscopists. *Am J Med* 107:214–218.
30. Painter J, Saunders DB, Bell GD, et al. (1999) Depth of insertion at flexible sigmoidoscopy: implications for colorectal cancer screening and instrument design [see comments]. *Endoscopy* 31:227–231.
31. Selby JV, Friedman GD. (1989) US Preventive Services Task Force. Sigmoidoscopy in the periodic health examination of asymptomatic adults [review]. *JAMA* 261:594–601.
32. Zarchy TM, Ershoff D. (1994) Do characteristics of adenomas on flexible sigmoidoscopy predict advanced lesions on baseline colonoscopy? [see comments]. *Gastroenterology* 106:1501–1504.
33. Read TE, Read JD, Butterly LF. (1997) Importance of adenoma 5 mm or less in diameter that are detected by sigmoidoscopy. *N Engl J Med* 336:8–12.
34. Schoen RE, Carle D, Cranston L, et al. (1998) Is colonoscopy needed for the nonadvanced adenoma found on sigmoidoscopy? *Gastroenterology* 115:533–541.

Chapter 6 / Promrat, Aziz, and Wu

35. Levin TR, Palitz A, Grossman S, et al. (1999) Predicting advanced proximal colonic neoplasia with screening sigmoidoscopy. *JAMA* 281:161–167

36. Sciallero S, Bonelli L, Aste H, et al. (1999) Do patients with rectosigmoid adenomas 5 mm or less in diameter need total colonoscopy? *Gastrointest Endosc* 50:314–321.

37. Selby JV, Friedman GD, Quesenberry CPJ, Weiss NS. (1992) A case-control study of screening sigmoidoscopy and mortality from colorectal cancer [see comments]. *N Engl J Med* 326:653–657.

38. Newcomb PA, Norfleet RG, Storer BE, Surawicz TS, Marcus PM. (1992) Screening sigmoidoscopy and colorectal cancer mortality [see comments]. *J Natl Cancer Inst* 84:1572–1575.

39. Muller AD, Sonnenberg A. (1995) Protection by endoscopy against death from colorectal cancer. *Arch Intern Med* 155:1741–1748.

40. Byers T, Levin B, Rothenberger D, Dodd GD, Smith RA. (1997) American Cancer Society guidelines for screening and surveillance for early detection of colorectal polyps and cancer: update 1997. American Cancer Society Detection and Treatment Advisory Group on Colorectal Cancer. *CA Cancer J Clin* 47:154–160.

41. Rasmussen M, Kronborg O, Fenger C, Jorgensen OD. (1999) Possible advantages and drawbacks of adding flexible sigmoidoscopy to hemoccult-II in screening for colorectal cancer. A randomized study [see comments]. *Scan J Gastroenterol* 34:73–78.

42. Berry DP, Clarke P, Hardcastle JD, Vellacott KD. (1997) Randomized trial of the addition of flexible sigmoidoscopy to fecal occult blood testing for colorectal neoplasia population screening. *Br J Surg* 84:1274–1276.

43. Fletcher RH, Farraye FA. (1999) Screening flexible sigmoidoscopy: effectiveness is not enough [editorial; comment]. *Gastroenterology* 117:486–488.

44. Winawer SJ, Zauber AG, Ho MN, et al. (1993) Prevention of colorectal cancer by colonoscopic polypectomy. The National Polyp Study Workgroup [see comments]. *N Engl J Med* 329:1977–1981.

45. Rex DK, Chak A, Vasudeva R, et al. (1999) Prospective determination of distal colonic findings in average-risk patients with proximal colon cancer. *Gastrointest Endosc* 49:727–730.

46. Rex DK, Cutler CS, Lemmel GT. (1997) Colonoscopic miss rates of adenomas determined by back-to-back colonoscopies. *Gastroenterology* 112:24–28.

47. Rex DK, Johnson DA, Lieberman DA, Burt RW, Sonnenberg A. (2000) Colorectal cancer prevention 2000: screening recommendations of the American College of Gastroenterology. *Am J Gastroenterol* 95:868–877.

48. Glick S, Wagner JL, Johnson CD. (1998) Cost-effectiveness of double-contrast barium enema in screening for colorectal cancer. *Am J Roentgenol* 170:629–636.

49. Rex DK, Rahmani EY, Haseman JH. (1997) Relative sensitivity of colonoscopy and barium enema for detection of colorectal cancer in clinical practice. *Gastroenterology* 112:17–23.

50. Blakeborough A, Sheridan MB, Chapman AH. (1997) Complications of barium enema examinations: a survey of UK consultant radiologists 1992 to 1994. *Clin Radiol* 52:142–148.

51. McFarland EG, Brink JA. Helical CT. (1999) Colonography (virtual colonoscopy): the challenge that exists between advancing technology and generalizability. *Am J Roentgenol* 173:549–559.

52. Fenlon HM, Ferrucci JT. (1999) First International Symposium on Virtual Colonoscopy: Meeting Summary. *Am J Roentgenol* 173:565–569.

53. Hara AK, Johnson CD, Reed JE, et al. (1997) Detection of colorectal polyps with CT colography: initial assessment of sensitivity and specificity. *Radiology* 205:59–65.

108   **Part III / Screening for Gastrointestinal Cancers**

54. Rex DK, Vining D, Kopecky KK. (1999) An initial experience with screening for colon polyps using spiral CT with and without CT colography (virtual colonoscopy). *Gastrointest Endosc* 50:309–313.
55. Fenlon HM, Nunes DP, Schroy PC III, et al. (1999) A comparison of virtual and conventional colonoscopy for the detection of colorectal polyps. *N Engl J Med* 341:1496–1503.
56. Sonnenberg A, Delco F, Bauerfeind P. (1999) Is virtual colonoscopy a cost-effective option to screen for colorectal cancer? *Am J Gastroenterol* 94:2268–2274.
57. St John DJ, Young GP, Alexeyeff MA, et al. (1993) Evaluation of new occult blood tests for detection of colorectal neoplasia [see comments]. *Gastroenterology* 104:1661–1668.
58. Rockey DC. (1999) Occult gastrointestinal bleeding [review]. *N Engl J Med* 341:38–46.
59. Allison JE, Tekawa IS, Ransom LJ, Adrain AL. (1996) A comparison of fecal occult-blood tests for colorectal-cancer screening [see comments]. *N Engl J Med* 334:155–159.
60. Laken SJ, Petersen GM, Gruber SB, et al. (1997) Familial colorectal cancer in Ashkenazim due to a hypermutable tract in APC. *Nat Genet* 17:79–83.
61. Powell SM, Petersen GM, Krush AJ, et al. (1993) Molecular diagnosis of familial adenomatous polyposis [see comments]. *N Engl J Med* 329:1982–1987.
62. Laken SJ, Papadopoulos N, Petersen GM, et al. (1999) Analysis of masked mutations in familial adenomatous polyposis. *Proc Natl Acad Sci USA* 96:2322–2326.
63. Vasen HF, Watson P, Mecklin JP, Lynch HT. (1999) New clinical criteria for hereditary nonpolyposis colorectal cancer (HNPCC, Lynch syndrome) proposed by the International Collaborative group on HNPCC. *Gastroenterology* 116:1453–1456.
64. Rodriguez-Bigas MA, Boland CR, Hamilton SR, et al. (1997) A National Cancer Institute Workshop on Hereditary Nonpolyposis Colorectal Cancer Syndrome: meeting highlights and Bethesda guidelines [see comments]. *J Natl Cancer Inst* 89:1758–1762.
65. Wijnen JT, Vasen HF, Khan PM, et al. (1998) Clinical findings with implications for genetic testing in families with clustering of colorectal cancer. *N Engl J Med* 339:511–518.
66. Frayling IM, Beck NE, Ilyas M, et al. (1998) The APC variants I1307K and E1317Q are associated with colorectal tumors, but not always with a family history. *Proc Natl Acad Sci USA* 95:10,722–10,727.
67. Rozen P, Shomrat R, Strul H, et al. (1999) Prevalence of the I1307K APC gene variant in Israeli Jews of differing ethnic origin and risk for colorectal cancer [see comments]. *Gastroenterology* 116:54–57.
68. U.S. Preventive Services Task Force. (1996) *U.S. Preventive Services Task Force: Guide to Clinical Preventive Services*, 2nd edition. Baltimore: Williams and Wilkins, pp. 89–103.
69. Nelson DB, Mcquaid KR, Bond JH, Lieberman DA. (1999) Population based colonoscopy screening for colorectal cancer is feasible and safe: preliminary results from the VA Cooperative Colonoscopy Screening Trial [abstract]. *Gastrointest Endosc* 49:AB65.
70. Anonymous. (1999) Screening for colorectal cancer-United States, 1997. *MMWR Morb Mortal Wkly Rep* 48:116–121.
71. Schroy PC, Heeren T, Bliss CM, et al. (1999) Implementation of on-site screening sigmoidoscopy positively influences utilization by primary care providers [see comments]. *Gastroenterology* 117:304–311.
72. Lurie JD, Welch HG. (1999) Diagnostic testing following fecal occult blood screening in the elderly. *J Natl Cancer Inst* 91:1641–1646.

Chapter 6 / Promrat, Aziz, and Wu

73. Fuchs CS, Giovannucci EL, Colditz GA, et al. (1994) A prospective study of family history and the risk of colorectal cancer [see comments]. *N Engl J Med* 331:1669–674.

74. St John DJ, McDermott FT, Hopper JL, et al. (1993) Cancer risk in relatives of patients with common colorectal cancer. *Ann Intern Med* 118:785–790.

75. Winawer SJ, Zauber AG, Gerdes H, et al. (1996) Risk of colorectal cancer in the families of patients with adenomatous polyps. National Polyp Study Workgroup [see comments]. *N Engl J Med* 334:82–87.

76. Ahsan H, Neugut AI, Garbowski GC, et al. (1998) Family history of colorectal adenomatous polyps and increased risk for colorectal cancer. *Ann Intern Med* 128:900–905.

77. Weinberg DS, Newschaffer CJ, Topham A. (1999) Risk for colorectal cancer after gynecologic cancer. *Ann Intern Med* 131:189–193.

7 Screening for Hepatocellular Carcinoma

Kirti Shetty, MD, Khalid Aziz, MD, and George Y. Wu, MD, PhD

KEY PRINCIPLES

- Hepatocellular carcinoma (HCC) is an extremely prevalent malignancy worldwide, with a recent documented increase in its incidence reported in the United States.
- High-risk groups for the development of HCC have been well defined. These include those with cirrhosis, chronic viral hepatitis, and the metabolic liver diseases.
- Screening for HCC is designed to detect the malignancy at an early and potentially treatable stage.
- The accepted screening strategy for HCC includes 6-monthly testing of serum alpha-fetoprotein levels, and high-resolution ultrasonography.
- Even though screening is expensive, studies demonstrate that in a carefully selected patient population, it is a cost-effective approach and is comparable to other well-established screening practices.

INTRODUCTION

Hepatocellular carcinoma (HCC) is the fourth most common malignancy worldwide, accounting for as many as half a million deaths annually *(1,2)*. Although it has been considered a disease of the developing world, it is now being increasingly recognized as an important contributor to the morbidity and mortality of those with chronic liver disease in the West. As new and more effective treatment modalities become avail-

From: *Cancer Screening: A Practical Guide for Physicians*
Edited by: K. Aziz and G. Y. Wu © Humana Press Inc., Totowa, NJ

112 Part III / Screening for Gastrointestinal Cancers

able for HCC, it is important for us to identify these cancers at an earlier, treatable stage.

EPIDEMIOLOGY

Geographic Factors

The frequency of HCC shows a dramatic geographic variation *(3)*. Based on incidence rates reported by cancer registries worldwide, three incidence-based regions may be delineated (Table 1):

> **Group 1:** High-incidence areas (50–100 cases/100,000 population/yr). These include countries in sub-Saharan Africa and Southeast Asia, with Mozambique having the highest incidence in the world (98–100/ 100,000 population/yr)
> **Group 2:** Moderate-incidence areas (10–50/100,000 population/yr). These include Japan, southern Europe (Italy, Spain, Greece), and the Middle East.
> **Group 3:** Low-incidence areas (<5/100,000 population/yr). These encompass much of northern Europe and North America.

A recent study *(4)* analyzed the trends in the incidence of HCC in the United States, utilizing three separate databases. The incidence of histologically proven HCC was found to have increased from 1.4 per 100,000 population for the period from 1976 to 1980, to 2.4 per 100,000 for the period 1991 to 1995. This increased incidence was particularly marked among younger persons (aged 40–60 yr) and resulted in an overall increase of 41% in the disease-specific mortality rate. The reasons for the increase are unclear, but they are thought to be related to the burgeoning caseload of occult and recently diagnosed hepatitis C infection in the United States.

The clinical characteristics of HCC show some interesting and important variations among different geographic regions *(5)*. Patients in high-incidence areas are often infected with the hepatitis B virus (HBV) perinatally, leading to cancer development in the third or fourth decade of life, with rapid progression of tumor growth. These tumors are also more likely to present with elevated serum α-fetoprotein levels, at a higher median range. In low-incidence areas, HCC is most often a disease of later life and occurs as a complication of clinically obvious cirrhosis.

Gender and Racial Predominance

Hepatocellular carcinoma is more common in males than females. In high-incidence areas, the male–female ratio is approximately 7 to 1. In the United States, this ratio is 3 to 1. In the recently concluded study

Chapter 7 / Screening for Hepatocellular Carcinoma

Table 1
Worldwide Incidence of HCC

Region	Rate per 100,000 population/yr
High-incidence areas	50–100
Southeast Asia, sub-Saharan Africa	
Moderate-incidence areas	10–50
Japan, southern Europe	
Low-incidence areas	<10
United States, northern Europe	

mentioned earlier *(4)*, the overall increase in the incidence of HCC was found to be less pronounced among women than men.

Within geographic regions, a racial and ethnic variation is noted. In South Africa, the black population has a high incidence of the disease, whereas the frequency within the white population is similar to that in Western Europe. In the United States, blacks are affected twice as often as whites. Of note, approximately one-quarter of the cases of HCC within the United States occur among a heterogeneous population that is comprised of Hispanics, Native Americans, Pacific Islanders, and Asians. This group has the highest risk for HCC within the United States (7.4/100,000 population) *(4)*. However, the proportion of cases of HCC represented by this group has remained constant over the past two decades, making it unlikely that the observed rise in incidence of HCC is attributable to this cohort alone.

Familial clustering is known to occur *(6)*, especially among families infected with HBV. Geographical clustering may rarely occur, with contaminated water sources being implicated. This has been described in the Nantong area of China, as well as along the Arkansas River in the United States.

BIOLOGY OF HCC

Hepatocellular carcinoma is a unique malignancy in that it is preceded by a defined pathological involvement of the target organ in most, if not all, cases. Several etiological factors have been described in the pathogenesis of HCC. More than one of these factors may be present in a given individual, suggesting synergism among these agents.

Hepatitis B Virus Infection

Worldwide, it is estimated that HBV infection accounts for almost 80% of all cases of HCC. This association has been found to be strongest in the ethnic Chinese and black Africans. In high-incidence areas, 60–70% of those with HCC are positive for the hepatitis B surface antigen (HBsAg), and more that 90% have antibody to the hepatitis B core antigen (anti-HBc), indicating present or past infection *(3)*.

In the United States, less than 20% of HCC patients have anti-HBc in serum and only a small fraction are HBsAg positive *(7,8)*. The seroprevalence of HBV is relatively low, with an estimated 1–1.25 million persons harboring a silent HBV infection *(9)*. Data from the National Institutes of Health indicate that the annual probability of HCC development in those with HBV-related chronic hepatitis is 0.5%, and among those with cirrhosis, it is 2.4% *(10)*.

The exact mechanism by which HBV causes cancer is debated. The integration of HBV into the host genome is believed to cause genetic mutations leading onto cancer development *(11–13)*. In addition, the chronic inflammation and increased cell turnover caused by the virus may act as a promoter of carcinogenesis.

At this time, our understanding of this complex process suggests that genome integration may be less crucial to the development of HCC than is the inflammation and regeneration caused by chronic hepatitis.

Hepatitis C Virus Infection

It is now increasingly clear that hepatitis C virus (HCV) is responsible for a significant number of cases of HCC. In southern Europe, as many as 50–75% of patients with HCC are positive for the HCV antibody *(14)*. A recent study from Japan *(15)*, where HBV and HCV infection are equally prevalent, indicated that the incidence of HCC was 2.7 times higher in those with chronic hepatitis C than in those with chronic hepatitis B. In cases of posttransfusion hepatitis, where exposure to HCV may be accurately determined, it has been estimated that the latent period for the development of HCC is approximately two to three decades *(16)*.

The mechanism by which HCV causes HCC is controversial. In contrast to HBV, HCV-associated HCC rarely occurs in the absence of cirrhosis *(15)*. This suggests that liver inflammation, injury, and regeneration play an important role in carcinogenesis.

Several other factors, when combined with HCV, appear to have a synergistic effect in leading to HCC. Most notable among these is concomitant HBV infection, which in one study *(17)* was demonstrated to confer a relative risk of 82 for the development of HCC compared to seven in those with HCV alone. Excessive alcohol use also increases the risk *(18)*, as does the rare acquired condition porphyria cutanea tarda, which may be sometimes associated with chronic hepatitis C *(19)*.

Cirrhosis

Cirrhosis underlies most cases of HCC. However, significant numbers of HCC arise in noncirrhotic livers, and one recent study suggests that these may account for as many as 50% of cases *(20)*. Even in the absence of cirrhosis, evidence of liver injury and regeneration is usually present. An important exception to this is the fibrolamellar variant of HCC, which arises in the absence of cirrhosis.

The generally accepted theory explaining the progression of cirrhosis to cancer is based on the development of macroregenerative nodules within the cirrhotic liver *(21–23)*. Areas of cellular atypia develop within these nodules, leading to dysplasia and then foci of HCC. It is well recognized that the etiology of the cirrhosis is an important determinant of malignant potential. The highest frequencies of HCC occur in cirrhosis resulting from viral hepatitis (HBV and HCV infection), hereditary hemochromatosis, and $\alpha 1$-antitrypsin deficiency. The risk is thought to be lower in primary biliary cirrhosis, Wilson's disease, and autoimmune hepatitis *(3)*.

Metabolic Disorders

HEREDITARY HEMOCHROMATOSIS

This genetic disorder characterized by hepatic and systemic iron overload is known to be strongly associated with HCC. Some studies have suggested that the relative risk of developing HCC in those with cirrhosis is as high as 200, with an overall incidence of 45% *(24)*. HCC rarely develops in the absence of cirrhosis. Of late, investigators have focused on the role of hepatic iron-free foci. These are nodules that are free of iron against a background of hepatocytes loaded with iron. Dysplastic changes are often seen within these nodules, and one study found a significant risk of subsequent development of HCC in these individuals *(25)*.

$\alpha 1$-ANTITRYPSIN DEFICIENCY

$\alpha 1$-Antitrypsin (AAT) deficiency, especially in its homozygous ZZ state, has been found to be associated with HCC. A case-control autopsy study from Sweden compared the rates of cirrhosis and HCC in AAT-deficient subjects with matched controls. A relative risk of 8 for cirrhosis and 20 for HCC was defined *(26)*.

GLYCOGEN STORAGE DISEASES

These disorders are unique because they do not present against a background of cirrhosis and because they represent the one example of hepatic adenomas progressing to malignant tumors *(27)*. Of these diseases, the best-described associations with HCC exist for type I (von Gierke's disease) and type III (Cori Forbes disease).

The Porphyrias

The hereditary porphyrias are uncommonly associated with HCC *(5)*. However, porphyria cutanea tarda (PCT), an acquired condition, is thought to predispose to HCC. It is often associated with HCV infection, and the relative contributions of each condition to the development of HCC are difficult to distinguish in most clinical studies.

Hereditary Tyrosinemia

This is a rare metabolic disease associated with severe liver disease, usually causing death in the first decade of life. Approximately 40% of patients develop HCC.

Wilson's Disease

Hepatocellular carcinoma is rare in this disorder, although a dozen cases have been described in the literature *(28)*.

Alcohol and Toxins

Excessive alcohol ingestion is considered a risk factor for HCC, when combined with other factors, and as a causative agent for the development of cirrhosis. However, there is little evidence to suggest that alcohol *per se* is carcinogenic.

Environmental Toxins

Aflatoxin B is a mycotoxin derived from *Aspergillus flavus,* a contaminant of improperly stored grain. This toxin has been found to produce a mutation of the p53 tumor suppressor gene and may potentiate the oncogenic potential of the hepatitis B virus *(29)*.

Other toxins linked to HCC include Thorotrast, used as an intravenous contrast agent for a short period in the post-World War II period, and androgenic steroids when taken by males for the enhancement of athletic performance. The link between estrogens and HCC is more tenuous. Women who use oral contraceptives and who have experienced pregnancies have been found to have a slightly higher incidence of HCC.

Miscellaneous

Membranous obstruction of the inferior vena cava is a rare congenital anomaly, which has been found to predispose to HCC in African and Japanese populations. HCC develops in approx 45% of affected individuals. However, this etiological entity appears to account for only a small proportion of the total number of HCC cases in these regions *(30)*.

Chapter 7 / Screening for Hepatocellular Carcinoma

RATIONALE FOR SCREENING

Certain prerequisites for a successful screening program have been defined by the World Health Organization *(31,32)*. HCC developing against a background of chronic liver disease meets the majority of these requirements.

The Disease Must be Common, with Significant Morbidity and Mortality

Hepatocellular carcinoma, as discussed in earlier sections, is an extremely prevalent condition worldwide. Untreated, the survival rates for HCC are dismal (1% at 2 yr) *(33)*.

The Target Population Should be Easily Identifiable

The risk factors for developing HCC are well defined. These include chronic viral hepatitis, cirrhosis, and hemochromatosis. However, it should be recognized that a proportion of those with HCC do not have cirrhosis, and in the United States, only 30–40% of reported HCC cases may be accounted for by HBV and HCV infection *(4)*.

The Disease Must Have an Established Natural History Such That Intervention at a Predefined Stage Would Provide an Improved Outcome

As with other malignancies, HCC has a variable growth rate. Three patterns of growth have been described: tumors with no, or very slow, growth; tumors with constant growth; tumors with declining growth *(34)*. Each of these groups accounts for approximately one-third of nodules. The tumor doubling time, assessed through ultrasonography, varies between 27 and 605 d, with a median of 180 d. This is the reason for employing a twice-yearly surveillance schedule.

The rationale behind screening for HCC is based on the assumption that tumors detected through surveillance are more amenable to treatment than symptomatic tumors. However, there is a paucity of data proving this. In one study from Japan, 65% of HCC detected through a surveillance program were less than 2 cm in size, and the overall 3-yr survival rate of all patients was relatively high at 41%, suggesting that early detection and treatment improved overall survival *(35)*. A recent study from Hong Kong *(36)* compared HCC characteristics and treatment outcomes in two categories of patients: those in whom the tumor was detected through surveillance and those who were symptomatic. The symptomatic cohort had a significantly larger tumor size, with higher proportions presenting with bilobar involvement and metastatic

118 Part III / Screening for Gastrointestinal Cancers

disease. Operability rates and cumulative survival were significantly better in the surveillance cohort. However, other studies have been disappointing and have failed to demonstrate any meaningful benefit *(37)*. This apparent anomaly may be attributable to the fact that favorable tumor characteristics may not translate into a higher rate of resectability. In most surgical series, the resection rate varied from 29 to 54% *(38–40)*. Recently published data suggest that liver transplantation provides good results in those with small tumors against a background of cirrhosis *(41)*. Orthotopic liver transplantation (OLT) is a promising option, but its utilization is likely to be limited by the reality that the areas of the world with the least accessibility to medical technology are also the ones most affected by HCC.

The Screening Tests Must Have a High Sensitivity and Specificity

As will be discussed in following sections, the standard screening tests for HCC, which include serum AFP testing and abdominal ultrasound, have far from acceptable levels of accuracy. This is a significant limiting factor in their utilization.

The Screening Tests Must Be Acceptable to the Target Population

The acceptability of serum α-fetoprotein (AFP) and ultrasonography may be inferred indirectly from the numbers of subjects lost to follow-up during a surveillance program. Studies have demonstrated that noncompliance rates are lower in those with liver disease (3–18%) than in asymptomatic HBV carriers (23%) *(38,40)*. Unfortunately, no studies exist examining the compliance rates with the involved, and often invasive, workup required for positive screening tests.

Effective Therapy Must Exist Such That Surveillance Would Decrease Disease-Specific Mortality

Therapeutic options for HCC include hepatic resection, OLT, and local destruction of the tumor. Hepatic resection (partial or total hepatectomy) offers optimal therapy. Unfortunately, only a small proportion of those with HCC has a potentially resectable tumor on diagnosis. The postresection tumor recurrence rate is very high (approaching 25%/yr).

Orthotopic liver transplantation has increasingly been considered a suitable alternative to resection *(41)*. With small tumors, post-OLT recurrence is significantly lower than with resection. OLT is probably the best treatment for those with decompensated cirrhosis, unable to

Chapter 7 / Screening for Hepatocellular Carcinoma 119

tolerate a hepatectomy. However, this therapy is significantly limited by the shortage of donor organs and the lack of transplant programs in much of the developing world.

Other options include local destruction of the tumor by injection with acetic acid or absolute alcohol and chemoembolization with chemotherapeutic agents *(13)*. These approaches have not been shown to confer significant survival benefit when used alone, but may be useful adjuncts to OLT or hepatic resection.

The only way to demonstrate improved survival in a population that is screened is to conduct randomized, controlled studies comparing mortality rates in cohorts with and without surveillance. To date, the only large randomized trial of screening studied 14,794 HBV carriers in Shanghai, China who were randomized to AFP determinations every 6 mo vs no surveillance *(13)*. Ultrasonography was offered to those with elevated AFP levels. No survival benefit could be demonstrated despite the fact that 18% of the tumors detected were less than 3 cm. However, interpretation of these results is complicated by the fact that most patients did not have adequate access to definitive treatment, a significant concern in medically underserved areas.

In North America, two large published series have examined this issue. The first of these screened approx 75% of the native Alaskan population for the hepatitis B surface antigen *(42)*. The 1400 HBV carriers thus detected were screened over a 5-yr period, using AFP as the only screening test. Twenty tumors were detected, of which 10 were resectable. At the end of 5 yr, only four tumors were found to have recurred. Using a slightly different approach in an urban Canadian population, Zoli et al. *(38)* screened both the general population and known HBV carriers. Of the 14 tumors detected, 6 were resected. However, only three patients survived more than 2 yr from diagnosis.

These data demonstrate that outcomes are highly variable and are dependent on not only the geographic regions where screening occurs but also on the treatment options available.

METHODS OF SCREENING

Two main strategies exist for the screening of HCC: population-based screening, which involves screening everyone in the general population, and clinic-based programs, in which selected groups judged to be at risk for HCC are screened.

Blood Tests

α-Fetoprotein is a tumor marker, which was used in the first reported surveillance studies in HCC. The sensitivity of AFP varies widely, depending on various factors. The most important of these is the level of AFP that should trigger further investigation. For example, if the threshold level of AFP is raised from 20 to 100 mg/L, the sensitivity of the test falls from 39 to 13% while the specificity increases *(39)*.

Another factor impacting on the sensitivity of AFP is the coexistence of HBV infection. In one study comparing the utility of AFP in detected HCC, the specificity was found to be only 50% in HBV-positive patients, compared with 78% in HBV-negative patients *(43)*.

Complicating the interpretation of AFP levels is the fact that AFP may be elevated in conditions other than HCC. The most important of these conditions is active viral hepatitis, when the raised AFP often, but not always, parallels an increase in transaminases. Isoelectric focusing of sera may identify variant forms of AFP more commonly associated with tumor. Pregnancy as well as yolk sac and other gastrointestinal mucosal malignancies may also cause false-positive elevations of AFP *(3)*.

Studies have demonstrated that serum AFP levels persistently above 20 mg/L confer a relative risk of HCC of approx 14. Fluctuating levels are associated with an intermediate relative risk of 6. Conversely, serum AFP levels may be normal or only modestly raised in the presence of HCC.

Three large, well-designed studies have evaluated the utility of AFP as a screening tool for AFP. These studies report a sensitivity of 39–64%, a specificity of 76–91%, and a positive predictive value of 9–32% *(32)*.

Radiological Tests

The three radiological methods used to study the liver are ultrasonography, computerized tomography (CT), and magnetic resonance imaging (MRI). Of these, the best studied as a screening tool is the abdominal ultrasound (US).

Ultrasound has several advantages as a screening test. It is relatively inexpensive, easily available even in developing countries, and is safe. The accuracy of US has been well defined in both healthy (noncirrhotic) hepatitis B surface antigen carriers and in those with cirrhosis. Its sensitivity was 71 and 78%, respectively, with a positive predictive value of 14 and 73%, respectively *(32)*. CT and MRI scanning do not appear to be feasible options as screening tests, given their high costs.

Confirmatory Tests

These include CT, spiral CT, MRI, lipiodol–CT, and hepatic angiography. For lesions greater than 3 cm, the sensitivity and specificity of contrast-enhanced CT are 68 and 81%, respectively. Smaller tumors are

Chapter 7 / Screening for Hepatocellular Carcinoma 121

better detected by either MRI (81% sensitivity for tumors less than 2 cm) or spiral CT scan (87% sensitivity for tumors less than 1 cm). Lipiodol–CT scanning involves administration of the lipid compound lipiodol, which has been shown to be selectively retained in foci of HCC. Sensitivities of 93–97% have been reported for this technique.

Computed tomography scanning, especially with the newer spiral techniques, has been demonstrated to have a very high sensitivity for small lesions. A recent study on explanted livers assessed pretransplantation radiological imaging in cirrhotic patients. US, CT, and hepatic angiography were found to have sensitivities of 80, 86.6, and 90%, respectively.

Tissue Diagnosis

The use of biopsy to confirm the presence of HCC is controversial. A small but well-described risk of seeding of the tumor along the needle tract has been used to discourage indiscriminate needle biopsies. Also, it is difficult to distinguish well-differentiated HCC from cirrhotic nodules. Therefore, needle biopsies should be employed judiciously when considerable doubt exists as to the diagnosis, and further management is likely to be influenced by the biopsy findings.

Unfortunately, most of the surveillance studies described to date have not evaluated the financial costs or medical burdens imposed by the workup of false-positive tests. Without such data, it is difficult to analyze the acceptability of surveillance to the target population.

SUMMARY

In summary, the best screening approach to HCC appears to be a combination of AFP and ultrasonography (*see* Algorithm 1). The recommended screening interval is 6 mo. If the AFP is consistently greater than 20 mg/L, the screening interval should be reduced to 3 mo. However, no guidelines exist as to whether a normal ultrasound in the presence of an elevated AFP should lead to further investigations to exclude HCC.

The population to be targeted for screening should include those deemed to be at high risk, as summarized in Table 2.

COST-EFFECTIVENESS OF SCREENING

To become a part of standard medical practice, a screening strategy must not only be considered effective from a clinical standpoint but also in terms of a cost–benefit analysis. To date, four published studies have studied the costs of HCC screening. Kang et al. *(44)* analyzed the data

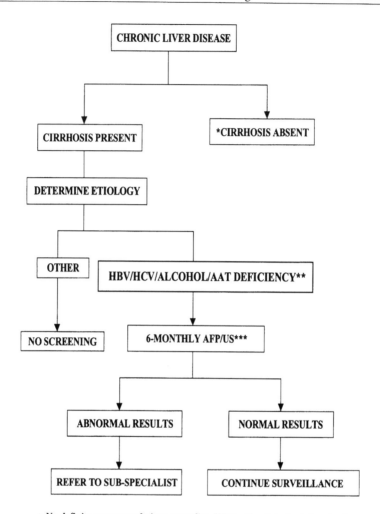

No definite recommendations regarding HBV without cirrhosis (see text)
* *Alpha 1 antitrypsin deficiency*
** *Alpha fetoprotein/ultrasound*

Algorithm 1. Screening for hepatocellular carcinoma.

from the surveillance of HBV carriers, using both ultrasound and AFP. They concluded that the cost of detecting each tumor would be $11,800. However, their projected tumor growth rates are somewhat at variance from those seen in other surveillance studies. A Japanese study *(45)* evaluated the efficacy of a mass-screening program. The cost per tumor detected was $25,000. A recent study from Hong Kong *(36)* estimated that the annual cost of screening chronic hepatitis B and C carriers in order to detect one HCC was only $1167. This cost rose modestly to

Chapter 7 / Screening for Hepatocellular Carcinoma

Table 2
Screening Strategies for HCC

Screening recommended	*Screening not required*
Cirrhosis	Cirrhosis
Viral hepatitis	Autoimmune hepatitis
Heredity hemochromatosis	PBC
Alcoholic	Wilson's disease
AAT deficiency	
Porphyria cutanea tarda	Hereditary porphyrias
	Chronic hepatitis C w/o cirrhosis
	Heredity hemochromatosis w/o cirrhosis
Family history of HCC	Poor surgical candidates
Chronic hepatitis B w/o cirrhosis	

$1667 if only treatable tumors were taken into account. However, in this study, the incidence of HCC was somewhat higher (142 cases out of the 2000 carriers screened) than in other studies, therefore enhancing the cost-effectiveness of surveillance. Sarasin et al. *(46)* used a decision-analysis model to estimate the costs of screening selected individuals with Child's grade cirrhosis. This study subdivided patients into groups based on their age, cancer risk, and cirrhosis-related mortality. In the best-case scenario involving young patients with a high cancer incidence and low mortality, biannual screening provided a gain in life expectancy of 9 mo (8.5%). However, in those with the worst-case scenario, surveillance actually decreased life expectancy by 9 d. The important point that emerged from this analysis is that patient selection is crucial to the cost-efficiency of a surveillance program in HCC. In the "ideal" patient selected by this study, the cost per year gained ranged from $26,000 to $55,000, with a mean gain in life expectancy ranging from 3 to 9 mo. Analyses of surveillance data from breast and cervical cancers show that regular screening prolongs the life of a 50-yr-old woman by 2 and 3 mo, respectively *(47,48)*. The costs per life-year gained range between $21,700 and $134,100 for breast cancer and between $2300 and $33,600 for cervical cancer. In colon cancer screening, the cost per life-year gained is approx $25,320 *(49)*. From this comparative literature, we may infer that although HCC screening is expensive, its costs are very comparable to those incurred by other cancer surveillance programs.

INDICATIONS FOR CONSULTING THE SUBSPECIALIST

A gastroenterologist or hepatologist should probably be involved in the care of most patients with cirrhosis, chronic viral hepatitis, and the metabolic liver diseases, to aid in therapeutic decisions as well as in determining appropriate evaluation and listing for liver transplantation. However, there are several specific scenarios that would require specialist interventions:

1. Abnormal screening tests. These may include either elevated AFP levels or an abnormal ultrasound. In the presence of these indicators, the decision to pursue further involved diagnostic workup may be best left to the specialist.
2. Uncertainty regarding whether screening is indicated. As discussed in previous sections, the cancer risk in several chronic liver diseases is controversial, with a constant flux of opinions.
3. Abrupt deterioration in clinical condition. The sudden appearance of decompensated liver disease, such as new-onset ascites, encephalopathy, or hyperbilirubinemia, may herald the development of HCC, even in patients with unremarkable screening tests. These patients will require a complete investigation.
4. Development of extrahepatic manifestations. HCC is associated with several paraneoplastic manifestations. These include erythrocytosis, hypoglycemia, hypercholesterolemia, and various dermatological conditions such as porphyria cutanea tarda. The unexplained onset of these conditions in a high-risk patient should prompt a referral to a specialist for further workup.

CONTROVERSIAL AREAS

1. Our previous discussion has demonstrated that the costs of a screening program for HCC are certainly comparable to those for other cancers. However, HCC screening is far from an inexpensive strategy. This, coupled with the lack of any demonstrable survival benefits from a screening program, has led some to doubt whether screening for HCC is a cost-effective option. This is an issue that can only be resolved by a randomized, controlled trial. Unfortunately, it is unlikely that such a study will ever be carried out, given the ethical problems inherent in including an unscreened population. At the present time, we will have to depend on decision analyses, as well on the indirect evidence obtained from controlled trials on the treatment of small HCCs.
2. The patient population that should be screened for HCC remains a controversial issue. It is well accepted that cirrhosis and chronic viral hepatitis both predispose to HCC. Ideally, all patients with viral hepatitis B and C should be screened for HCC. However, in a low-incidence

Chapter 7 / Screening for Hepatocellular Carcinoma 125

region such as the United States, this may not be a cost-effective approach. Because the incidence of HCV-related HCC is rare in the absence of cirrhosis, it seems reasonable to assess all those with chronic hepatitis C for cirrhosis (ideally with a liver biopsy), and then pursue surveillance studies in only those with cirrhosis. HBV-related HCC does, however, occur frequently and those with HBV, especially males over the age of 40, should probably be subjected to screening, even in the absence of cirrhosis. However, this approach has never been critically evaluated in a clinical study.

3. The age at which surveillance should begin remains ill-defined. HCC occurring against a background of HBV infection is uncommon before the age of 30. However, no definite age cutoff has been proposed for the initiation of screening studies. Similarly, there is no upper age limit at which screening is discontinued, although clinical judgment would indicate that surveillance be stopped at the point when predicted life expectancy is limited.

It is possible that as our understanding of HCC evolves, we will be better able to target screening to high-risk populations, namely males, those of advancing age, and those infected with specific genotypes of hepatitis C, although the latter issue remains to be better defined *(50)*.

Prevention strategies for HCC are being evolved. Universal Hepatitis B vaccination in a high-incidence area such as Taiwan has demonstrably reduced the incidence of HCC *(51)*. Unfortunately, large-scale vaccination programs have not been implemented in other endemic areas such as Africa.

Therapies such as interferon, aimed at eliminating the hepatitis C virus, have been reported to decrease the incidence of HCC, even in nonresponders. However, most of the studies examining this issue have been retrospective, and their study designs preclude any definite conclusions. At the present time, the role of interferon therapy in the prevention of HCC is unclear and awaits further study *(52)*.

Other chemopreventive agents such as oltipraz and polyprenoic acid are undergoing clinical trials at this time. If their promise is realized, our approach to the management of HCC is likely to be dramatically altered in the future.

REFERENCES

1. Bosch FX, Ribes J, Borras J. (1999) Epidemiology of primary liver cancer. *Semin Liv Dis* 19:271–285.
2. Parkin DM, Muir CS, Whelan SL, et al. (1992) Cancer incidence in five continents. *IARC Sci Pub* 6:882–883.
3. Di Bisceglie AM. (1999) Malignant neoplasms of the liver. In: Schiff ER, Sorrell MF, Maddrey WC, eds. *Schiff's Diseases of the Liver*, 8th edition. Philadelphia: Lippincott-Raven, pp. 1281–1304.

126 **Part III / Screening for Gastrointestinal Cancers**

4. El-Sera, HB, Mason AC. (1999) Rising incidence of hepatocellular carcinoma in the United States. *N Engl J Med* 340:745–750.
5. Parkin DM, Pisani P, Ferlay J. (1999) Estimates of the worldwide incidence of twenty-five major cancers in 1990. *Int J Cancer* 80:827–841.
6. Heyward WL, Lanier AP, Bender TR, et al. (1983) Early detection of primary hepatocellular carcinoma by screening for alpha-fetoprotein in high-risk families. *Lancet* 2(8360):1161,1162.
7. Di Bisceglie AM, Order S., Klien JL, et al. (1991) The role of chronic viral hepatitis in hepatocellular carcinoma in the United States. *Am J Gastroenterol* 86:335–338.
8. Yu MC, Ton, M, Coursaget P, et al. (1990) Prevalence of hepatitis B and C viral markers in black and white patients with hepatocellular carcinoma in the United States. *J Natl Cancer Inst* 82:1036–1041.
9. McQuillan GM, Townsend TR, Fields HA, et al. (1989) Seroepidemiology of hepatitis B virus infection in the United States:1976 to 1980. *Am J Med* 87:5S–10S.
10. Hoofnagle JH. (1988) The natural history of hepatocellular carcinoma, pp. 393–395. In: Di Bisceglie AM, moderator, *Hepatocellular Carcinoma. Ann Intern Med* 108:390–401.
11. Zuckerman AJ, Harrison TJ. (1987) Hepatitis B virus chronic liver disease and hepatocellular carcinoma. *Postgrad Med J* 63(Suppl 2):13–19.
12. Hsia CC, Axiotis CA, Di Bisceglie AM, Tabor E. (1992) Transforming growth factor in human hepatocellular carcinoma and co-expression with hepatitis B surface antigen in adjacent liver. *Cancer* 70:1049–1056.
13. Di Bisceglie AM, Carithers RL, Gores GJ. (1998) Hepatocellular carcinoma. *Hepatology* 28:1161–1165.
14. Bruix J, Barrera JM, Calvet X, et al. (1989) Prevalence of antibodies to hepatitis C virus in Spanish patients with hepatocellular carcinoma and hepatic cirrhosis. *Lancet* II:4–6.
15. Takano S, Yokosuk, O, Imazeki F, Tagawa M, Omatam M. (1995) Incidence of hepatocellular carcinoma in chronic hepatitis B and C: a prospective study of 251 patients. *Hepatology* 21:650–654.
16. Tong MJ, El-Farra NS, Reikes AR, Co RL. (1995) Clinical outcomes after transfusion-associated hepatitis C. *N Engl J Med* 332:1463–1466.
17. Kew MC, Yu M., Kedda, et al. (1997) The relative roles of hepatitis B and C viruses in the etiology of hepatocellular carcinoma in southern African Blacks. *Gastroenterology* 112:184–187.
18. Yamauchi M, Nakahara M, Maezawa Y, et al. (1993) Prevalence of hepatocellular carcinoma in patients with alcoholic cirrhosis and prior exposure to hepatitis C. *Am J Gastroenterol* 88:39–43.
19. Salata H, Cortes JM, de Salamanca RE, et al. (1985) Porphyria cutanea tarda and hepatocellular carcinoma: frequency of occurrence and related factors. *J Hepatol* 1:477–487.
20. Nzeako UC, Goodman ZD, Ishak KG. (1996) Hepatocellular carcinoma in cirrhotic and noncirrhotic livers. A clinico-histopathologic study of 804 North American patients. *Am J Clin Pathol* 105:65–75.
21. Thiese ND., Schwartz M, Miller C, et al. (1992) Macroregenerative nodules and hepatocellular carcinoma in forty-four sequential adult liver explants with cirrhosis. *Hepatology* 16:949–955.
22. Kondo F, Ebara M, Sugiura N, et al. (1990) Histological features and clinical course of large regenerative nodules: evaluation of their precancerous potentiality. *Hepatology* 12:592–598.

Chapter 7 / Screening for Hepatocellular Carcinoma 127

23. Thiese ND. (1996) Cirrhosis and hepatocellular neoplasia: more like cousins than like parent and child [editorial]. *Gastroenterology* 111:526–528.

24. Deugnie YM, Guyader D, Crantock L, et al. (1993) Primary liver cancer in genetic hemochromatosis: a clinical, pathological, and pathogenetic study of 54 cases. *Gastroenterology* 104:228.

25. Deugnier YM, Charalambous P, le Quilleuc D, et al. (1993) Preneoplastic significance of hepatic iron free foci in genetic hemochromatosis. *Hepatology* 18:1363–1369.

26. Eriksson S, Carlson J, Velez R. (1986) Risk of cirrhosis and primary liver cancer in alpha 1-antitrypsin deficiency. *N Engl J Med* 314:736–739.

27. Haagsm, EB, Smit GP, Niezen-Knoning KE, et al. (1997) Type IIIb glycogen storage disease associated with end-stage cirrhosis and hepatocellular carcinoma. *Hepatology* 25:537–540.

28. Cheng WSC, Govindrajan S, Redeker AG. (1992) Hepatocellular carcinoma in a case of Wilson's disease. *Liver* 12:42–45.

29. Ross RK, Yuan J, Yu MC, et al. (1992) Urinary aflatoxin biomarkers and risk of hepatocellular carcinoma. *Lancet* 339:943–946.

30. Kew MC, McKnight A., Hodkinson J.et al. (1989) The role of membranous obstruction of the inferior vena cava in the etiology of hepatocellular carcinoma in southern African blacks. *Hepatology* 9:121–125.

31. Wilson JM, Junger, J. (1968) *Principles and Practice of Screening for Disease.* WHO Public Paper, Geneva: WHO, p. 34.

32. Collie, J, Sherman M. (1998) Screening for hepatocellular carcinoma. *Hepatology* 27:273–278.

33. Stuart KE, Anand AJ, Jenkins RL. (1986) Hepatocellular carcinoma in the United States. Prognostic features, treatment outcome and survival. *Cancer* 77:2217–2222.

34. Barbara L, Benzi G, Gaiani S, et al. (1992) Natural history of small untreated hepatocellular carcinoma in cirrhosis: a multivariate analysis of prognostic factors of tumor growth rate and patient survival. *Hepatology* 16:132–137.

35. Oka H, Kuriola N, Kim K, et al. (1990) Prospective study of early detection of hepatocellular carcinoma in patients with cirrhosis. *Hepatology* 12:680–687.

36. Yuen M-F, Cheng C-C., Lauder IJ, et al. (2000) Early detection of hepatocellular carcinoma increases the chances of treatment: Hong Kong experience. *Hepatology* 31:330–335.

37. Colombo M, De Franchis R., Del Ninno E, et al. (1991) Hepatocellular carcinoma in Italian patients with cirrhosis. *N Engl J Med* 325:675–680.

38. Zoli M, Magalotti D, Bianchi G., et al. (1996) Efficacy of a surveillance program for early detection of hepatocellular carcinoma. *Cancer* 78:977–985.

39. Sherman M, Peltekian KM, Lee C. (1995) Screening for hepatocellular carcinoma in chronic carriers of hepatitis B virus: incidence and prevalence of hepatocellular carcinoma in a North American urban population. *Hepatology* 22:432–438.

40. Oka H, Tamori A, Kuroki T, et al. (1994) Prospective study of alpha-fetoprotein in cirrhotic patients monitored for development of hepatocellular carcinoma. *Hepatology* 19:61–66.

41. Mazzaferro V, Regalia E, Doci R, et al. (1996) Liver transplantation for the treatment of small hepatocellular carcinomas in patients with cirrhosis. *N Engl J Med* 334:693–698.

42. McMahon BJ, Alberts SR, Wainwright RB, et al. (1990) Hepatitis B-related sequelae: prospective study of 1400 hepatitis B surface antigen-positive Alaska native carriers. *Arch Intern Med* 150:1051–1054.

128 Part III / Screening for Gastrointestinal Cancers

43. Lee H-S, Chung YH, Kim CY. (1991) Specificities of serum alpha-fetoprotein in HbsAg+ and HbsAg– patients in the diagnosis of hepatocellular carcinoma. *Hepatology* 14:68–72.
44. Kang JY, Lee TP, Yap I, et al. (1992) Analysis of cost-effectiveness of different strategies for hepatocellular carcinoma in screening for hepatitis B virus carriers. *J Gastroenterol Hepatol* 7:463–468.
45. Mima S, Sekiya C, Kanagawa H, et al. (1994) Mass screening for hepatocellular carcinoma: experience in Hokkaido, Japan. *J Gastroenterol Hepatol* 9:361–365.
46. Sarasin FP, Giostra E, Hadengue A. (1996) Cost effectiveness of screening for detection of small hepatocellular carcinoma in Western patients with Child-Pugh Class A cirrhosis. *Am J Med* 1:422–434.
47. Eddy DM. (1991) Screening for breast cancer. In: Eddy DM, ed., *Common Screening Tests*. Philadelphia: American College of Physicians, pp. 229–254.
48. Eddy DM. (1990) Screening for cervical cancer. *Ann Int Med* 113;214–226.
49. Lieberman DA. (1995) Cost-effectiveness model for colon cancer screening. *Gasteoenterology* 109:1781–1790.
50. Bruno S, Silini E, Crosignani A, et al. (1997) Hepatitis C virus genotypes and risk of hepatocellular carcinoma in cirrhosis: a prospective study. *Hepatology* 25:754–758.
51. Chang M, Chen C, Lai M, et al. (1997) Universal hepatitis B vaccination in Taiwan and the incidence of hepatocellular carcinoma in children. *N Engl J Med* 337;1855–1859.
52. Kowdley KV. (1999) Does Interferon therapy prevent hepatocellular carcinoma in patients with chronic hepatitis C? *Gastroenterology* 117:738–740.

8 Screening for Oropharyngeal Cancer

Krishnamoorthy Srinivasan, MS, SLO
and Mohan Kameswaram, MS, FRCS, MAMS

KEY PRINCIPLES

- Oral and oropharyngeal malignancies are uncommon in the United States and other Western countries. However, the incidence is very high in India, East Africa, and Far East Asia.
- Prognosis for early cancer is excellent, but advanced cancer has not only high mortality but is also associated with poor quality of life, as extensive facial surgery is usually required with many functional disabilities.
- There is a very high incidence of synchronous or metachronous cancer in the aerodigestive tract in patients with oropharyngeal carcinoma, which is a major threat to their long-term survival after curative therapy for oropharyngeal cancer.
- Several risk factors have been identified in the etiology of oropharyngeal cancer and include cigaret smoking, alcohol, betel nut chewing, and immunocompromised state.
- Although screening involves only a simple oral examination, it is often neglected and the majority of the cases present at an advanced stage.
- A thorough examination of the oral cavity is recommended as part of routine physical examination particularly in the high-risk patients.

INTRODUCTION

Oral and oropharyngeal malignancies, although not very common, are assuming importance because of the increasing incidence in

From: *Cancer Screening: A Practical Guide for Physicians*
Edited by: K. Aziz and G. Y. Wu © Humana Press Inc., Totowa, NJ

129

130   Part III / Screening for Gastrointestinal Cancers

immunocompromised patients and patients who are migrating from high-incidence areas to low-incidence areas. The prognosis is generally poor, as there is almost always a delay in the reporting of these cases *(1)*. Furthermore, a significant percentage of patients initially cured of oropharyngeal carcinoma go on to develop new primary tumors in the aerodigestive tract, which are the major threat to long-term survival after successful therapy of the first cancer *(2,3)*. In addition, patients who have undergone surgery for oropharyngeal carcinoma have significant residual cosmetic and functional debilities, with marked reduction in the quality of life.

EPIDEMIOLOGY

The types of malignancies in the oropharynx are as follows:

1. Squamous-cell carcinoma—70%.
2. Non-Hodgkin's lymphoma—25%.
3. Minor salivary gland tumors—5%.

The incidence of oral and oropharyngeal cancer shows a definite geographical variation, because of a different pattern of tobacco use (smoking or chewing) and other substance abuse *(4–7)*. In the United States, the incidence is about 4% of all new cancer cases, where smokers outnumber chewers, but in Bombay, the incidence is about 50% of all cancers where the betel nut is commonly chewed *(7)*.

In the United States approx 30,000 new cases of oropharyngeal cancer are diagnosed each year, with a 5-yr survival rate of 55% for American whites and 34% for American blacks. The incidence of oropharyngeal cancer is similar in the United States, the United Kingdom, and Canada *(8,9)*.

More than 90% of all oropharyngeal cancers occur in patients over the age of 45. Incidence increases with age until about age 65, when the rate levels off at 45–50 cases per 100,000 population *(10)*. As with other head and neck tumors, male predominance is common, with a male-to-female ratio of 4:1, because of the greater use of tobacco by men. Compared with nonusers, alcohol users are 3.6 times more likely to have oropharengeal cancer, 5.8 times for tobacco users, and 19 times for users of both alcohol and tobacco *(11)*.

BIOLOGY OF OROPHARYNGEAL CARCINOMA

Squamous-Cell Carcinoma

Squamous-cell carcinoma (SCC) is the most common malignancy in the head and neck region and constitutes 70% of oropharyngeal malig-

Chapter 8 / Screening for Oropharyngeal Cancer 131

nancies. Lymph-node metastasis is early and may be the presenting feature, as this area is richly supplied with lymphatics. In searching for occult primary cancer in the CUP syndrome (carcinoma of unknown primary), the most common sites are the nasopharynx, tonsils, and the base of the tongue. Several environmental, viral, and genetic factors have been implicated in the pathogenesis of oropharyngeal carcinoma. These include the following:

BETEL NUT

The two most important factors that act synergistically in the etiology of SCC are tobacco and alcohol in the Western countries, whereas betel nut chewing is the major factor in India, East Africa, Far East Asia, and the South Pacific. The betel nut is used daily by 600 million people worldwide *(12)*. The betel nut is chewed alone or as part of the betel package (paan). The betel nut is the fruit of betel or *Areca catechu*, whereas paan is a fresh mature betel leaf with the undersurface smeared with lime, made up into a package that contains cuttings of the betel nut, catechu, and, at times, tobacco, along with many other sweetening and flavoring agents. The International Agency for Research on Cancer has classified the betel nut as a Group A carcinogen when used with tobacco *(13)*. The betel nut acts synergistically with tobacco to produce oral cancer *(14–16)*. Approximately 30% of oral cancers in Southeast Asia are caused by betel nut use. In Taiwan, the rate of oral cancer is four times that of Japan and 2.6 times that of the United States *(17)*. Of those Taiwanese who develop oral cancer, 88% chew betel nuts on a daily basis.

Submucous fibrosis (SF) is a premalignant condition, which is common in individuals who chew betel nut or use paan. In a study of 186 betel nut chewers, 71 patients had signs and symptoms of SF and 10 patients had SCC. All the patients with SCC had typical signs of SF, which was confirmed on biopsy specimen obtained from unaffected parts of the mouth *(18)*. The chewing of Khat (betel nut soaked in tobacco), primarily in the Middle East and East Africa (Yemen, Sudan), is associated with a very high incidence of SCC *(19)*. SCC of the hard palate is endemic in parts of Asia, particularly in Andhra Pradesh (India), where reverse chutta (homemade cigar), smoking with the burning end held in the mouth, is a common practice *(1)*.

ALCOHOL AND TOBACCO EXPOSURE

Tobacco initiates a linear dose-response carcinogenic effect in which duration is more important than the intensity of exposure. The major carcinogenic activity of cigaret smoke resides in the tar fraction, which contains a complex mixture of interacting cancer initiators, promoters, and cocarcinogens. Smoking seems to be the primary factor in the complex causality equation for these cancers. However, alcohol is an important promoter of carcinogenesis and is a contributive factor in at least 75% of oropharyngeal cancers *(4)*. Alcohol potentiates the carcinogenic effect of tobacco at every level of tobacco use, and the causative effect is most striking at the highest levels of exposure to both *(20)*. Carcinogens present in the tar are insoluble in saliva but are highly soluble in alcohol and easily absorbed in the oropharynx *(21)*. In heavy smokers, approx 15 yr must pass before the risk is approximately back to the level of people who never smoked *(22)*. Smoking marijuana appears to confer an even greater risk for SCC than does cigaret smoking *(23,24)*. Marijuana smoke has a four times higher tar burden and 50% higher concentrations of benzpyrene and aromatic hydrocarbons than are present in tobacco smoke.

Genetic Factors

Genetic factors also seem to play a significant role in this disease. Although a large portion of the population uses tobacco, only a small fraction of individuals will develop tobacco-induced malignancies. One hypothesis is that a substantial portion of the variation in human susceptibility to tobacco-induced cancers is the result of the presence of a genetic polymorphism among the exposed population. This polymorphism results in the altered function of detoxification enzymes, DNA repair proteins, tumor-suppressor genes and/or proto-oncogenes. Previous work by various groups has implicated DNA polymorphism in the STM1, P1A1, and p53 genes as risk factors for the development of tobacco-induced carcinoma of the lung. Similarly, SCC of the oropharynx has an extremely strong epidemiological link to combined tobacco and ethanol exposure *(25)*. A 20–30% incidence of synchronous and/or metachronous cancers has been reported in patients with SCC of the upper aerodigestive tract *(26)*.

Miscellaneous Factors

In the past, syphilis, poor oral hygiene, chronic gingivitis, and ill-fitting dentures have been implicated in the etiology of oral cancer, but recent reports have failed to show this association *(27–29)*.

In an interesting study in a group of 200 patients with head and neck cancer, 11 had no history of smoking or alcohol use. Of these, 10 patients had used mouthwash at least twice a day for more than 20 yr. Nine had used the same brand of mouthwash and eight used the mouthwash undiluted. The proprietary mouthwashes implicated in this study contained 14–28% alcohol *(30)*.

Chapter 8 / Screening for Oropharyngeal Cancer 133

VIRAL INFECTION

Epidemiological studies have shown that herpes simplex virus 1 (HSV-1) can act as a mutagen in the development of SCC. Patients with oral SCC have increased levels of HSV-1 IgA and IgM antibodies that are of prognostic significance. However, their role in the carcinogenesis has recently been questioned because HSV-1 gene products appear in oral SCC tissues only in a small number of cases *(31,32)*. Recently, the human papilloma viruses 8 and 16 have shown to be associated with SCC *(33)*.

IMMUNOSUPPRESSION

Another group of patients in whom SCC is increasingly recognized is the patients on immunosuppressant medications following organ transplantation and human immunodeficiency virus (HIV) injection. The incidence of oropharyngeal cancer in this population is 7.6 times greater than the normal population *(34,35)*.

Lymphoma

Lymphoma of the head and neck region can arise in nodal or extranodal sites. Hodgkin's disease is rare in the oropharynx, but non-Hodgkin's lymphoma constitutes 15–20% of the tumors. Etiology is largely unknown. However autoimmune disorders such as Sjögren's syndrome, congenital and acquired immunodeficiencies, and chronic Epstein–Barr virus infection have been implicated *(1,36)*.

SALIVARY GLAND TUMORS

The majority of tumors of the major salivary glands are benign, whereas the majority of minor salivary glands are malignant. The vast majority of them are adenoid cystic carcinoma arising either in the tonsils or soft palate *(1)*. These tumors are similar to nonmelanoma skin cancer and lip cancer in their epidemiological association with ultraviolet-B and ionizing radiation exposure *(37,38)*. There seems to be no association between tobacco and salivary gland tumors *(39)*.

RATIONALE FOR SCREENING

Despite the fact that over 90% of the oropharyngeal malignancies occur in a region of the body, which is easily visible to the patient and the physician, there is almost always a delay of 6–8 mo before a diagnosis of oropharyngeal carcinoma is made *(1)*. This delay should be avoided or minimized, because the outcome is evidently better with early treatment. A simple examination, with the knowledge of prema-

134 Part III / Screening for Gastrointestinal Cancers

lignant conditions and the awareness of the high-risk group, should be able to detect the majority of the cases. Four of the seven warning signs of cancer (which are promoted by the American Cancer Society) pertain to the upper aerodigestive tract. These include the following:

1. A sore in the oropharynx that does not heal.
2. A lump in the neck.
3. Difficulty in swallowing.
4. Persistent hoarseness.

All of these factors can easily be included in the examination by taking a few extra minutes and effort.

METHODS OF SCREENING

Clinical Examination

Unlike several other cancers, screening for oropharyngeal cancer does not require intricate, time-consuming, or expensive procedure. Simple examination of the oral cavity by any trained health care provider can result in the detection of early-stage cancer as well as premalignant lesions. In Sri Lanka, primary health care workers were trained in the oral examination, and they sent 660 patients with suspected cancer to the referral center, of which only 10% had no lesion and 58% were confirmed as having oral cancer *(40)*.

In a study of 672,000 veterans, 814 oral cancers were detected when oral examination was included as part of the initial visit. The study concluded that the primary care physician should be able to detect and refer cases of suspected malignancies of the oropharynx by a thorough oral examination in high-risk patients (chronic tobacco and alcohol users over age 40). The detection rate can be as high as 1 in every 200–250 individuals examined *(41)*.

The detection rate for early-stage disease increased from 20 to 33% over a 3-yr period in a regional oral cancer detection program when investigators stressed the importance of routine oral examination *(42)*.

Visual oral examination, including palpation of the tongue, floor of the mouth, salivary glands, and lymph nodes of the neck, should be a routine part of the physical examination. The red patch (erythroplakia) is more often associated with malignancy than the white patch (leukoplakia). The other forms of mucosal changes should be examined to rule out trauma (from teeth) and a clinical judgment should be made regarding the relevance of these lesions. Any lump in the neck should be thoroughly examined to rule out the possibility of it being a secondary node. Dysphagia and hoarseness of the voice persisting for more than 15 d

Chapter 8 / Screening for Oropharyngeal Cancer

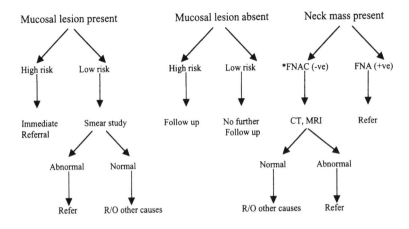

* Fine needle aspiration cytology

Algorithm 1. Patients for routine examination.

should be referred to the subspecialist for indirect laryngoscopy (*see* Algorithm 1).

Although no randomized clinical trials show the efficacy of early detection, as measured by improvement in survival or decrease in mortality, until proven otherwise, it must be assumed that early detection and treatment will improve prognosis in oral cancer.

FURTHER WORKUP

Any nonhealing sore should be considered potentially malignant and a smear should be sent for cytology. Mouth rinse using toluidine blue has shown to increase the sensitivity and specificity of smear cytology and occasionally multiple primary cancers in the mouth can be identified that were missed on clinical examination *(26)*. Likewise, any suspicious swelling or node in the neck should be subjected to aspiration biopsy. This test is especially helpful in differentiating between a simple cyst and a cystic degeneration in a metastatic node. The risk of cancer seeding has not been reported with this procedure and the specificity and sensitivity of this test is over 90% *(43)*.

Ultrasound or computed tomography may be required to differentiate between cystic or solid tumor in the neck and can also be used to perform lymph node aspiration cytology accurately.

If oral or oropharyngeal cancer is identified, evaluation of the larynx, hypopharynx, esophagus, and lungs should be performed to rule out multiple primary cancers. Yearly aerodigestive surveillance should be continued after satisfactory treatment of the index cancer.

INDICATIONS FOR CONSULTATION WITH SUBSPECIALIST

A nonhealing oral ulcer or any abnormal mucosal lesions particularly in the high-risk patients should be referred immediately to a subspecialist for smear cytology. Patients with persistent hoarseness for more than 15 d, progressive dysphagia, or odynophagia especially associated with loss of weight or loss of appetite for more than 1 mo in the older age group likewise should be referred to the appropriate subspecialist for further workup. Patients who are found to have a neck mass should have a thorough oral exam. These patients will need referral to a subspecialist if any suspicious looking area is found in the oral cavity. Mouth rinse using toluidine blue may be helpful in doubtful cases. Ultrasound or computed tomography guided biopsy of the neck mass is recommended for patients in whom no abnormality is seen on the oral exam.

SUMMARY

Oropharyngeal cancer is an ideal cancer for screening. It is a disease with known risk factors, an asymptomatic phase with identifiable clinical features, a simple inexpensive screening modality, and effective therapy for early cancer. Despite all these favorable factors, there is a significant delay in the diagnosis of these cancers with a marked reduction in the survival and quality of life because of extensive disfiguring facial surgery in advanced cases. The incidence and mortality rate for oral cancer is nearly double that of cervical cancer; still conducting a pelvic examination and Pap smear appears more acceptable than looking in the mouth. It is strongly recommended that physicians should include oral examination as an essential part of every physical examination.

REFERENCES

1. Hibbert J (ed). (1997) *Scott-Brown's Otolaryngology. Laryngology and Head and Neck Surgery.* 6th edition.
2. Lippman SM, Hong WK. (1992) Retinoid chemoprevention of upper aerodigestive tract carcinogenesis. In: Devita VT, Hellman S, Rosenberg SA, eds. *Important Advances in Oncology.* Philadelphia: Lippincott, pp. 93–109.
3. Vikram B. (1984) Changing patterns of failure in advanced head and neck cancer. *Arch Otolaryngol* 110:564.
4. Blot WJ, McLaughlin JK, Winn DM, et al. (1988) Smoking and drinking in relation to head and pharyngeal cancer. *Cancer Res* 48:3282.
5. Depue RH. (1986) Rising mortality from cancer of the tongue in young white males [letter]. *N Engl J Med* 315:647.
6. Devesa SS, Blot WJ, Stone BJ, et al. (1995) Recent cancer trends in the United States. *J Natl Cancer Inst* 87:175–182.

Chapter 8 / Screening for Oropharyngeal Cancer 137

7. Squier CA. (1984) Smokeless tobacco and oral cancer:A cause for concern? *CA Cancer J Clin* 34:242.

8. Boring CC, Squires TS, Tong T. (1993) Cancer statistics 1993. *CA Cancer J Clin* 43:7.

9. Wingo PA, Tong T, Bolden S. (1995) Cancer statistics 1995. *CA Cancer J Clin* 45:18–30.

10. Ries LAG, Miller GA, Hankey BF, Kosary CL, Harras A, Edward BK. (1994) *SEER Cancer Statistic Review 1973–1991. Tables and Graphs.* Washington, DC: National Institute of Health, p. 2798.

11. Stevens MH, Gardner JW, Parkin JL, et al. (1983) Head and neck cancer survival and lifestyle change. *Arch Otolaryngol* 109(11):746–749.

12. International Agency for Research on Cancer. (1987) Tobacco chewing and some related nitrosamines. In: *Monographs of Evaluation of Carcinogenic Risk of Chemicals to Humans.* Vol. 37. Lyon: IARC, pp. 141–200.

13. Nelson BS, Heischober B. (1999) Betel nut: a common drug used by naturalized citizens from India, Far East Asia, and the South Pacific Islands. *Ann Emerg Med* 34(2):238–243.

14. Hirayama T. (1966) An epidemiological study of oral and pharyngeal cancer in Central and South East Asia. *Bull WHO* 34:41–69.

15. Thomas SJ, MacLennan R. (1992) Slaked lime and betel nut cancer in Papua New Guinea. *Lancet* 340:577,578.

16. Ashby J, Styles JA, Boyland E. (1979) Betel nuts, arecaidine, and oral cancer [letter]. *Lancet* 1:112.

17. Wang F. (1997) Taiwan's love-hate relationship with betel nuts. *Taiwan News* 20:1,2.

18. Seedat HA, Van Wyk CW. (1988) Betel chewing and dietary habits of chewers without and with submucus fibrosis and with concomitant oral cancer. *S Afr Med J* 77(11):572–575.

19. Soufi HE, Kameswaran M, Malatani T. (1991) Khat and oral cancer. *J Laryngol Otol* 105(8):643–645.

20. Kabat GC, Wynder EL. (1989) Types of alcoholic beverage and oral cancer. *Int J Cancer* 43:190.

21. Prout MN, Sidari JN, Witzburg RA , Grillone GA, Vaughan CW. (1997) Head and neck cancer screening among 4611 tobacco users older than 40 years. *Otolaryngol Head Neck Surg* 116(2):201–208.

22. Cann CI, Fried MP, Rothman KJ. (1985) Epidemiology of squamous cell cancer of the head and neck. *Otolaryngol Clin N Am* 18:367.

23. Caplan GA, Brigham BA. (1990) Marijuana smoking and carcinoma of the tongue. Is there an association? *Cancer* 66:1005.

24. Donald PJ. (1986) Marijuana smoking—possible cause of head and neck carcinoma in young patients. *Otolaryngol Head Neck Surg* 94:517.

25. Henner WS, Williams JEM. (2000) Genetic polymorphism and individual variation in susceptibility to cancer of the oropharynx. Oregon Health Sciences University Grant No. 825282.

26. Mashberg A, Barsa P. (1984) Screening for oral and oropharengeal squamous carcinomas. *CA Cancer J Clin* 35(5):262–268.

27. Trieger N, Ship II, Taylor GW, Weisberger D. (1958) Cirrhosis and other predisposing factors in carcinoma of the tongue. *Cancer* 11:357.

28. Myer I, Abbey LM. (1970) The relationship of syphilis to primary carcinoma of the tongue. *Oral Surg* 30:678–681.

29. Wynder EL, Bross IJ, Felman R. (1957) A study of the etiological factors of cancer of the mouth. *Cancer* 10:1300–1323.

Part III / Screening for Gastrointestinal Cancers

30. Weaver A, Fleming SM, Smith DB, Park A. (1979) Mouthwash and oral cancer. Carcinogen or coincidence. *J Oral Surg* 37:50.
31. Shillitoe EJ, Greenspan D, Greenspan JS, Silverman S Jr. (1986) Five year survival of patients with oral cancer and its association with antibody 2 herpes simplex virus. *Cancer* 58:2256.
32. Shillitoe EJ, Hwang CB, Silverman S Jr., Greenspan JS. (1986) Examination of oral cancer tissue for the presence of proteins ICP4, ICP5, ICP6 and ICP8 of herpes simplex virus type 1. *J Natl Cancer Inst* 76:371.
33. De Villers EM, Weidauer H, Otto H, zur Hausen M. (1985) Papillomavirus. DNA in human tongue carcinomas. *Int J Cancer* 36:575.
34. Bhuvanesh S, Balwally AN, Shah AR, Rosenfeld RN, Har-El G, Lucente FE. (1996) Upper aero-digestive tract squamous cell carcinoma. The human immunodeficiency virus connections. *Arch Otolaryngol Head Neck Surg* 122:639–643.
35. Jain AB, Yee LD, Nalensic MA, et al. (1998) Comparative incidence of Denovo non-lymphoid malignancies after liver transplantation under tacrolimus using SEER data. *Transplantation* 15:66(9):1193.
36. Levine AM. (1994) Lymphoma complicating immunodeficiency disorders. *Ann Oncol* 5:29.
37. Belsky JL, Tachikawa C, Cihak RW, Yamamoto T. (1972) Salivary gland tumors in the atom bomb survivors. Hiroshima-Nagasaki 1957–1970. *JAMA* 219:864.
38. Spitz MR, Sider JG, Newell GR, Batsakis JG. (1988) Incidence of salivary gland cancer in the United States relative to ultravoilet radiation exposure. *Head Neck Surg* 10:305.
39. Henderson BE, Louie E, Soohoo JJ, Buell P, Gardner MB. (1977) Risk factors associated with nasopharyngeal carcinoma. *N Engl J Med* 295:1101.
40. Warnakulasuriya S, Pindborg JJ. (1990) Reliability of pre-cancer screening by primary health care workers in Sri Lanka. *Commun Dent Health* 7:73–79.
41. Mashberg A, Barsa P. (1995) Screening for oral and oropharengeal squamous carcinomas. *CA Cancer J Clin* 34:262–268.
42. Prout M. (1990) Follow up studies on head and neck screening. Unpublished.
43. Kline TS (ed). (1988) *Handbook of Fine Aspiration Biopsy Cytology*, 2nd edition. New York: Churchill Livingstone, pp. 6.

IV SCREENING FOR UROGENITAL CANCERS

9 Screening for Prostate Cancer

Peter C. Albertsen, MD

KEY PRINCIPLES

- The benefits of one-time or repeated screening with either a digital rectal examination and/or testing for prostate-specific antigen (PSA), followed by some form of aggressive therapy has not yet been proved.
- Both the digital rectal examination and serum PSA measurement have both false-positive and false-negative results.
- Testing for serum PSA will likely lead to additional invasive testing, including a transrectal ultrasound and biopsy.
- Treatment with radical prostatectomy, radiation therapy, brachytherapy, or some combination of these treatments is necessary to realize any benefit from the discovery of prostate cancer by screening tests.
- Aggressive treatments for prostate cancer are associated with several risks, including incontinence, bowel and bladder irritability, impotence, and a very small, but definite risk of early death.
- Early detection and treatment of prostate cancer may avert future cancer associated illness and death from prostate cancer.
- Men most likely to benefit from screening and treatment are men in their sixth and seventh decades as compared with men older than 70 yr of age.
- Routine screening for prostate cancer without a discussion of these issues is inappropriate.

EPIDEMIOLOGY

Incidence

Adenocarcinoma of the prostate is the most common nonskin cancer of American men. The American Cancer Society estimates that within

From: *Cancer Screening: A Practical Guide for Physicians*
Edited by: K. Aziz and G. Y. Wu © Humana Press Inc., Totowa, NJ

the United States 179,300 cases of prostate cancer were diagnosed in 1999 *(1)*. During the two decades spanning 1973–1992, the age-adjusted prostate cancer incidence rate for all men increased dramatically *(2)*. The rate increased linearly between 1973 and 1986, but accelerated between 1987 and 1992 following the introduction of testing with prostate-specific antigen (PSA). During the 5 yr preceding 1992, the age-adjusted incidence rate of prostate cancer increased 84% from 102.9 per 100,000 men to 189.4 per 100,000 men. The two largest increases were observed in 1990 and 1991.

Since 1992, there has been a precipitous drop in the number of new cases of prostate cancer, so that by 1995, the most current year for which accurate data are available, the incidence rates appear to be returning to rates present before the introduction of widespread testing for PSA (Fig. 1) *(3)*. The shapes of the incidence curves are similar for African-Americans and whites, although the peak incidence for African-Americans was 1 yr later than whites. The incidence of prostate cancer in African-Americans is twice that among whites.

Despite widespread screening efforts targeted at men age 50–65 yr, the age-adjusted incidence rates still suggest that prostate cancer is a disease of older men. For the two decades leading up to 1993, the age-adjusted incidence rates were highest for men age 75 yr and older, followed by the rate among men age 65–74 yr *(4)*. Since 1993, the age-adjusted rate has decreased sharply among men age 75 yr and older, so that the highest age-adjusted rate of prostate cancer now occurs among men age 65–74 yr. Prostate cancer is relatively uncommon among men under age 65 yr, but the annual age-adjusted rate among this group of men has more than tripled between 1989 and 1992. Since 1992, the rate has declined slightly.

For a good portion of the 1980s the mean age at diagnosis was approx 72 yr for whites and 70 yr for African-Americans *(4)*. Since the introduction of PSA testing, the mean age at diagnosis has fallen. As of 1994, the mean age at diagnosis among whites was 69 yr and among blacks it was 67 yr. These statistics suggest that prostate cancer in the late 1990s is now being diagnosed approx 2.5 yr earlier than a decade ago.

Since the introduction of widespread testing for PSA, the number of new cases of moderately differentiated disease has increased dramatically. Between 1974 and 1984, the number of incident cases of well, moderately, and poorly differentiated disease were roughly comparable. Between 1984 and 1989 the age-adjusted incidence of well-differentiated and poorly differentiated tumors increased slowly, while the age-adjusted incidence of moderately differentiated disease grew more

Chapter 9 / Screening for Prostate Cancer

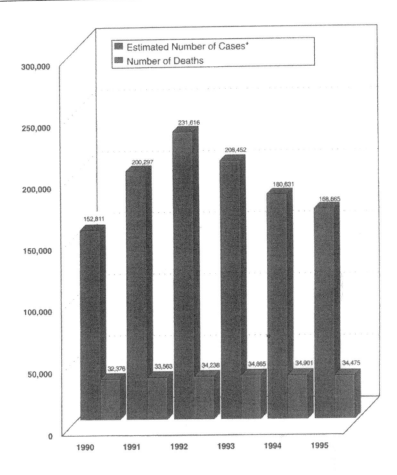

Fig. 1. Incidence of prostate cancer. Estimates obtained by multiplying the age-specific incidence rates for the 11 SEER registries by the U.S. population for each year. (From Stanford JL, Stephenson RA, Coyle LM, Cerhan J, Correa R, Eley JW, et al. [1999] *Prostate Cancer Trends 1973–1995, SEER Program*, Bethesda, MD: National Cancer Institute.)

rapidly. After 1989, there was a dramatic increase in the number of moderately differentiated tumors such that the number of these new cases was two to three times higher than the number of well-differentiated and poorly differentiated tumors. Since 1991, moderately differentiated tumors have represented over half of the newly diagnosed cases, whereas well-differentiated and poorly differentiated tumors account for approx 20% of new cases each.

Before 1986, the diagnosis of localized prostate cancer accounted for the majority of the increase in incident cases. Only modest increases were detected for regional and distant-stage cases. After this point, the stage-specific incidence rates began to increase exponentially for all stages, with the exception of distant-stage disease. From 1986 to 1991, the incidence of localized disease increased 75%, and the incidence of regional and unstaged disease rose 144 and 161%, respectively (2). Since 1991, the age-adjusted incident rates for distant disease have fallen dramatically, so that they are now approximately half the value they were at the start of the decade. Decreasing rates of distant disease most likely reflect the widespread use of PSA testing. Whereas the decreasing rates of distant disease are a significant indicator that testing for PSA identifies prostate cancer at an earlier stage, this decrease does not necessarily imply that prostate cancer mortality will fall also. Currently available mortality estimates have not demonstrated a convincing fall in prostate cancer deaths and, therefore, the efficacy of aggressive prostate cancer screening and treatment remains to be proven.

MORTALITY

The mortality rate from prostate cancer has also changed during the past two decades. In 1999, an estimated 37,000 men died from this disease (1). After increasing steadily from 1973 to1990, the mortality rate from prostate cancer fell by 6.3% during the period 1991–1995 (4). The rate for men under age 75 yr fell 7.4%, whereas the rate for men 75 yr and older, a group that accounts for two-thirds of all prostate cancer deaths, fell 3.8%. This is the first reported fall in the mortality rate from this cancer since the 1930s, when cancer statistics were first collected. Whether this decline in prostate cancer mortality can be attributed to early diagnosis and screening is the subject of much controversy and debate.

In absolute terms, 33,565 men died of prostate cancer in 1991 and 34,901 men died of prostate cancer in 1994 (4). When viewed in relative terms, however, the data suggest a different trend. Among white men, the age-adjusted mortality rate rose from 20.3 per 100,000 men in 1973 to 24.7 per 100,000 men in 1991. Rates among African-Americans were more than twice as high. Since then, rates have declined. The National Cancer Institute recently reported data showing that the prostate cancer death rate in the United States fell between 1991 and 1995. The overall decline was from 26.5 to 17.3 deaths per 100,000 men in the population (5). The percentage decline was greatest for young, white males and smallest for older men and African-American men (Fig. 2). The differences between the absolute and relative age-adjusted rates are explained by the increasing number of men dying from prostate cancer, but the even greater increase in the number of older men who are still alive in

Chapter 9 / Screening for Prostate Cancer

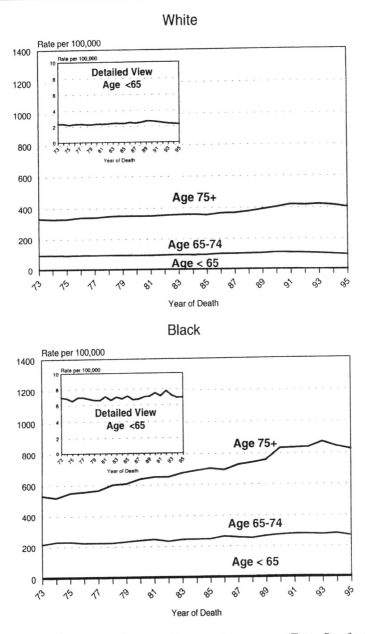

Fig. 2. Age-adjusted mortality rate from prostate cancer. (From Stanford JL, Stephenson RA, Coyle LM, Cerhan J, Correa R, Eley JW, et al. [1999] *Prostate Cancer Trends 1973–1995, SEER Program*, Bethesda, MD: National Cancer Institute.)

the US population. The greater increase in the size of the population at risk (the denominator) has been proportionally more rapid than the

146   Part IV / Screening for Urogenital Cancers

increase in the number of men dying from prostate cancer (the numerator). This has resulted in a recent, small age-adjusted decline during the past year.

THE BIOLOGY OF PROSTATE CANCER

Prostate cancer encompasses a wide spectrum of clinical outcomes. Some patients suffer a rapid progression of their disease, but others live with their disease for many years, ultimately succumbing to competing medical hazards. Because of the varying outcomes, physicians cannot easily determine whether the interventions they propose are likely to alter the natural course of this disease. Unlike some cancers where death is a virtual certainty in the absence of treatment, the natural history of prostate cancer is much more varied. Of several variables tested, tumor histology and tumor volume appear to be the best predictors of clinical outcome.

We recently reported long-term outcomes of a competing risk analysis of 767 men diagnosed between 1971 and 1984 who were managed expectantly for clinically localized prostate cancer (6). Our study design consisted of a case series analysis of patients identified through the Connecticut tumor registry who satisfied several criteria. First, we searched for men with long-term follow-up extending for 10–20 yr after diagnosis to capture the impact of prostate cancer and competing medical hazards. Second, we looked for men age 55–74 yr at diagnosis to identify a group of men who had an average life expectancy of more than 10 yr. Third, we recovered the original histology slides of these patients to permit reanalysis using contemporary Gleason grading standards. Finally, we assembled a patient cohort sufficiently large to permit stratification by the biospy. Gleason score and age at diagnosis are factors known to be important determinants of outcome.

The results of our study are presented in Fig. 3. Few men (4–7%) with Gleason 2 to 4 tumors identified by prostate biopsy had progression leading to death from prostate cancer within 15 yr of diagnosis. A majority of the younger men are still alive, but they face the possibility of death from prostate cancer in the future. In contrast, most of the older men with Gleason 2 to 4 tumors identified by biopsy at diagnosis have died from competing medical hazards rather than prostate cancer.

Compared with men with well-differentiated tumors, men with Gleason 5 and 6 tumors identified by prostate biopsy experienced a somewhat higher risk of death from prostate cancer when managed expectantly (6–11% and 18–30%, respectively). Of the younger men with Gleason 5 and 6 tumors, more than half are still alive after 15 yr,

Chapter 9 / Screening for Prostate Cancer 147

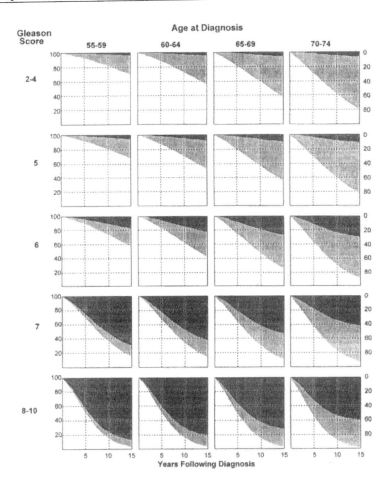

Fig. 3. Survival (white lower band) and cumulative mortality from prostate cancer (dark gray upper band) and other causes (light gray middle band) up to 15 yr after diagnosis stratified by age at diagnosis and Gleason score. The percentage of men alive can be read from the left-hand scale and the percentage of men who have died from prostate cancer or from other causes during this interval can be read from the right-hand scale. (From ref. 6 with permission.)

whereas a majority of the older men have died from competing medical hazards.

Men with Gleason scores 7 and 8–10 tumors identified by prostate biopsy experienced a very high rate of death from prostate cancer regardless of their age at diagnosis (42–70% and 60–87%, respectively). Very few of these men of any age are still alive. Most have died from prostate cancer, except for approximately one-third of the oldest men, who died from competing medical hazards.

148   Part IV / Screening for Urogenital Cancers

The volume of prostate cancer at the time of diagnosis is the other key variable that consistently predicts long-term clinical outcomes. Prior to the advent of testing for PSA, clinicians relied on the digital rectal examination and imaging studies such as the bone scan and computerized tomography to assess the extent of disease. The advent of testing for PSA has enabled clinicians to identify disease much earlier than previously imagined.

McNeal and colleagues have demonstrated that tumors less than 0.5 cm^3 frequently occur in older men, but rarely extend beyond the confines of the prostate. Tumors greater than 3.0 cm^3 often demonstrate seminal vesicle invasion and loss of normal histology features. Tumors that are 6.0 cm^3 or larger are rarely curable, even with aggressive management. In a large autopsy series, McNeal and colleagues showed that tumors containing poorly differentiated histology features, specifically patterns 4 and/or 5, often grow to sufficient size to metastasize *(7)*.

Stamey et al. have shown that many prostate cancers grow at a very slow rate *(8)*. Half of all prostate cancers take more than 5 yr to double in size, as compared with breast cancers, which can double in size every 3 mo. Most men over age 50 yr with prostate cancers smaller than 0.5 cm^3 at the time of diagnosis will not live long enough for their cancers to achieve sufficient size to metastasize. Most clinicians now utilize that standard sextant biopsy technique to evaluate men who are suspected of having prostate cancer. Stamey et al. have determined that patients with one or more cores containing more than 3 mm of tumor are likely to have a prostate volume greater than 0.5 cm^3 *(9)*.

Although serum PSA levels are not sufficiently reliable to predict tumor burden for individual patients, serum PSA levels do correlate with tumor volume when evaluating large groups of men. In a classic analysis of over 10,000 men age 50 yr and older participating in a screening program for prostate cancer, Catalona et al. reported that only 45% of men with a PSA score greater than 10 ng/mL had disease localized to the prostate *(10)*. Recently, Partin et al. combined information provided by serum PSA level, Gleason score, and clinical stage to generate a series of normograms to predict local tumor extension and capsular penetration *(11)*.

RATIONALE FOR SCREENINIG

Screening for prostate cancer is controversial. The controversy stems in part from the different perspectives of health care policy analysts, practicing clinicians, patients, health care insurers, and government agencies. Those who advocate screening emphasize the significant

Chapter 9 / Screening for Prostate Cancer

morbidity and mortality associated with prostate cancer. They believe that the current level of experimental evidence supports the concept that aggressive intervention dramatically improves survival among men diagnosed with early-stage disease compared with a more conservative approach, which deals with the clinical manifestations of the natural progression of this disease *(12,13)*. Those who oppose prostate cancer screening emphasize the lack of experimental evidence supporting the theory that early detection and treatment of this disease substantially lowers cause-specific mortality. They point to the significant morbidity associated with current treatment efforts and conclude that screening is unethical because there is a high probability that screening may cause more harm than good *(14,15)*.

Physicians screen for prostate cancer with the purpose of identifying and curing those cancers that result in significant patient morbidity and mortality. No one advocates screening for indolent disease. To establish the validity of a screening program, however, screening advocates must satisfy five criteria *(16)*. First, the disease in question must represent a substantial public health burden. The large number of incident cases and deaths from prostate cancer each year indicate that this is so. Public health officials, however, are also quick to point out that prostate cancer is responsible for significantly less excess mortality when compared to other diseases such as heart disease or even other cancers such as lung cancer or breast cancer. Therefore, even if prostate cancer screening demonstrates that it can save lives, advocates would still need to compete with other disease advocates for limited health care dollars.

Second, to be effective, screening programs must identify disease in an asymptomatic, localized phase. Research suggests that digital rectal examinations frequently identify cancer only after it has extended beyond the prostate capsule *(17)*. The advent of testing for PSA, however, has permitted much earlier detection of this disease. Potosky et al. have demonstrated that the rising incidence of prostate cancer reported during the past decade is a direct result of increased detection with transurethral resection and, more recently, a result of the increased use of PSA testing *(2)*. However, the ability to diagnose localized prostate cancer raises other concerns. Specifically, how many incidental, nonfatal cancers are identified by a screening program versus how many potentially fatal cancers are missed?

Third, a good screening test must have reasonable values for sensitivity and specificity. These concepts will be reviewed in the next section. It is important to remember, however, that screening test characteristics depend not only on the screening test but also on the population of patients being tested. As men age, the prior probability of prostate cancer increases, but the percentage of patients who have localized prostate cancer decreases. The confounding effect of benign prostate hypertrophy also leads to decreased test performance characteristics in older men. Richie et al. demonstrated these effects in a report concerning a large screening program using digital rectal examination and PSA *(18)*.

Fourth, to be a candidate for a screening program, the potential of curing the disease in question must be significantly greater in the early stages than in more advanced stages. In the case of clinical prostate cancer, this criterion is often assumed to be true because the 10-yr cause-specific survival of men with localized disease is much higher than the relative survival of men with regional extension or distant metastases. Unfortunately, the contribution of aggressive therapy to improved survival is unknown. The lack of control groups in case series analyses raises the question of whether patients treated with endocrine manipulation alone, without surgery or radiation, may do just as well. Without knowing the relative efficacy of radical prostatectomy, radiation therapy, brachytherapy, or hormonal manipulation in isolation, it is impossible to assess the relative contribution of each to a patient's longevity. Similar assumptions concerning the diagnosis and management of breast cancer were eventually proven to be false *(19)*.

The fifth and most important criterion to validate a screening program requires that screen-detected patients experience an improved outcome compared with those patients who have not been screened. Evidence to support this criterion should ideally come from randomized trials. Any other study design risks the potential for selection bias, lead-time bias, and length-time bias. Any or all three of these biases can confound data from case series analyses and lead to erroneous conclusions *(20)*. As a result of these biases, Sackett et al. have commented that "early diagnosis will always appear to improve survival, even when therapy is worthless"*(21)*. To address this issue, two large trials are currently being conducted in the United States and in Europe to determine whether screening for prostate cancer using serum prostate-specific antigen will lower the death rate from prostate cancer.

METHODS FOR SCREENING PROSTATE CANCER

Digital Rectal Examination

Despite a lack of evidence from controlled studies that the digital rectal examination reduces disease-specific mortality, physicians have relied on this examination for the past century *(22,23)*. To perform a digital rectal examination, a physician should ask a patient to bend at the

Chapter 9 / Screening for Prostate Cancer

waist or climb on the examination table in a knee–chest position. The physician then inserts a gloved finger inside the rectum and palpates the posterior aspect of the prostate gland. This can also be performed with the patient in a lateral decubitus position, but this makes the examination more difficult. The gland should be symmetric in size, should not be fixed to the pelvic side wall, and should have a consistency similar to the thenar eminence of a contracted thumb. If the gland is of average size, the physician should be able to feel the entire posterior aspect of the prostate. The seminal vesicles can be palpated in men with relatively small glands, whereas only the apical portion is palpable in men with relatively large glands. Although occasionally uncomfortable, the test itself is not associated with any significant risks and requires little time to perform. Because a digital rectal examination is usually included as part of a standard physical examination, this screening test rarely incurs any additional financial cost.

In relatively unselected groups of men over age 50 yr, between 7 and 15% will have suspicious results on digital rectal examination. Abnormalities that can be palpated include areas of induration, marked asymmetry, and a discrete nodule within the prostate. Unfortunately, interpreter reliability for this test is modest even when performed by experienced urologists (24,25). The true sensitivity and specificity of the digital rectal examination remains unknown because previous studies have not systematically biopsied all men with prostate glands that were normal on palpation or used long-term observation of all men who were screened with this examination. Data from community-based studies suggest that the positive predictive value of digital rectal examination for prostate cancer is 15–30% and varies little with the age of the patient (26). Digital rectal examination appears to have a cancer detection rate of approx 1–2% when used as a solitary screening tool in men who are older than 50 yr of age. When an abnormality of the prostate is detected on rectal examination, the probability of finding a clinically significant prostate cancer on biopsy doubles and the probability of finding a tumor with extracapsular extension increases three- to ninefold. Unfortunately, a normal digital rectal examination does not exclude the possibility of prostate cancer primarily because the test lacks sensitivity.

Serum Prostate-Specific Antigen

Since the late 1980s, physicians have shown a growing enthusiasm for testing for PSA as a method of screening for prostate cancer. This enthusiasm is based on the observation that serum PSA levels are elevated in virtually all men with clinically apparent prostate cancer.

Unfortunately, PSA is not specific to prostate cancer but can also reflect other prostate conditions such as benign prostate hypertrophy and prostatitis.

Prostate-specific antigen is a protease secreted almost exclusively by prostatic epithelial cells. The prostate lumen contains the highest concentrations of PSA in the body. Several barriers, including the prostate basement membrane, the intervening stroma, the capillary basement membrane, and the capillary endothelial cell, prevent PSA from entering the bloodstream. Blood levels of PSA are increased when this normal glandular structure is disrupted. PSA circulates in the body in several molecular forms. In the ejaculate, PSA exists in a free form. In the bloodstream, however, PSA is conjugated to a number of protease inhibitors.

α-1 Anti-chymotrypsin and α-2 macroglobulin are the most prevalent PSA complexes present in the serum. When PSA is bound with α-1 anti-chymotrypsin, immunoassays can detect the two epitopes that remain unmasked. In contrast, when PSA is bound with α-2 macroglobulin, all the epitopes are masked and, therefore, PSA cannot be measured by currently available immunoassays. These findings are important because the free form of PSA exists in a lower proportion in those men with prostate cancer than in those men without prostate cancer.

Serum PSA can be measured by several commonly available assays. Levels greater than 4.0 ng/mL are usually considered abnormal for most of these assays. Whereas an elevated PSA level can indicate the presence of prostate cancer, other conditions can also produce an abnormal result. Benign prostate hypertrophy, a condition common in older men, can often lead to modest elevations of serum PSA. Acute prostatitis can lead to even higher levels that can remain elevated for several weeks. Other causes of elevated serum PSA levels include transrectal biopsy and prostate surgery. Digital rectal examination will not cause a significant elevation in PSA. Age-specific and race-specific thresholds for abnormal PSA values have been proposed, but these standards have not achieved wide acceptance *(27,28)*.

Because prostate biopsies are rarely performed on men with normal serum PSA values, the true sensitivity and specificity of testing for serum PSA remain unknown. The test has a reported sensitivity of up to 80% in detecting prostate cancer in screened men, but it lacks specificity *(29)*. False-positive results frequently occur among men with benign prostate hypertrophy or prostatitis. Approximately 25–46% of men with benign prostate hypertrophy have elevated PSA values *(30)*. PSA values may also fluctuate by as much as 30% for physiologic reasons. The

Chapter 9 / Screening for Prostate Cancer

positive predictive value of PSA in screening studies ranges from 28 to 35% *(31,32)*. This means that approximately one-third of men with an elevated PSA will be found to have prostate cancer and two-thirds will not. Participants in these studies were either patients seen in urology clinics or community volunteers, raising the concern that the positive predictive value may be lower when screening occurs in primary care settings.

An abnormal PSA is seen in about 15% of men who are older than 50 yr of age, but this proportion increases substantially as men age. Serum PSA levels between 4 and 10 ng/mL increase the odds of having clinically significant prostate cancer from 1.5- to threefold and the odds of extracapsular extension increase three- to fivefold *(33)*. Although PSA levels higher than 10 ng/mL may still reflect benign prostate hyperplasia, the odds of finding prostate cancer with extracapsular extension are increased 20-fold. For most cases of prostate cancer, men who have PSA levels greater than 10 ng/mL have a high probability of having extracapsular extension and, therefore, are much less likely to be cured using aggressive surgical or radiation techniques.

In an effort to improve the sensitivity and specificity of screening for prostate cancer using PSA, several researchers have proposed measuring serum PSA in its free and conjugated forms. Catalona et al. recently conducted a multicenter trial that evaluated men with total serum PSA levels between 4.0 and 10.0 ng/mL and negative digital rectal examinations *(34)*. Of 773 men who were evaluated, 379 (49%) were ultimately found to have prostate cancer. As expected, the total PSA was significantly higher in the men with cancer, whereas the ratio of free/total was higher in those men with negative biopsies (Tables 1 and 2). Unfortunately, when the cutoff values for the ratio of free/total PSA are set at a level to yield a sensitivity of 90–95%, the specificity of this assay is only approx 20–30% *(35)*. Furthermore, results from different assay manufacturers yield significant variations in serum level determinations. Accordingly, measuring conjugated serum PSA has yet to gain wide acceptance.

DIAGNOSTIC ALGORITHM

As a result of the controversy surrounding the use of serum PSA testing as a screening test for prostate cancer, the American College of Physicians has made the following recommendation concerning how this test should be utilized in medical practice. They suggest that "rather than screening all men for prostate cancer as a matter of routine, physicians should describe the potential benefits and known harms of screen-

Table 1
Probability of Detecting Prostate Cancer Using Serum PSA

Serum PSA (ng/mL)	Probability of cancer
<2	1%
2–4	15%
4–10	25%
>10	>50%

Table 2
Probability of Detecting Prostate Cancer Using Percent Free PSA if a Patient's Serum PSA is Between 4–10 ng/mL

Percent free PSA	Probability of cancer
0–10%	56%
10–15%	28%
15–20%	20%
20–25%	16%
>25%	8%

ing, diagnosis and treatment; listen to the patient's concerns; and then individualize the decision to screen" *(33)*. Men at high risk for developing prostate cancer are those men over the age of 50 yr and men age 40 yr and older who have at least one first-degree relative diagnosed with prostate cancer. African-American men also appear to have a higher risk of developing prostate cancer and, therefore, may choose to start screening at age 40 yr.

After discussing the risks and benefits of screening, physicians usually recommend both a digital rectal examination and a serum PSA level. (*See* Algorithm 1.) If either of these tests is positive, urologists usually recommend a transrectal ultrasound accompanied by a transrectal biopsy. A PSA level 4.0 ng/mL or greater is usually considered abnormal and will often prompt a recommendation for transrectal ultrasound and biopsy. Men in their sixth decade may consider undergoing a biopsy if their serum PSA value is over 3.0 ng/mL, whereas men in their eighth decade may consider delaying a biopsy until their PSA is greater than 5.0 ng/mL. These recommendations reflect the fact that as men age, they often develop benign prostate hypertrophy. Men taking finasteride, an oral 5 α-reductase inhibitor, should be aware that this

Chapter 9 / Screening for Prostate Cancer

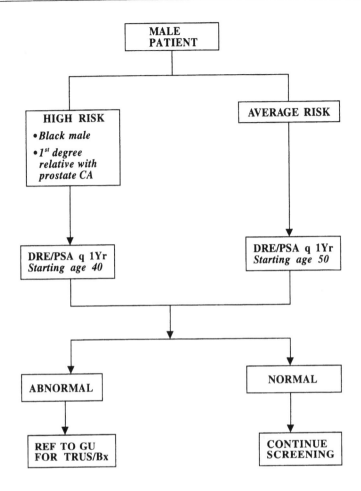

Algorithm 1. Diagnostic algorithm.

drug lowers the serum PSA level. To correct for this, men should double the measured serum PSA level before deciding whether the value is normal or abnormal for them. Men with minimally elevated values may wish to repeat serum PSA testing after 3–6 mo to determine whether an elevated value persists. Men who undergo transrectal ultrasound and prostate biopsy usually have six cores of tissue sampled. If any of these cores demonstrates prostate cancer, the patient will be counseled concerning appropriate treatment alternatives. Those men who do not show any evidence of prostate cancer are usually advised to undergo additional annual testing to determine whether their PSA levels are rising or remain stable. Men with rising PSA levels are more likely to harbor clinically significant prostate cancer.

COST-EFFECTIVENESS

Several researchers have published decision models designed to analyze the costs of prostate cancer screening and treatment. These models have yielded different results because there is no consensus concerning the natural progression of disease and the efficacy of treatment.

Krahn et al. developed a sophisticated decision-analytic cost–utility model comparing four screening strategies against a strategy of not screening *(35)*. They explored several combinations of digital rectal examination, transrectal ultrasound, and serum PSA testing in a single episode of screening. They did not consider a series of annual or repeated screens. The authors were primarily interested in addressing two questions:

1. Given the available evidence, what is the net clinical benefit and the economic burden of screening for prostate cancer?
2. Are there identifiable subgroups that might achieve a greater benefit from screening? In their model, they assumed that all localized cancers would be treated with radical prostatectomy. For the outcome of their model, they calculated life expectancy, quality-adjusted life expectancy, and cost–utility ratios for unselected and high-prevalence populations.

Their model provides several insights concerning the cost effectiveness of screening for prostate cancer. First, in unselected men between the ages of 50 and 70 yr, screening with PSA and digital rectal examination prolonged unadjusted life expectancy. Men age 50 were estimated to achieve, on average, a net benefit of 0.6 d; for men age 60, it was 1.1 d, and for men age 70, it was 1.7 d. Unfortunately, when the morbidity of radical prostatectomy was considered, the net benefit from a population perspective showed a diminished quality-adjusted life expectancy. Second, they found that screening with digital rectal examination alone yielded no reduction in mortality at any age. Third, high-prevalence populations achieve the same results, increased life expectancy, but losses in quality-adjusted life expectancy. Fourth, all screening protocols increased costs dramatically. Their results were sensitive only to assumptions concerning the efficacy of radical prostatectomy in curing prostate cancer.

Responding to criticisms of the Krahn model and an earlier decision-analytic model published by Fleming et al., Barry and colleagues developed an extensive cost-effectiveness analysis of PSA screening *(36–40)*. When constructing their model, they made several assumptions that were favorable to screening protocols. First, they assumed that all cancers confined to the prostate are cured by radical prostatectomy regardless of tumor grade. Second, they assumed that prognosis is driven entirely by tumor grade and not by the extent of capsular penetration.

Chapter 9 / Screening for Prostate Cancer 157

Third, they used relatively high rates of grade-specific metastatic and cancer-specific death rates. Finally, they assumed a high prevalence of cancers in the screened population. Based on these assumptions, they calculated that men age 65 yr achieve, on average, a net benefit of 16 d, undiscounted and without a quality of life adjustment. This decreased to 10 d by age 70 and to 6 d by age 75. They also calculated that a Medicare benefit for a screening program based on serum PSA would cost over $2 billion during the first year alone.

Hanley and McGregor analyzed prostate cancer screening for the health ministry of the Province of Quebec, Canada *(41)*. Because no randomized controlled trials of screening or treatment have been completed, they assessed the efficacy of screening by comparing the case fatality rates for patients undergoing radical prostatectomy against patients not undergoing screening or surgery. Two population-based studies suggest that the prostate cancer fatality rate among men up to 85 yr old who do not undergo operations for screen-detected prostate cancer is approx 22%. Two substantial surgical series suggest that the prostate cancer fatality rate for patients undergoing surgery is approx 15%. They conclude that in a population subjected to regular screening, the number of cancer deaths averted for every 100 operations would be the difference between these two case fatality rates. A sensitivity analysis suggests that this value may by as low as 1% and as high as 9%. Using current estimates of the efficacy of radical prostatectomy, Hanley and McGregor project that for every 100 men with screen-detected prostate cancer, on average one and, at the extreme, nine cancer deaths are averted. The remaining 91–99 operations would result in no benefit to the patient.

Concerning the costs associated with such a program, Hanley and McGregor conclude that the costs of screening and treatment would be approx $214,000 (Canadian) per year of life saved. This is substantially higher than the $40,000 to $50,000 per life-year associated with the end-stage renal disease program, a common benchmark for cost-effectiveness ratios.

CONTROVERSY REGARDING PROSTATE CANCER SCREENING

Unfortunately, definitive evidence of whether screening for prostate cancer with either a digital rectal examination or testing for serum prostate-specific antigen improves health is currently unavailable. Several trials in progress are scheduled for completion early in the next decade. For now, controversy centers on an appropriate policy in the interim.

158 Part IV / Screening for Urogenital Cancers

Although scientific evidence for this is lacking, proponents of screening argue that universal screening has the potential to save lives. They believe that the potential benefits of screening outweigh the risks and that waiting for better evidence will result in unnecessary deaths from prostate cancer. Critics argue that before embarking on an ambitious screening program, the benefits of screening must be proven. Furthermore, to expose men to the significant known risks of complications that are associated with screening and treatment of this disease before the benefits of treatment are demonstrated is inappropriate.

Randomized trials provide the best methodology for determining the efficacy of screening and treatment. After reviewing data from case series analyses, clinicians are often too quick to credit medical intervention for successful outcomes and blame tumor biology for disease progression. Furthermore, when faced with a decision of administering or withholding therapy, physicians generally wish to err on the side of having done everything possible.

These uncertainties must be acknowledged when physicians counsel patients. Physicians should neither recommend nor discourage screening for prostate cancer without ensuring that patients have complete information regarding the risks and benefits of screening and treatment. Physicians should also attempt to understand their patient's personal preferences. Once informed about the uncertainties surrounding prostate cancer screening, some patients find it difficult to make their decision and prefer instead to seek their doctor's advice. Offering an opinion in response to a patient's request is appropriate, but the response should consider the individual patient's risk of developing clinically significant disease. Physicians who uniformly either encourage or discourage PSA testing do not serve their patient's best interests. As with much of clinical medicine, the interpretation of the information concerning prostate cancer screening that is available in brochures or videotapes must be tailored to the individual patient. This interpretation is probably best done in the context of an ongoing relationship with a primary care provider or a urologist.

REFERENCES

1. Landis SH, Murray T, Bolden S, Wingo PA. (1999) Cancer statistics, 1999. *CA Cancer J Clin* 49:9–31.
2. Potosky AL, Miller BA, Albertsen PC, Kramer BS. (1995) The role of increasing detection in the rising incidence of prostate cancer. *JAMA* 273:548–552.
3. Wingo PA, Landis S, Ries LAG. (1997) An adjustment to the 1997 estimate for new prostate cancer cases. *CA Cancer J Clin* 47:239–242.
4. Ries LAG, Kosary CL, Hankey BF, Miller BA, Clegg L, Edwards BK, (eds). (1998) *SEER Cancer Statistics Review, 1973-1995.* Bethesda, MD: National Cancer Institute.

Chapter 9 / Screening for Prostate Cancer

5. Mettlin CJ, Murphy GP. (1998) Why is the prostate cancer death rate declining in the United States? *Cancer* 82:249–251.
6. Albertsen PC, Hanley JA, Gleason DF, Barry MJ. (1998) Competing risk analysis of men aged 55 to 74 years at diagnosis managed conservatively for clinically localized prostate cancer. *JAMA* 280:975–980.
7. McNeal JE, Bostwick DG, Kindrachuk RA, et al. (1986) Patterns of progression in prostate cancer. *Lancet* 1(8472):60–63.
8. Stamey TA, Yang N, Hay AR, et al. (1987) Prostate specific antigen as a serum marker for adeno-carcinoma of the prostate. *N Eng J Med* 317:909–916.
9. Stamey TA, Freiha FS, McNeal JE, et al. (1993) Localized prostate cancer. Relationship of tumor volume to clinical significance for treatment of prostate cancer. *Cancer* 71:933–938.
10. Catalona WJ, Smith DS, Ratliff TL, Basler WJ. (1993) Detection of organ-confined prostate cancer is increased through prostate-specific antigen based testing. *JAMA* 270:948–954.
11. Partin AW, Kattan MW, Subong EN, et al. (1997) Combination of prostate-specific antigen, clinical stage, and Gleason score to predict pathological stage of localized prostate cancer. A multi-institutional update. *JAMA* 277:1445–1451.
12. Catalona WJ. (1993) Screening for prostate cancer: Enthusiasm [editorial]. *Urology* 42:113–115.
13. Walsh PC. (1994) Prostate cancer kills: strategy to reduce deaths. *Urology* 44:463–466.
14. Kramer BS, Brown ML, Prorok PC, Potosky Al, Gohagan JK. (1993) Prostate cancer screening: what we know and what we need to know. *Ann Intern Med* 119:914–923.
15. Chodak GW. (1993) Questioning the value of screening for prostate cancer in asymptomatic men. *Urology* 42:116–118.
16. Hulka BS. (1998) Cancer screening. Degrees of proof and practical application. *Cancer* 62:1776–1780.
17. Thompson IM, Rounder JB, Teague JL, Peek M, Spence CR. (1987) Impact of routine screening for adenocarcinoma of the prostate on stage distribution. *J Urol* 137:424–426.
18. Richie JP, Catalona WJ, Ahmann FR, et al. (1993) Effect of patient age on early detection of prostate cancer with serum prostate-specific antigen and digital rectal examination. *Urology* 42:365–374.
19. Adair F, Berg J, Joubert L, Robbins GF. (1974) Long term follow-up of breast cancer patients. The 30 year report. *Cancer* 33:1145–1150.
20. Morrison AS. (1991) Intermediate determinants of mortality in the evaluation of screening. *Int J Epidemiol* 20:642–650.
21. Sackett DL, Hayens RB, Guyatt GH, Tugwell P. (1991) *Clinical Epidemiology: A Basic Science for Clinical Medicine*. Boston: Little, Brown.
22. Gerber GS, Thompson IM, Thisted R, Chodak GW. (1993) Disease-specific survival following routine prostate cancer screening by digital rectal examination. *JAMA* 269:61–64.
23. Friedman GD, Hiatt RA, Quesenberry CP, Selby JV. (1991) Case-control study of screening for prostatic cancer by digital rectal examinations. *Lancet* 337:1526–529.
24. Smith DS, Catalona WJ. (1995) Interexaminare variability of digital rectal examination for early detection of prostate cancer. *Urology* 45:70–74.
25. Varenhorst E, Berglund K, Lofman O, Pedersen K. (1993) Inter-observer variation in assessment of the prostate by digital rectal examination. *Br J Urol* 72:173–176.
26. Pederson KV, Carlsson P, Varenhorst E, Lofman O, Berglund K. (1990) Screening for carcinoma of the prostate by digital rectal examination in a randomly selected population. *Br Med J* 300:1041–1044.

160   **Part IV / Screening for Urogenital Cancers**

27. Oesterling JE, Jacobsen SJ, Cooner WH. (1995) The use of age-specific reference ranges for serum prostate specific antigen in men 60 years old or older. *J Urol* 153:1160–1163.
28. Catalona WJ, Hudson MA, Scardino PT, et al. (1994) Selection of optional prostate specific antigen cutoffs for early detection of prostate cancer: receiver operating characteristic curves. *J Urol* 52:2037–2042.
29. Brawer MK. (1999) Prostate-specific antigen:Current status. *CA Cancer J Clin* 49:264–281.
30. Oesterling JE. (1991) Prostate specific antigen: a critical assessment of the most useful tumor marker for adenocarcinoma of the prostate. *J Urol* 145:907–923.
31. Catalona WJ, Smith DS, Ratliff TL, et al. (1991) Measurement of prostate-specific antigen in serum as a screening test for prostate cancer. *N Eng J Med* 324:1156–1161.
32. Garnick MB. (1993) Prostate cancer: screeing, diagnosis, and management. *Ann Intern Med* 118:804–818.
33. Coley CM, Barry MJ, Mulley AG. (1997) Screening for prostate cancer. *Ann Intern Med* 126:480–484.
34. Catalona WJ, Partin AW, Slawin KM, et al. (1998) Use of the percentage of free prostate-specific antigen to enhance differentiation of prostate cancer from benign prostatic disease: a prospective multicenter clinical trial. *JAMA* 279:1542–1547.
35. Krahn MD, Mahoney JE, Eckman MH, et al. (1994) Screening for prostate cancer: a decision analytic view. *JAMA* 272:773–780.
36. Fleming C, Wasson JH, Albertsen PC, Barry MJ, Wennberg JE. (1993) A decision analysis of alternative treatment strategies for clinically localized prostate cancer. *JAMA* 269:2650–2658.
37. Barry MJ, Fleming C, Coley CM, et al. (1995) Should Medicare provide reimbursement for prostate-specific antigen testing for early detection of prostate cancer? Part I: Framing the debate. *Urology* 4:2–13.
38. Coley CM, Barry MJ, Fleming C, et al. (1995) Should Medicare provide reimbursement for prostate-specific antigen testing for early detection of prostate cancer? Part II: Early detection strategies. *Urology* 46:125–141.
39. Barry MJ, Fleming C, Coley CM, et al. (1995) Should Medicare provide reimbursement for prostate-specific antigen testing for early detection of prostate cancer? Part III: Management strategies and outcomes. *Urology* 46:277–289.
40. Barry MJ, Fleming C, Coley CM, et al. (1995) Should Medicare provide reimbursement for prostate-specific antigen testing for early detection of prostate cancer? Part IV: Estimating the risks and benefits of an early detection program. *Urology* 46:445–461.
41. Hanley JA, McGregor M. (1995) *Screening for Cancer of the Prostate: An Evaluation of Benefits, Unwanted Health Effects and Costs.* Montreal: CETS.

10 Screening for Testicular Cancer

*Charles G. Petrunin, MD
and Craig R. Nichols, MD*

KEY PRINCIPLES

- Although a relatively uncommon malignancy, testicular cancer represents the most common cancer in adolescent males.
- Testicular cancer is one of the most curable cancers.
- Several risk factors for the development of testicular cancer have been identified; these include cryptorchidism, past history of unilateral testicular malignancy, and history of testicular cancer in first-degree relatives.
- Screening for the testicular cancer is controversial; patients should be informed about the risks and counseled about the option for screening.

INTRODUCTION

Testicular cancer is a rare malignancy (just over 1% of all malignancies in males), yet it represents the most common malignancy in men from the ages of 25 to 35 yr. Testicular cancer is an intriguing disease because of the historical significance associated with it. Thirty years ago when testicular cancer was diagnosed at an advanced stage, it was almost always fatal *(1)*. With the advent of cisplatin and the development of its therapeutic niche, testicular cancer has not only become a chemotherapeutic success, but it has also become a standard that subsequent trials have tried to achieve *(2)*. Because of effective therapy, early-stage disease is treated with exceptional overall survival. Aggressive therapy for advanced disease, although successful, carries more risk of delayed toxicity; thus, testicular cancer is a malignancy for which effective screening can have a significant impact.

From: *Cancer Screening: A Practical Guide for Physicians*
Edited by: K. Aziz and G. Y. Wu © Humana Press Inc., Totowa, NJ

EPIDEMIOLOGY

The American Cancer Society reported 7400 new cases of testicular cancer in 1999, with approx 300 expected deaths *(3)*. Testicular cancer, of which 95% are germ-cell tumors, is the most common malignancy in males in the second and third decades of life. The incidence declines steadily after age 40. The disease is remarkably more common in the Caucasian population as compared to Africans, Hispanics, and Asians *(4)*. The age-adjusted incidence of germ-cell tumors over the last 40 yr has nearly doubled in Scandinavia, the United Kingdom, Canada, and the United States *(5)*. The reason for this increase is not yet well understood. There are three discrete peaks of incidence according to age: infancy, age 25–35, and over age 50. Each peak corresponds to a specific tumor-cell type: Embryonal carcinoma and teratoma predominates in infants; seminoma, embryonal cell carcinoma, teratoma, and teratocarcinoma occur primarily in young adults; and spermatocytic seminoma or lymphoma present mainly in older adults.

RISK FACTORS

The major predisposing risk factor for the development of testicular cancer is cryptorchidism. In men with a history of cryptorchidism, 80–85% of testicular cancers occur in the cryptorchid testicle and 15–20% occur in the contralateral testicle *(6)*. The risk of cryptorchid-associated tumor is highest when the retained testis is within the abdomen versus the inguinal canal and if the corrective orchidopexy is performed after the age of 6 *(7)*. A previous history of unilateral testicular cancer is also an important factor and nearly 3% of patients with a history of unilateral testicular cancer will develop malignancy in the contralateral testis *(8)*.

Other risk factors include sedentary lifestyle with a probably higher than average scrotal heat, obesity, and excess estrogen exposure in the uterus *(9–11)*. There is a two times greater risk of developing in a son whose father has testicular cancer and an even higher risk for brothers of cancer victims, suggesting maternal and *in utero* factors *(12)*. Increased incidence of testicular cancer has been reported in Klinefelter's and Down's syndrome *(13,14)*. Testicular cancer is reported to be more common in immunosuppressed individuals (human immunodeficiency virus [HIV] or chemically induced) supporting the immune system surveillance in the hypothesis in the development of cancer *(15)*.

CLASSIFICATION AND BIOLOGY OF TESTICULAR TUMOR

Ninety-five percent of testicular cancers are of germ-cell origin, of which seminoma is the most common type. Prognosis and treatment

Chapter 10 / Screening for Testicular Cancer   163

Table 1

Classification of Testicular Tumors

Germ-cell tumors	Nongerm-cell tumors
Seminomatous germ-cell tumors	Stromal tumors
Seminoma	Leydig (interstitial) cell tumors
Typical	Sertoli cell tumors
Anaplastic	Granulosa-theca cell tumors
	Gonadoblastoma
Nonseminomatous germ-cell tumors	Adenexal/paratesticular tumors
Embryonal cell carcinoma	Mesothelioma
Teratoma	Sarcoma
Mature, immature, containing	Adenocarcinoma
malignant transformation	Lymphoma
Choriocarcinoma	Carcinoid
Yolk-sac tumors	
Mixed germ-cell tumors	

World Health Organization Classification

depend on the cell type and stage of the disease. Recent advances in treatment have resulted in a 92% overall 5-yr survival *(16)*. Even among the small proportion of patients (12%) with advanced disease at diagnosis, 5-yr survival is close to 70% *(17)*. The classification and biology of testicular tumors are given in Tables 1 and 2, respectfully *(18,19)*.

CLINICAL PRESENTATION

The most common complaint in a patient with a testicular malignancy is testicular swelling or fullness *(20)*. Classically, the swelling or mass is painless, but by no means should a painful, tender testicular mass be discarded as a nonmalignant process *(21)*. Pain that may be associated with testicular malignancy can be diffuse and indolent or rarely can be localized and acute, mimicking testicular torsion, particularly if there is intratumoral hemorrhage or infarction. Signs and symptoms consistent with epididymitis or orchitis occur in as many as 25% of patients with testicular neoplasms and it is not uncommon for a patient to undergo unsuccessful antibiotic therapy before the definitive diagnosis is made *(22)*. Nonspecific symptoms because of advanced retroperitoneal spread or metastasis may be the presenting feature in some patients. Many patients may present because of paraneoplastic syndromes associated with testicular cancer; these include gynecomastia, infertility, and hyperthyroidism *(23)*.

Table 2
Common Characteristics and Biology of Testicular Tumors

	Seminoma	Embryonal cell	Choriocarcinoma	Yolk sac	Teratoma
% of all GCT	40%	25%	<1%	<1%	30%
Age at presentation	30–40		15–30		
Metastatic at diagnosis	30%		60%		
Visceral Mets at presentation	<5%		Common for choriocarcinoma		
Focal necrosis and hemorrhage	Rare		Common		
Elevated HCG	10%	None	>90%	Rare	50%
Elevated α-feto protein	Never	30%	None	85%	40%
Marker negative	90%	70%	Rare	<10%	10%
Central nervous system involvement	Rare		Common		
Curable with therapy					
Stage I	>99%		>99%		
Stage II	>95%		>95%		
Stage III	>90%		50–90%		

SCREENING (*SEE* ALGORITHM 1)

Testicular Examination

SCREENING AVERAGE-RISK POPULATION

The two screening tests proposed for testicular cancer are the physician's palpation of the testes and self-examination of the testes by the patient. The American Cancer Society recommends a cancer checkup that includes testicular examination every 3 yr for men over 20 and annually for those over 40 *(24)*. It has been demonstrated that education about testicular cancer and self-examination may enhance knowledge and self-reported claims of performing testicular examination *(25,26)*. Few studies, however, have examined whether education or self-examination instructions actually increase the performance of self-examination. It is also unclear whether persons who detect testicular abnormalities seek medical attention promptly. Patients with testicu-

Chapter 10 / Screening for Testicular Cancer

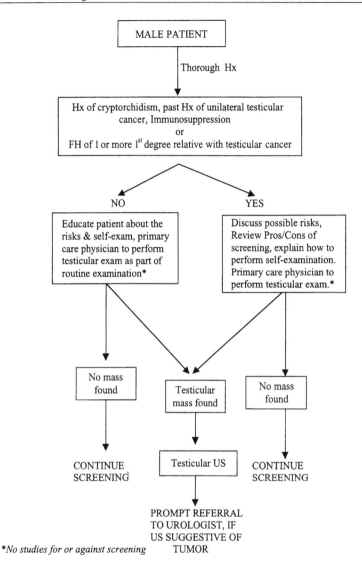

Algorithm 1.

lar symptoms may wait as long as several months before contacting a physician *(27)*.

Finally, no studies have been conducted to test whether persons who perform testicular self-examination are more likely to detect early-stage tumors or have better survival than those who do not practice self-examination *(28)*. Published evidence that self-examination can detect testicular cancer in asymptomatic persons is limited to a small number of case reports *(29)*.

166 Part IV / Screening for Urogenital Cancers

Current cure rates for testicular cancer are greater than 80% *(28,30)*. Survival, however, is still better for patients with Stage I cancer than in those with more advanced disease, and the treatment of early cancer has less cost and morbidity. There is evidence that once testicular symptoms have appeared, it signifies more advanced disease and lower survival *(27,31,32)*. Thus, it makes sense that testicular cancer screening should be encouraged despite the lack of evidence that it will detect early-stage tumor, and adolescent and young adult males should be advised to seek prompt medical attention if they notice a scrotal abnormality.

SCREENING HIGH-RISK POPULATION

The appropriate management and follow-up of patients with a history of an undescended testicle is controversial *(33,34)*. No studies have been performed to evaluate the benefits of formal screening of men with a history of cryptorchidism. It is known that orchiopexy at puberty does not reduce malignant transformation and it is uncertain whether earlier orchiopexy prior to school age, which is now common practice, will prevent development of testicular cancer *(33)*. The American Academy of Family Physicians recommends a clinical testicular examination for men age 13–39 yr who have a history of cryptorchidism, orchiopexy, or testicular atrophy *(35)*. Patients with an increased risk of testicular cancer (those with a history of cryptorchidism or atrophic testes) should be informed of their increased risk and counseled about the options for screening. Such patients may then opt to be screened or to perform testicular self-examination.

WORKUP OF TESTICULAR MASS

Ultrasonography

If a palpable testicular or scrotal mass is discovered, scrotal ultrasound is widely considered as the imaging of choice. The majority of the palpated scrotal masses are benign, and the predominant role of imaging is to identify masses requiring further investigations. A well-performed ultrasound examination can usually distinguish between testicular and nontesticular masses *(36)*. Ultrasound has been reported to have a sensitivity of 95% for the diagnosis of testicular cancers, but specificity is around 50%, because of a large number of benign conditions that mimic malignancy *(37)*. Magnetic resonance imaging (MRI) has not been shown to have significant clinical advantage over ultrasound for imaging of the scrotum in several studies. However, if the ultrasound is indeterminate for a testicular tumor because of background hemorrhage, MRI may be able to distinguish scrotal hematoma from the tumor *(38–40)*.

Chapter 10 / Screening for Testicular Cancer 167

If a testicular cancer is found, an abdominal, pelvic, and chest computed tomagraphy is recommended to assess metastatic lesions.

Tumor Markers

Several tumor markers have been proven useful in the diagnosis of testicular cancer but only α-fetoprotein (AFP) and β-human chorionic gonadotropin (hCG) have demonstrated clinical utility (41). Elevated levels of AFP are found in embryonal, endodermal sinus tumor, and hCG is positive in seminoma and choriocarcinoma (42). Nonseminomatous germ-cell tumors are positive for AFP in 65%, hCG in 63%, and either marker in 80–90% of all cases. However, these markers are not helpful in routine screening (41–44) because of their low sensitivity, low specificity, and low prevalence of testicular cancer in the general population.

INDICATIONS FOR REFERRAL TO A SUBSPECIALIST

Any patients with a strong clinical suspicion of testicular malignancy, including a suggestive testicular ultrasound, should be promptly referred to urology for further diagnostic workup. Male patients, particularly in the younger age group, with carcinoma of unknown primary should have a thorough testicular exam and should be evaluated by a medical oncologist and urologist if any abnormality is detected.

Patients who present with symptoms suggestive of epididymitis or orchitis should be examined and carefully followed up to rule out any possibility of testicular carcinoma. They should be further evaluated by testicular ultrasound and referred to a subspecialist if symptoms persist or their examination is suggestive of testicular carcinoma (22).

Patients with a history of cryptorchidism, atrophic testes, or family history of testicular cancer should be followed very closely and should have a yearly testicular examination. Immediate referral to a subspecialist is warranted if any suspicious abnormality is found on the clinical examination.

SUMMARY

Testicular cancer is one of the most curable of the solid tumors and is an excellent model for multimodality treatment of solid cancers. However, there is significant mortality and morbidity associated with advanced disease. There is no direct evidence on which to base a recommendation for or against screening for testicular cancer by either physician examination or patient self-examination, as no screening studies have been done. Primary care physicians have the responsibility to

168 Part IV / Screening for Urogenital Cancers

include the testicular examination as part of their routine examination, to educate young males about the frequency of testicular cancer in their age group, and to explain how to perform self-examination.

REFERENCES

1. Li M, Whitmore W, Golbey R, Grabstald H. (1960) Effects of combined drug therapy on metastatic cancer of the testis. *JAMA* 174:145.
2. Einhorn L. (1997) Testicular cancer: an oncological success story. *Clin Cancer Res* 3:2630.
3. *Cancer Facts and Figures.* (1999) American Cancer Society, New York.
4. Spitz M, Side J, Pollack E, Lynch H, Newell G. (1986) Incidence and descriptive features of testicular cancer among United States whites, blacks, and hispanics, 1973–1982. *Cancer* 58:1785.
5. Weir H, Marrett L, Moravan V. (1999) Trends in the incidence of testicular germ cell cancer in Ontario by histologic subgroup, 1964–1996. *CMAJ* 160:201.
6. Vogt HB, McHale MS. (1992) Testicular cancer: role of primary care physicians in screening and education. *Postgrad Med* 92:93–101.
7. Gilbert J, Hamilton J. (1940) Incidence and nature of tumors in ectopic testes. *Surg Gynecol Obstet* 71:31.
8. Osterlind A, Berthelsen J, Abildgaard, N. (1987) Incidence of bilateral germ cell cancer in Denmark 1960-1984: preliminary findings. *Int J Androl* 10:203.
9. Aker O, Ekbom A, Hsieh CC, et al. (1996)Testicular nonseminoma and seminoma in relation to perinatal characteristics. *J Natl Cancer Inst* 66:627–631.
10. Braun MM, Ahlbom A, Floderus B, et al. (1995) Effect of twinship on incidence of cancer of the testis, breast, and other sites. *Cancer Causes Control* 6:519–524.
11. Thonneau P, Ducot B, Bujan J, et al. (1996) Heat exposure as a hazard to male infertility. *Lancet* 346:204,205.
12. Sonneveld DJ, Sleijfer DT, Schrafford Koops H, et al. (1999) Familial testicular cancer in a single-centre population. *Eur J Cancer* 35(9):1368–1373.
13. Nichols C, Heerema N, Palmer C, et al. (1987) Klinefelter's syndrome associated with mediastinal germ cell neoplasms. *J Clin Oncol* 5:1290.
14. Dieckmann K., Rube C, Henke R. (1997) Association of Down's syndrome and testicular cancer. *J Urol* 157:1701.
15. Lyter DW, Bryant J, Thackeray R, et al. (1995) Incidence of human immunodeficiency virus-related and nonrelated malignancies in a large cohort of homosexual men. *J Clin Oncol* 13:2540–2646.
16. Wingo PA, Tong T, Bolden S. (1995) Cancer statistics, 1995. *CA Cancer J Clin* 45:8–30.
17. Ries LAG, Miller BA, Hankey BF, et al. (eds.) (1994) *SEER Cancer Statistics Review, 1973–1991: Tables and Graphs.* Bethesda: National Cancer Institute.
18. Mostofi, F, Sesterhenn, I. (1994) Revised international classification of testicular tumors. In: Jones W, Harnden P, Appleyard I, eds. *Germ Cell Tumors III*, Oxford: Pergamon, p. 153.
19. Bosl G, Bajorin D, Sheinfeld J, Motzer, R. (1997) Cancer of the testis. In: DeVita V, et al., eds. *Cancer: Principles and Practice of Oncology*, 5th edition, Philadelphia: Lipincott-Raven, p. 1397.
20. Loeher P, Birch R, William, S, et al. (1987) Chemotherapy of metastatic seminoma:The southeastern cancer study group experience. *J Clin Onc* 5:1212.
21. Sesterhenn I, Wiess R, Mostofi F, et al. (1992) Prognosis and other clinical correlates of pathologic review in stage I and II testicular carcinoma. A report from the Testicular Cancer Intergroup Study. *J Clin Onc* 10:69.

Chapter 10 / Screening for Testicular Cancer 169

22. Small E, Torti, F. (1995) Testes: management of specific malignancies. In: Abeloff M, Armitage J, Lichter A, Niederhuber J, eds. *Clinical Oncology*, New York: Churchill/Livingston, p. 1493.

23. Doherty A, Bower M, Christmas T. (1997) The role of tumor markers in the diagnosis and treatment of testicular germ cell cancers. *Br J Urol* 79:247.

24. Schottenfeld D, Warshauer ME. (1982) Testis. In: Schottenfeld D, Fraumeni JF, eds. *Cancer Epidemiology and Prevention.* Philadelphia: WB Saunders, pp. 947–957.

25. Marty PJ, McDermott RJ. (1986) Three strategies for encouraging testicular self-examination among college-aged males. *J Am Coll Health* 34:253–258.

26. Ostwald SK, Rothenberger J. (1985) Development of a testicular self-examination program for college men. *J Am Coll Health* 33:234.

27. Bosl GJ, Vogelzang NJ, Goldman A, et al. (1981) Impact of delay in diagnosis on clinical stage of testicular cancer. *Lancet* 2:970–972.

28. Westlake SJ, Frank JW. (1987) Testicular self-examination: an argument against routine teaching. *Fam Pract* 4:143–148.

29. Garnick MB, Mayer RJ, Richie JP. (1980) Testicular self-examination [letter]. *N Engl J Med* 1302:297.

30. Williams SD, Birch R, Einhorn LH, et al. (1987) Treatment of disseminated germ-cell tumors with cisplatin, bleomycin, and either vinblastine or etoposide. *N Engl J Med* 316:1435–1440.

31. Field TE. (1964) Common errors occurring in the diagnosis of testicular neoplasms and the effect of these errors on prognosis. *J Roy Army Med Corps* 110:152–155.

32. Post GJ, Belis JA. (1980) Delayed presentation of testicular tumors. *S Med J* 73:33–35.

33. Hawtrey CE. (1990) Undescended testis and orchiopexy: recent observations. *Pediatr Rev* 11:305–308.

34. Giwercman A, Bruun E, Frimodt-Moller C, Skakkebaek NE. (1989) Prevalence of carcinoma in situ and other histopathological abnormalities in testes of men with a history of cryptorchidism. *J Urol* 142:998–1002.

35. American Academy of Family Physicians. (1994) *Age Charts for the Periodic Health Examination.* Kansas City, MO: American Academy of Family Physicians.

36. Carroll BA, Gross DM. (1983) High frequency scrotal sonography. *Am J Roentgenol* 140:511–515.

37. Tackett RE, Ling D, Catalona WJ, Melson GL. (1986) High-resolution sonography in diagnosing testicular neoplasms: clinical significance of false positive scans. *Scan J Uro* 135:494–496.

38. Baker LL, Hajek PC, Burkhard TK, et al. (1987) Magnetic resonance imaging of the scrotum: pathologic conditions. *Radiology* 163:93–98.

39. Seidenwurm D, Smathers RL, Lo RK, et al. (1987) Testes and scrotum: MR imaging at 1.5T. *Radiology* 164:393–398.

40. Thurnher S, Hricak H, Carrol PR, et al. (1988) Imaging of testis: comparison between MR imaging and US. *Radiology* 167:631–636.

41. Johnson JO, Mattrey RF, Phillipson J. (1990) Differentiation of Seminomatous and nonseminomatous testicular tumors with MR imaging. *Am J Roentgenol* 154:539–543.

42. Mostofi FK, Sesterhenn IA. (1985) Pathology of germ cell tumors of the testis. *Prog Clin Biol Res* 203:1–34.

43. Catalona WJ. (1982) Current management of testicular tumors. *Surg Clinics N Am* 62:1119–1127.

44. Kurman RJ, Scardino PT, McIntire KR, et al. (1977) Cellular localisation of alpha fetoprotein and human chorionic gonadotropin in germ cell tumors of the testis using an indirect immunoperoxidase technique (a new approach to classification utilizing tumor markers). *Cancer* 40:2136–2151.

V   DERMATOLOGICAL CANCERS

11 Screening for Skin Cancer

Marti J. Rothe, MD, Tracy L. Bialy, BA and Jane M. Grant-Kels, MD

KEY PRINCIPLES

- Approximately half of all cancers are skin cancers.
- One million new skin cancers are diagnosed each year in the United States; approx 4% are cutaneous malignant melanoma. Nearly 90% of skin cancer deaths are from malignant melanoma. In the United States, one person dies of melanoma every hour.
- Early detection and education are leading to a leveling off or decrease in the incidence and mortality rates of cutaneous malignant melanoma.
- Total-body skin examinations are required for patients at high risk for skin cancer.
- Primary care physicians can improve their ability to diagnose skin cancer with intensive education.
- Periodic surveillance by the subspecialist may be necessary for patients at high risk for skin cancer.

EPIDEMIOLOGY

It is estimated that 1 million new cases of skin cancer are diagnosed each year in the United States. Basal-cell carcinoma (BCC) accounts for approx 80%, squamous-cell carcinoma (SCC) approx 16%, and cutaneous malignant melanoma (CMM) approxly 4% of new skin cancers *(1)*. BCC is the most common cancer affecting individuals of European descent whose ancestors migrated to the United States or Australia; SCC is only one-fifth as common as BCC, but it is among the most frequently diagnosed cancers in the United States and the second most

From: *Cancer Screening: A Practical Guide for Physicians*
Edited by: K. Aziz and G. Y. Wu © Humana Press Inc., Totowa, NJ

173

common cancer in Australia *(2)*. A report in 1998 identified CMM as the 4th most common cancer in Australia and New Zealand, the 10th in the United States, Canada, and Scandinavia, and the 18th in Great Britain *(3)*. CMM is the sixth most common cause of estimated new cancer cases in the United States for 1999 among males and seventh among females, accounting for 4% and 3%, respectively, of new cases *(4)*. In the United States, CMM is more common than any noncutaneous cancer among 25–29 yr olds *(5)*. Epidemiological data are more precise for CMM than nonmelanoma skin cancer (NMSC) because the diagnosis of the former but not the latter is routinely reported to tumor registries.

INCIDENCE OF CUTANEOUS MALIGNANT MELANOMA

Marked increases in the incidence of CMM have been observed. It has been estimated that the incidence in Caucasians has increased from 3% to 7% per year from the mid-1960s to the mid-1990s *(6)*. Calculations based on data from the Surveillance, Epidemiology, and End Results (SEER) program of the National Cancer Institute show an increase in the incidence of CMM in the United States of 120.5% from 1973 to 1994 *(7)*. Increased education and awareness appear to result in earlier detection and a greater increase in thin than thick tumors. In the United States, a 500% increase from the period of 1973–1977 to 1983–1987 was reported in the diagnosis of *in situ* CMM compared to a 52% increase in the diagnosis of invasive CMM *(8)*. However, data suggest that the increased incidence is not solely the result of increased surveillance and detection of clinically insignificant tumors. Advanced disease has also increased. From 1973 to 1994, localized disease increased 223.8% among males and 133.7% among females, whereas regional or distant disease rose 75% among males and 23.5% among females *(7)*. From 1988 to 1994, annual increases of 3.3, 3.9, and 4.6% of tumors <1 mm, 1–2.99 mm, and ≥3 mm in depth, respectively, yield a cumulative increase of 22, 26, and 31%, respectively *(9)*.

Stabilization or decrease incidence rates of CMM have been reported over the past few years. For example, in the United States from 1990 to 1994, rates stabilized or declined for females younger than 60 yr old and males younger than 50 yr old, whereas rates increased for older age groups *(7)*. The incidence in the United States of invasive tumors decreased two consecutive years from 14.1 per 100,000 in 1991 to 13.8 per 100,000 in 1993 *(8)*. In Scotland, the incidence of CMM in women has stabilized since 1986 but has continued to increase in men *(10)*. In the Netherlands, the age-adjusted incidence of invasive CMM increased steadily during the 1980s for both men and women; during the

Chapter 11 / Screening for Skin Cancer

1990s, the incidence stabilized for men and the rate of increase slowed in women *(11)*.

SKIN CANCER RISK FACTORS

Skin cancer is exceedingly more common in Caucasians than other races, although NMSC not infrequently affects Hispanics and acral lentiginous melanoma is the most common type of CMM affecting Asians and blacks. Both NMSC and CMM are more common in men than women. NMSC most commonly affects chronically sun-exposed sites, including the head and neck, trunk, and upper extremities. CMM most commonly affects sites of intermittent intense sun exposure, the trunk in men and the lower extremity in women. Risk factors for NMSC and CMM include a history of significant sun exposure, light colored eyes, skin, and hair, tendency to sunburn easily and tan poorly, personal or family history of skin cancer, male sex, advancing age, immunodeficiency, such as status post organ transplantation or from human immunodeficiency virus (HIV) infection (SCC more commonly affects immunodeficient patients than BCC), defective repair of ultraviolet-induced DNA damage in xeroderma pigmentosum, exposure to ionizing radiation, and psoralen and ultraviolet A radiation therapy for psoriasis (association is greatest for patients who have had 250 or more treatments and the risk for developing SCC is greater than for developing BCC or melanoma). *(See* Algorithm 1.) There are additional unique risk factors for the development of CMM, such as a personal history of atypical moles or multiple moles. The relative importance of risk factors for CMM is enumerated in Table 1 *(12,13)*.

PROGNOSIS OF SKIN CANCER (TABLE 2)

Approximately 50–60% of patients with NMSC are at risk for developing a subsequent NMSC within 5 yr *(14)*. The frequency of multiple primary CMM is 1–8%, with 30% of patients presenting with multiple primary tumors concurrently, 63% developing additional primary tumors subsequent to the diagnosis of the first primary CMM, and 7% having multiple primary tumors both concurrently and subsequently *(15)*.

The prognosis for BCC is excellent. Only 0.0028% of BCCs metastasize. Metastatic disease is more common in men than women and usually arises from large neglected tumors. Five-year survival for metastatic BCC is less than 33% *(14)*. Patients with basal-cell nevus syndrome, a rare sporadic or autosomal dominant condition characterized by multiple BCCs, jaw cysts, palmoplantar pits, and a wide variety of other anomalies, may develop locally invasive or metastatic tumors.

High risk of malignancy	Low risk of malignancy
History of chronic sun-exposure and/or sunburns	Minimal lifetime sun exposure
History of bleeding, crusted, itchy lesion	Lesion asymptomatic
Fair-skin, blond or red hair, light eyes	Darker skin, dark hair, brown eyes
Family or personal history of skin cancer	No family or personal history of skin cancer

Algorithm 1. New or changing skin lesion. Plan: biopsy and submit to a dermatopathology lab.

Table 1

Relative Importance of Risk Factors for Development of Cutaneous Malignant Melanoma (CMM)

Risk factor	Relative risk
• Personal history of atypical moles, family history of melanoma, and >75–100 moles (familial atypical mole/melanoma syndrome)	35
• Personal history of NMSC	17
• Giant congenital nevus (>20 cm)	15–5
• Personal history of CMM	9–10
• Family history of CMM in first-degree relative	8
• Immunosuppression	8–6
• Personal history of atypical nevi (2–9) and no family history of CMM	7.3–4.9
• Personal history of 26-100 nevi	5.4–1.8
• Chronic tanning with UVA (including PUVA for psoriasis)	5.4
• Blistering sunburns (2–3 episodes)	3.8–1.7
• Freckling	3.0
• Fair skin, poorly tans	2.6
• One atypical nevus	2.3
• Red or blond hair	2.2

Relative risk is defined as degree of increased risk for person with risk factor as compared with person without risk; relative risk of 1 indicates no increased risk.
Source: Modified from refs. *12* and *13*.

Chapter 11 / Screening for Skin Cancer

Table 2
Skin Cancer Prognosis

	Risk factors for metastases
BCC	Large neglected tumors
	Basal-cell nevus syndrome
SCC	Depth >4 mm
	Diameter >2 cm
	Poorly differentiated histology
	Perineural, vascular, lymphatic invasion
	Tumors arising in burns, scars, osteomyelitis
	Immunodeficiency
CMM	Increasing tumor thickness
	Vertical growth phase
	Ulceration
	Acral lesions

Approximately 5% of SCCs metastasize within 5 yr. Risk factors for metastases include depth greater than 4 mm, diameter greater than 2 cm, poorly differentiated histology, perineural, vascular, and lymphatic invasion, tumors located on the lip, tumors arising in osteomyelotic foci, burns, and scars, and immunodeficiency. Five-year survival is approx 30% for patients with metastatic SCC *(14)*. In 1998, there were approx 1200 deaths from SCC *(1)*.

In the United States, nearly 90% of skin cancer deaths are from CMM and 7300 deaths from CMM were estimated for 1999 *(1)*. Mortality rates for CMM rose 38.9% from 1973 to 1994, but the change in mortality rates was greater for the period 1973–1977 than 1990–1994 *(7)*. Mortality rates are greater for males than for females and for older than younger individuals *(7)*. Mortality rates stabilized or decreased for all groups from 1990 to 1994, except for men 70 yr or older and women 60–69 yr old *(7)*. Thicker tumors are associated with greater risk for advanced disease and mortality. Five-year survival is 93–100% for tumors <0.76 mm in depth and 50% or less for tumors ≥4 mm *(16)*. For the period from 1989 to 1994, the 5-yr survival for CMM in the United States was 88% for white patients and 69% for black patients *(4)*.

BIOLOGY OF SKIN CANCER

The pathogenesis of skin cancer is complex and a simplified scheme will be briefly summarized. Skin cancer is believed to develop as a consequence of DNA mutations induced by ultraviolet light (UVL).

UVL-induced mutations deleteriously affect tumor suppressor genes, such as p53 and CDKN2A, allowing clonal expansion of atypical cells. UVL also suppresses cell-mediated immune mechanisms of skin cancer surveillance *(17)*. Chronic low-dose exposure to UVL promotes the development of multiple mutations and clonal replication of keratinocytes. Intermittent high-dose exposure to UVL promotes multiple mutations and clonal replication of melanocytes *(18)*.

RATIONALE FOR SCREENING FOR SKIN CANCER

Skin cancer screening is advocated because early detection is believed to decrease morbidity and mortality. Because BCC is so rarely fatal, early detection impacts insignificantly on mortality. However, early diagnosis of BCC is effective in minimizing local tissue destruction by the tumor and allows for less complex surgical excision of the tumor, decreased size of the surgical defect, and improved cosmesis. Similarly, early detection of SCC reduces morbidity of the disease. Additionally, early detection of SCC is likely to be associated with decreased risk for regional and distant metastatic disease and improved mortality rates.

Early detection of CMM is considered essential because of the high mortality rate and the strong relationship between tumor thickness and mortality. CMMs diagnosed during periodic surveillance examinations are more likely to be smaller and thinner than those diagnosed at first presentation *(19)*. CMMs diagnosed at the American Academy of Dermatology (AAD)-sponsored annual screening programs from 1992 to 1994 were significantly more likely to be early tumors compared to 1990 SEER registry cases *(20)*. Although these results suggest that surveillance allows detection of thin tumors and, therefore, saves lives, there is the possibility that surveillance merely identifies clinically insignificant or biologically nonaggressive disease rather than tumors which would increase mortality if undetected and untreated. Studies assessing the relationship between early detection and mortality are limited *(21)*. Early detection programs in Scotland and Italy have been shown to lead to decreased mortality *(22,23)*. Skin self-examination has been suggested to reduce the mortality by 63% by reducing the incidence of CMM and the risk of advanced disease *(24)*.

METHODS OF SKIN CANCER SCREENING

Physical examination of the skin is the method by which individuals are screened for skin cancer. (*See* Algorithm 2.) Biopsy submitted to a dermatopathology laboratory is essential for histologic confirmation of suspicious lesions. History of risk factors for skin cancer and of new, changing, or symptomatic lesions aids the screening process. Total-body

Chapter 11 / Screening for Skin Cancer

Pearly papule or nodule with telangiectasia and central erosion and/or crust	BCC
Red scaling macule or minimally infiltrated papule	Actinic keratosis (AK)
Red scaling papule or plaque	Hyperplastic AK SCC *in situ* Superficial BCC
Red scaling plaque with irregular pearly border	Superficial BCC
Firm indurated area with yellow or ivory discoloration, telangiectasia, indistinct margins	Morpheaform BCC
Pearly lesion with irregular pigmentation	Pigmented BCC (rule out CMM)
Erythematous ulcerated and/or crusted nodule	SCC
Red nodule with central crusted crateriform ulcer	SCC—keratoacanthoma variant
Pigmented lesion that is asymmetrical, poorly circumscribed, variegated in color, diameter ≥6 mm or changing	CMM
- Irregular brown patch with pigment loss and papules and nodules on sun-damaged skin	Lentigo maligna melanoma
-Irregular, notched variegated plaque with brown, black, red, white, and/or blue coloration most often on the trunk or extremities	Superficial spreading melanoma
-Brown–black to blue–black or red nodule	Nodular melanoma
-Irregular brown lesion with asymmetry and variegated color on acral skin	Acral lentiginous melanoma
-Red nodule or red scaly patch	Amelanotic melanoma (2% of all CMM)

Algorithm 2. Differential diagnosis of common skin cancers.

photography of patients with atypical and/or multiple melanocytic nevi, epiluminescence microscopy, and computerized digital imaging are tools the subspecialist may utilize as adjuncts to the physical examination. Detection in the peripheral blood of biochemical markers for CMM is an experimental technique, which may be most useful in identifying advanced tumors and predicting response to medical therapy *(25)*.

PHYSICAL EXAMINATION

Physical examination for skin cancer surveillance should ideally be a total-body rather than partial skin examination. Complete skin examinations are 6.4 times more likely to detect CMM than partial examinations because many CMMs develop at sites usually covered by clothing *(26)*. Additionally, patients may present with multiple skin cancers concurrently, which may involve more than one anatomic site *(27)*. Special attention should be given to areas where lesions may be overlooked: nasolabial folds, external ear, postauricular skin, eyelids, fingernails and toenails, webspaces, soles, scalp, gluteal fold, and genitals. Sites of previous skin cancer should be assessed for evidence of recurrence. Patients at high risk for skin cancer should have surveillance by a dermatologist at 3- to 6-mo intervals, depending on the degree of risk. Opportunistic examinations of the skin may be performed by nondermatologists during physical examinations for nondermatologic concerns *(28)*. Patients at high risk for skin cancer should also perform periodic skin self-examination.

Accuracy of Physical Examination

Identification of suspicious lesions requires knowledge of the characteristic features of skin cancers and benign skin lesions (Figs. 1–12). A number of studies have been performed that evaluate how closely presumptive clinical diagnosis matches final histologic diagnosis. These studies include outcomes analysis of skin cancer screening clinics, retrospective reviews of specimens submitted to dermatopathology laboratories, and measures of the sensitivity and specificity of diagnostic criteria for CMM *(29,30)*.

Evaluations of outcomes from skin cancer screening clinics in British Columbia for 1994 and 1995 showed positive predictive values of 89% for actinic keratoses, 19% for atypical nevi, 43% for BCCs, and 17% for CMMs. Final histologic diagnoses for lesions misdiagnosed clinically during the screening include BCC (clinically misdiagnosed as actinic keratosis), seborrheic keratosis, actinic keratosis, dermatofibroma (clinically misdiagnosed as BCC), benign melanocytic nevus, blue nevus, and BCC (clinically misdiagnosed as CMM) *(31)*. A similar analysis of outcomes of skin cancer screening in New Haven, Connecticut in 1988 found positive predictive values of 43% for BCC, 14% for SCC, and 50% for SCC *in situ (32)*. The positive predictive value for CMM for the AAD annual screening programs from 1992 to 1994 was 17% *(20)*. A study from the Netherlands assessed accuracy of negative results from a screening program in 1990. Of 1551 individuals with negative screening, three NMSCs had been present at the time of the

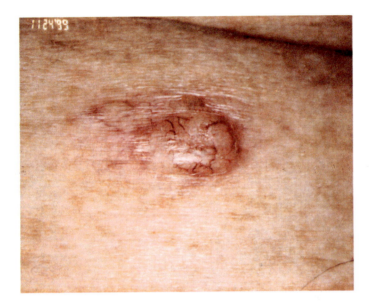

Fig. 1. Nodular BCC: a pearly nodule with telangiectasia and early central ulceration.

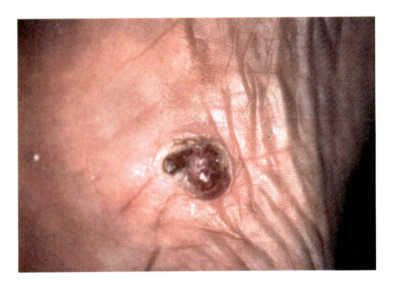

Fig. 2. Superficial BCC: a red plaque with pearly border that may mimic nummular eczema, psoriasis, or SCC *in situ*.

screen. The screening program was determined to have a sensitivity of 93.3%, specificity of 97.8%, and positive predictive value of 54% *(33)*.

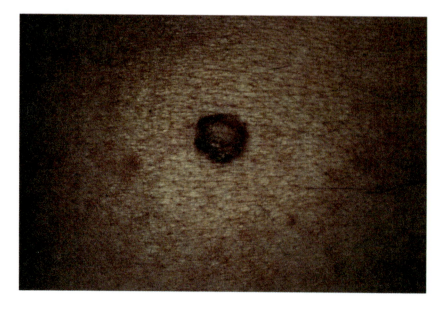

Fig. 3. Pigmented BCC: a BCC with brown-black pigmentation that may be confused clinically with melanocytic nevus, seborrheic keratosis, or melanoma.

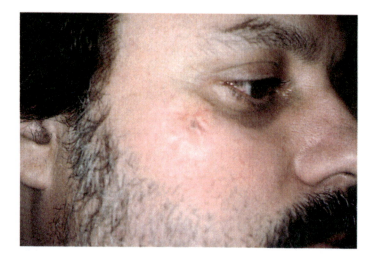

Fig. 4. Morpheaform BCC: a scarlike tumor that invades more deeply than other BCCs.

A retrospective review of 13,878 skin biopsy specimens submitted to New York University showed a clinical diagnostic accuracy for the diagnosis of CMM of approx 60% with a sensitivity of 81.1% and a

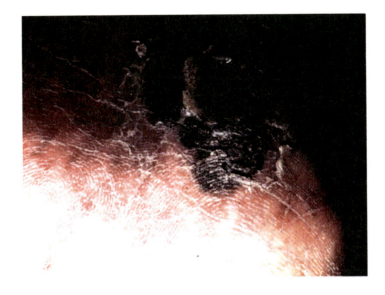

Fig. 5. SCC: hyperkeratotic and crusted plaques.

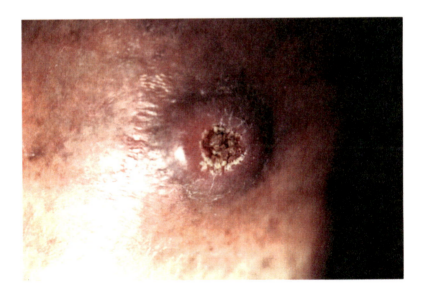

Fig. 6. Keratoacanthoma: a variant of SCC showing central keratin filled crater; previously this was thought to be a benign tumor.

specificity of 99.2% *(34)*. Thirty-three percent of 1784 histologically diagnosed CMMs submitted to the University of Texas Southwestern Medical Center dermatopathology laboratory were not suspected clini-

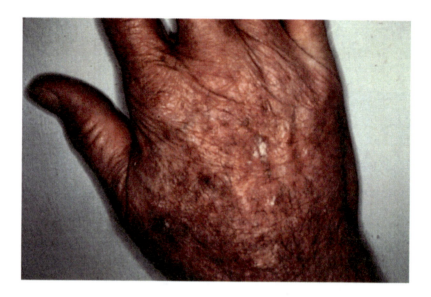

Fig. 7. Actinic (solar) keratoses: pink scaling papules affecting sun-exposed skin that may be more easily felt than seen; from <1% to <10% of actinic keratoses evolve into SCC.

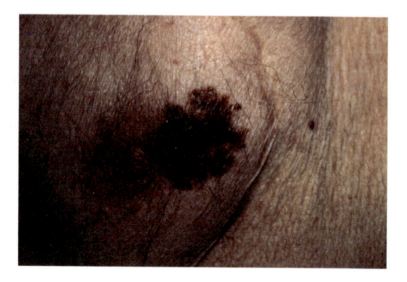

Fig. 8. Atypical melanocytic nevi: that multiple irregular pigmented papules that often affect the trunk and sun-protected sites such as the scalp and buttocks.

cally, yielding a diagnostic sensitivity of 67% *(35)*. A review of reports from a regional, nonhospital-based dermatopathology laboratory

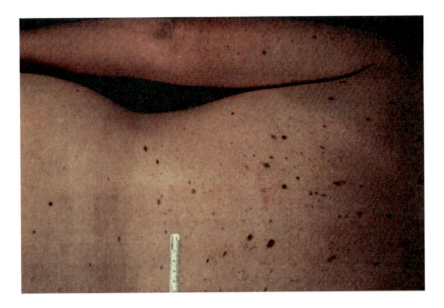

Fig. 9. Superficial spreading melanoma (SSM): a plaque showing asymmetry, border irregularity, color variegation, and diameter >6 mm; the upper back is the most common site in men and the lower legs in women.

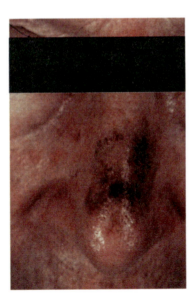

Fig. 10. Lentigo maligna melanoma: an irregular pigmented plaque with evidence of pigment loss (regression); common in the elderly on chronically sun-damaged skin of the head and neck, especially the nose and cheek, and shows a prolonged radial growth phase.

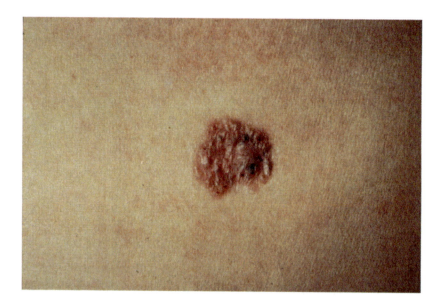

Fig. 11. Nodular melanoma: lesions may be deeply pigmented or amelanotic and demonstrate vertical growth.

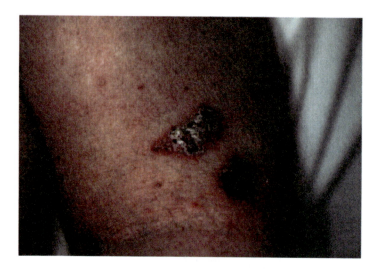

Fig. 12. Acral lentiginous melanoma: a deeply pigmented plaque that occurs on the palms, soles, or subungually; the most common CMM in Asians and blacks; delay in diagnosis is common and is associated with poor prognosis.

showed that a histologic diagnosis of malignancy was determined in 2.3% of 1946 biopsy specimens clinically diagnosed as benign

Chapter 11 / Screening for Skin Cancer 187

melanocytic nevi. Twelve CMMs, 30 BCCs, and three SCCs were diagnosed histologically *(36)*. A comparison of clinical diagnosis and histologic diagnosis of 44,258 specimens evaluated in the dermatopathology laboratory of the University of Graz showed a senstivity for the diagnosis of CMM of 70.1%, specificity of 99.4%, and positive predictive value of 60.7% *(37)*.

The accuracy of the ABCD (Asymmetry, Border irregularity, Color variegation, Diameter >6 mm) criteria for diagnosis of CMM has been assessed. One study determined a sensitivity of 92% *(38)*; another study determined a sensitivity of 100% and a specificity of 98.4% (39). A retrospective review of CMMs biopsies in Australia showed that 31% were ≤6 mm in diameter, bringing into question the utility of diameter as a diagnostic criterion *(40)*. A change in diameter is a more sensitive indicator.

Epiluminescence

Epiluminescence microscopy (ELM) and computerized digital imaging are tools that may improve the accuracy of the clinical diagnosis of CMM. ELM or skin-surface microscopy entails the application of immersion oil to the lesion and viewing the lesion through a hand-held dermatoscope. ELM reveals features not evident with the naked eye, which can clarify the diagnosis of pigmented lesions. ELM improves clinical diagnostic accuracy when utilized by trained, experienced clinicians, but it can confound the diagnosis when utilized by inadequately trained, inexperienced clinician *(41)*. Digital photography for the evaluation of pigmented lesions is evolving. One system based on assessment of color hues achieved clinical diagnostic accuracy of 92%, compared to 87% accuracy achieved without digital imaging *(42)*.

Total-Body Photography

Total-body photography is another adjunctive diagnostic aid that has been utilized most in the periodic surveillance of patients with atypical and/or multiple melanocytic nevi. Changes from baseline photographs can facilitate the early diagnosis of CMM. As well, the ability to follow pigmented lesions by comparing findings on periodic physical examination to baseline photographs decreases the unnecessary excision of atypical, but unchanged and benign nevi *(43)*.

GENETIC SCREENING

Genetic screening for skin cancer is experimental at this time. Approximately 10% of patients with CMM have a positive family history for CMM. Studies of families with atypical mole syndrome and melanoma have identified a melanoma susceptibility locus linked to chromosome 9p. Germline mutations in the tumor-suppressor gene CDKN2A have been identified in 40–50% of 9p-linked melanoma families *(44)*. Germline mutations of CDKN2A have also been identified in patients with familial and sporadic multiple primary melanoma *(45,46)*. Additional genes are likely to be implicated in CMM susceptibility. Screening for genetic markers for CMM is not routine at this time.

COST-EFFECTIVENESS

The cost-effectiveness of skin cancer screening has only been studied in a limited fashion. Medicare reimbursements for CMM and NMSC were more than $98 million in 1993 *(47)*. It is presumed that skin cancer screening will identify early malignancies requiring less expensive therapies than more advanced malignancies.

The estimated annual direct cost of treating newly diagnosed CMM in 1997 was $563 million. Approximately 90% of this cost was due to treatment of less than 20% of CMM patients, those with regional and distant metastases. Terminal care and interferon therapy are the most costly aspects of treatment for patients with advanced disease. Primary prevention (reduction of ultraviolet exposure) and secondary prevention (early detection) are suggested means for cost reduction *(48)*.

A cost-effectiveness analysis of skin cancer screening for a region in Italy showed 22.3 lives saved by early diagnosis from 1977 to 1985 and a savings of nearly $495,000 in treatment costs as opposed to the nearly $71,000 cost of the health campaign. The cost per year of lives saved was $400 *(49)*.

The most comprehensive cost-effectiveness analysis to date calculated that for every 1 million persons in a high-risk population screened, there is an increase of 1200 yr of life saved at a cost of $861 million and a cost-effectiveness ratio of $29,170 per year of life saved. This compares favorably to previously published reports of cost-effectiveness of $32,130 and $46,410 per year of life saved for annual mammography (55–65 yr old) and Pap smear every 3 yr, respectively *(47)*.

INDICATIONS FOR CONSULTING THE SUBSPECIALIST

With the exception of opportunistic examinations by physicians who are examining patients for nondermatologic conditions, skin cancer surveillance is best performed by the dermatologist. Most primary care physicians, whether in academic or nonacademic practices, do not perform complete skin examinations *(50,51)*. Furthermore, primary care

Chapter 11 / Screening for Skin Cancer 189

residents have been shown to misdiagnose benign and malignant tumors significantly more frequently than dermatology residents and dermatology attendings *(52)*. However, intensive educational intervention strategies can improve the ability of the primary care physician to recognize cutaneous malignancies *(53)*.

Patients with a history of atypical and/or multiple melanocytic nevi, with or without a personal or family history of CMM, may benefit from being followed in a pigmented lesion clinic. A pigmented lesion clinic is a multidisciplinary clinic which includes dermatologists, oncologists, and oncologic surgeons with expertise in nevi and CMM. The most up-to-date diagnostic and treatment techniques are available in these settings, as well as the expertise of a dermatologist subspecialist who has significantly greater experience and clinical diagnostic accuracy than even most other dermatologists. It has also been demonstrated that treatment for localized CMM is more cost-efficient when care is administered by a pigmented lesion clinic than by practitioners in the general community *(54)*.

SUMMARY

Primary care physicians are integral to the early detection of skin cancer. Although basal-cell and squamous-cell carcinomas account for the majority of cutaneous malignancies, cutaneous malignant melanoma accounts for the greatest mortality. Early detection and patient education has promoted stabilization of the incidence and mortality rates of cutaneous malignant melanoma. Total-body skin examination and self-examination for high-risk individuals are paramount. Subspecialists can aid in the diagnosis of skin cancer through total-body photography, epiluminescence, and skin biopsy interpreted by a dermatopathologist.

REFERENCES

1. Anon. (1999) 1999 Skin cancer fact sheet. *Cutis* 64:52D.
2. Stern RS. (1999) The mysteries of geographic variability in nonmelanoma skin cancer incidence. *Arch Dermatol* 135:843,844.
3. Serraino D, Fratino L, Gianni W, et al. (1998) Epidemiological aspects of cutaneous malignant melanoma. *Oncol Rep* 5:905–909.
4. Landis SH, Murray T, Bolden S, et al. (1999) Cancer statistics, 1999. *CA Cancer J Clin* 49:8–31.
5. Weinstock MA. (1997) Death from skin cancer among the elderly: epidemiological patterns. *Arch Dermatol* 133:1207–1209.
6. Armstrong BK, Kriker A. (1995) Skin cancer. *Dermatol Clin* 13:583–594.
7. Hall HI, Miller DR, Rogers JD, et al. (1999) Update on the incidence and mortality from melanoma in the United States. *J Am Acad Dermatol* 40:35–42.
8. Gloecklier-Ries LA, Kosary CL, Hankey BF, et al. (1997) *SEER Cancer Statistics Review, 1973-1994.* Bethesda, MD: National Cancer Institute, pp. 305–318.

9. Dennis LK. (1999) Analysis of the melanoma epidemic, both apparent and real: data from the 1973 through 1994 surveillance, epidemiology, and end results program registry. *Arch Dermatol* 135:275–280.
10. MacKie RM, Hole D, Hunter JA, et al. (1997) Cutaneous malignant melanoma in Scotland: incidence, survival, and mortality, 1979-94. The Scottish Melanoma Group. *Br Med J* 315:1117–1121.
11. van der Rhee HJ, van der Spek-Keijser LMT, van Westering R, et al. (1999) Increase in and stabilization of incidence and mortality of primary cutaneous malignant melanoma in western Netherlands, 1980-95. *Br J Dermatol* 140:463–467.
12. Robinson JK. (1997) Clinical crossroads: a 28-year-old fair skinned woman with multiple nevi. *JAMA* 278:1693–1699.
13. Robinson JK, Rigel DS, Amonette RA. (1998) What promotes skin self-examination? *J Am Acad Dermatol* 38:752–757.
14. Czarnecki D. (1998) The prognosis of patients with basal and squamous cell carcinoma of the skin. *Int J Dermatol* 37:656–658.
15. Johnson TM, Hamilton T, Lowe L. (1998) Multiple primary melanomas. *J Am Acad Dermatol* 39:422–427.
16. Richert SM, D'Amico F, Rhodes AR. (1998) Cutaneous melanoma: patient surveillance and tumor progression. *J Am Acad Dermatol* 39:571–577.
17. Grossman D, Leffell DJ. (1997) The molecular basis of nonmelanoma skin cancer: new understanding. *Arch Dermatol* 133:1263–1270.
18. Gilchrist BA, Eller MS, Geller AC, et al. (1999) The pathogenesis of melanoma induced by ultraviolet radiation. *N Engl J Med* 340:1341–1348.
19. Richert SM, D'Amico F, Rhodes AR. (1998) Cutaneous melanoma: patient surveillance and tumor progression. *J Am Acad Dermatol* 39:571–577.
20. Koh HK, Norton LA, Geller, 00AC, et al. (1996) Evaluation of the American Academy of Dermatology's National Skin Cancer Early Detection and Screening Program. *J Am Acad Dermatol* 34:971–978.
21. Weinstock MA. (1998) Mass population skin cancer screening can be worthwhile (if it's done right). *J Cutan Med Surg* 2:129–132.
22. MacKie RM, Hole D. (1992) Audit of public education campaign to encourage earlier detection of malignant melanoma. *Br Med J* 304:1012–1015.
23. Cristofolini M, Bianchi R, Boi S, et al. (1993) Effectiveness of the health campaign for the early diagnosis of cutaneous melanoma in Trentino, Italy. *J Dermatol Surg Oncol* 19:117–120.
24. Berwick M, Begg CB, Fine JA, et al. (1996) Screening for cutaneous melanoma by skin self-examination. *J Natl Cancer Inst* 88:17–23.
25. Reed JA, Albino AP. (1999) Update of diagnostic and prognostic markers in cutaneous melanoma. *Dermatol Clin* 17:631–643.
26. Rigel DS, Friedman RJ, Kopf AW, et al. (1986) Importance of complete cutaneous examination for the detection of malignant melanoma. *J Am Acad Dermatol* 14:857–860.
27. Czarnecki D, O'Brien T, Meehan C. (1994) Nonmelanoma skin cancer: numbers of cancers and their distribution in outpatients. *Int J Dermatol* 33:416,417.
28. Rigel DS. (1998) Is the ounce of screening and prevention for skin cancer worth the pound of cure? *CA Cancer J Clin* 48:236–238.
29. Whited JD, Grichnik JM. (1998) Does this patient have a mole or a melanoma? *JAMA* 279:696–701.
30. Grant-Kels JM, Bason ET, Grin CM. (1999) The misdiagnosis of malignant melanoma. *J Am Acad Dermatol* 40:539–548.
31. Engelberg D, Gallagher RP, Rivers JK. (1999) Follow-up and evaluation of skin cancer screening in British Columbia. *J Am Acad Dermatol* 41:37–42.

Chapter 11 / Screening for Skin Cancer 191

32. Bolognia JL, Berwick M, Fine JA. (1990) Complete follow-up and evaluation of a skin cancer screening in Connecticut. *J Am Acad Dermatol* 23:1098–1106.
33. Rampen FH, Casparie van Velsen JI, van Huytse BE, et al. (1995) False-negative findings in skin cancer and melanoma screening. *J Am Acad Dermatol* 33:59–63.
34. Grin CM, Kopf AW, Welkovich B, et al. (1990) Accuracy in the clinical diagnosis of malignant melanoma. *Arch Dermatol* 126:763–766.
35. Witheiler DD, Cockerell CJ. (1991) Histologic features and sensitivity of diagnosis of clinically unsuspected cutaneous melanoma. *Am J Dermatopathol* 13:551–556.
36. Reek MC, Chuang T-Y, Eads TJ, et al. (1999) The diagnostic yield in submitting nevi for histologic examination. *J Am Acad Dermatol* 40:567–571.
37. Wolf IH, Smolle J, Soyer HP, et al. (1998) Sensitivity in the clinical diagnosis of malignant melanoma. *Melanoma Res* 8:425–459.
38. Healsmith MF, Bourke JF, Osborne JE, et al. (1994) An evaluation of the revised seven-point checklist for the early diagnosis of cutaneous melanoma. *Br J Dermatol* 130:48–50.
39. McGovern TW, Litaker MS. (1992) Clinical predictors of malignant pigmented lesions: a comparison of the Glasgow seven-point checklist and the American Cancer Society's ABCDs of pigmented lesions. *J Dermatol Surg Oncol* 18:22–26.
40. Shaw HM, McCarthy WH. (1992) Small-diameter malignant melanoma: a common diagnosis in New South Wales, Australia. *J Am Acad Dermatol* 27:679–682.
41. Binder M, Schwarz M, Winkler A, et al. (1995) Epiluminescence microscopy. A useful tool for the diagnosis of pigmented skin lesions for formally trained dermatologists. *Arch Dermatol* 131:286–291.
42. Landau M, Matz H, Tur E, et al. (1999) Computerized system to enhance the clinical diagnosis of pigmented cutaneous malignancies. *Int J Dermatol* 38:443–446.
43. Rhodes AR. (1998) Intervention strategy to prevent lethal cutaneous melanoma: use of dermatologic photography to aid surveillance of high-risk persons. *J Am Acad Dermatol* 39:262–267.
44. Gruis NA, van der Velden PA, Bergman W, et al. (1999) Familial melanoma; CDKN2A and beyond. *J Invest Dermatol Symp Proc* 4:50–54.
45. Monzon J, Liu L, Brill H, et al. (1998) CDKN2A mutations in multiple primary melanomas. *N Engl J Med* 338:879–887.
46. Burden AD, Newell J, Andrew N, et al. (1999) Genetic and environmental influences in the development of multiple primary melanoma. *Arch Dermatol* 135:261–265.
47. Freedberg KA, Geller AC, Miller DR, et al. (1999) Screening for malignant melanoma: a cost-effectiveness analysis. *J Am Acad Dermatol* 41:738–745.
48. Tsao H, Rogers GS, Sober AJ. (1998) An estimate of the annual direct cost of treating cutaneous melanoma. *J Am Acad Dermatol* 38:669–680.
49. Cristofolini M, Bianchi R, Boi S, et al. (1993) Analysis of the cost-effectiveness ratio of the health campaign for the early diagnosis of cutaneous melanoma in Trentino, Italy. *Cancer* 71:370–374.
50. Federman DG, Concato J, Caralis PV, et al. (1997) Screening for skin cancer in primary care settings. *Arch Dermatol* 133:1423–1425.
51. Kirsner RS, Muhkerjee S, Federman DG. (1999) Skin cancer screening in primary care: prevalence and barriers. *J Am Acad Dermatol* 41:564–566.
52. Gerbert B, Maurer T, Berger T, et al. (1996) Primary care physicians as gatekeepers in managed care: primary care physicians' and dermatologists' skills at secondary prevention of skin cancer. *Arch Dermatol* 132:1030–1038.
53. Gerbert B, Bronstone A, Wolff M, et al. (1998) Improving primary care residents' proficiency in the diagnosis of skin cancer. *J Gen Intern Med* 13:91–97.
54. Fader DJ, Wise, CG, Normolle DP, et al. (1998) The multidisciplinary melanoma clinic: a cost outcomes analysis of specialty care. *J Am Acad Dermatol* 38:742–751.

VI — SCREENING FOR RESPIRATORY CANCERS

12 Screening for Lung Cancer

Michael J. McNamee, MD

KEY PRINCIPLES

- Lung cancer is the most frequent cause of cancer death in both men and women.
- It is plainly evident for several decades that more than 90% cases of lung cancer are caused by cigaret smoking and the most effective means of controlling lung cancer is prevention by reduction of tobacco use.
- No survival benefit in the screened population has been shown using presently available screening strategies, even in the high-risk patients.
- Several new techniques have shown promising results in the early detection of lung cancer, but further studies are needed.

EPIDEMIOLOGY

There is general agreement about several facts that have an impact on decisions about whether to utilize screening measures for the detection of lung cancer.

1. The United States began to experience an unprecedented epidemic of lung cancer in the latter half of the twentieth century, related to increases in cigaret smoking over the preceding 30 yr.
2. At least 90% of lung cancer is related to cigaret smoking. Other environmental exposures linked with lung cancer such as asbestos, radon, polycyclic aromatic hydrocarbons, chromium, nickel, and bis(choromethyl) ether are responsible for only a minority of cases.
3. The cure rate of lung cancer is 12% with an overall 5-yr survival of about 14%, increased only minimally over the past two decades despite

From: *Cancer Screening: A Practical Guide for Physicians*
Edited by: K. Aziz and G. Y. Wu © Humana Press Inc., Totowa, NJ

Table 1

Four Most Common Cancer Causes of Death

Primary site of cancer	No. of new cases (Estimated 1999)	No. of new deaths (Estimated 1999)	5-yr survival (%) (1989–1994)
Lung	171,600	158,900	14
Colorectal	129,400	56,600	63
Breast	176,300	43,700	85
Prostate	179,300	37,000	93

Source: Data from the American Cancer Society (Landis et al. [1999] *CA Cancer J Clin* 49:8). From Pulmonary Perspectives (ACCP) (1999) 16:3.

significant advances in diagnostic imaging, radiation therapy, and chemotherapy technologies. Lung cancer alone is responsible for more cancer deaths in the United States than the combined total from colorectal, breast, and prostate cancers (Table 1).

4. Males and females both exhibit a high risk of lung cancer from smoking, with lung cancer having surpassed breast cancer as the most common cause of cancer death in women. In 1964, the ratio of men to women dying of lung cancer was 7:1; more recently, it has fallen to 2:1, the lag resulting from widespread adoption of smoking by women a few decades later than by men. There is substantial evidence that women are more susceptible to harmful effects of cigaret smoking than are men.

5. Despite substantial public health efforts, smoking rates have not decreased to smoking cessation advocates expressed goals of 15%, with smokers continuing to represent about 25% of the population and with young people continuing to develop tobacco addiction.

6. Lung cancers detected at an early stage have much better 5-yr survival rates after successful surgical resection, as high as 70–80% for Stage I tumors. However only 15% of lung cancer is localized sufficiently to be resected reliably at the time of diagnosis (Stages I and II). Other factors such as performance status and histological subtype also affect survival.

7. Lung cancer mortality is especially high if the diagnosis is made as a result of the development of symptoms attributable to the cancer.

8. Despite the availability of potentially curative radiation therapy and chemotherapy, surgical resection is still regarded as the treatment of choice for cure of the non-small-cell carcinomas (squamous-cell carcinoma, adenocarcinoma, and large-cell undifferentiated carcinoma), necessitating early-stage diagnosis for success.

Chapter 12 / Screening for Lung Cancer 197

One could hardly imagine a confluence of circumstances better suited for screening than described by all of this: an easily definable at-risk population (chronic smokers) with far better survival rates with early-stage diagnosis and poor survival rates in symptomatic patients. One would intuit that this screening would be successful in saving the lives of some of the estimated 157,400 individuals who will die from the 170,000 lung cancer cases diagnosed in a single year. However, at the present time, government agencies, private philanthropic organizations, and medical societies (including the American Cancer Society, American College of Radiology, National Cancer Institute, U.S. Preventive Services Task Force, and the Canadian Task Force on the Health Examination) have not recommended routine screening for lung cancer. It is important that the primary care physician understand why screening for lung cancer has not been advocated, based on available scientific data, and why the approach to lung cancer has been vastly different from the approaches to colon cancer, breast cancer, and prostate cancer.

HISTORY OF LUNG CANCER SCREENING STUDIES

There has been general agreement that screening for small-cell lung carcinoma is ineffective, related to its short doubling time, early dissemination of disease, and propensity for central airway and mediastinal involvement. Screening efforts have therefore been directed at non-small-cell lung carcinomas, which represent 80% of primary lung cancers.

There have been three randomized, controlled studies in the United States designed to evaluate the effects of routine screening for lung cancer, primarily with the use of scheduled chest X-rays and sputum cytology studies. Yearly screening chest X-rays were recommended for smokers considered at high risk for lung cancer until the results of these studies were available. An understanding of the subject selection, design, and results of these studies is crucial to subsequent analysis of the validity of the conclusion not to recommend screening for lung cancer.

The most influential of these studies was the Mayo Clinic Project which enrolled 10,933 subjects from 1971 through 1976 *(1,2)*. The subjects were a high-risk group of men, over 45 yr of age, with a smoking history of at least one pack per day. Initial screening by chest X-ray and 3-d pooled sputum cytology was performed to determine prevalence of undiagnosed lung cancer at the onset and 91 cases were diagnosed. The case prevalence from ages 45 to 49 was 1 per 1000 (0.1%) and for ages over 65 was 17 per 1000 (1.7%). These cases were excluded from the longitudinal phase of the study. Subjects were also excluded if they had a life expectancy of less than 5 yr or were poor risks for potential pulmonary resection.

A total of 9211 study subjects (no cancer at onset, operable if necessary, with life expectancy >5 yr) were then randomized to control and screening groups and studied for 11 yr. There were 221 late-stage tumors diagnosed, 109 in the control group and 112 in the screened group. Overall, there was an excess of 46 cases of lung cancer diagnosed in the screened group, almost all early-stage and resectable, both squamous-cell carcinomas and adenocarcinomas. One would expect that there would be an increased number of early carcinomas in the screened group, followed by an increased number of late-stage (previously undetected) carcinomas in the control group; however, this latter pattern, expected in a successful screening intervention, never materialized in the 11-yr follow-up.

Analysis of the effects of screening was complicated by the fact that 116 cancers in the screened group were detected outside of screening and 44% of these were in the 25% of the screened group that did not comply with the screening schedule. Thus, some of the screened group functioned similarly to the control group. In addition, 30% of the lung cancers in the control group were found on what amounted to screening X-rays such as those done during routine physicals and for preoperative evaluation. Furthermore, 50% of the control group had yearly chest X-rays anyway and 80% had a chest X-ray over a 2-yr period for one reason or another. All of this served to narrow the difference between the screened and control groups, making it less likely that there would be a difference and significantly reducing the study's power to show any dramatic effect.

Screen-detected cancers (50% via sputum analysis and 35% via chest X-ray) had a >35% survival rate, compared with symptom-detected cancers, with a survival rate of 10%. These survival rate differences are consistent with those generally found throughout the medical literature. However, even intensive screening failed to detect many lung cancers before they were unresectable. There was no overall survival benefit from screening (cancer death rate 3.1 per 1000 person-years in the screened group compared with 3.0 in the control group), at least partly because there was no increase in late-stage cancers in the control group as would be expected from the progression of unscreened and undetected early cancers.

A recommendation not to screen routinely for lung cancer with either chest X-ray or sputum analysis followed the Mayo Clinic Project report *(3)*. However, dissatisfaction with the study design has continued to provoke controversy and statistical reanalyses *(4–8)*. It is not surprising

Chapter 12 / Screening for Lung Cancer

that repeated demonstration of far better survival rates for early stage tumors have fueled ongoing uncertainty. Furthermore, the finding of a prevalence of 0.83% of lung cancer is sufficient to allow for reasonable consideration of screening.

Similarly, the Memorial Sloan-Kettering lung cancer screening program enrolled 10,040 male smokers beginning in 1974 (9). Subjects were screened with annual chest X-rays with or without sputum cytology examination every 4 mo. The study was not designed to study chest X-ray screening primarily. Of the 288 cancers detected, 40% were diagnosed at Stage I with a 5-yr survival of 76%. This contrasted with an overall 35% 5-yr survival and a 20% 8-yr survival. Chest X-ray was more likely to detect cancer than sputum examination. Despite evidence for early-stage detection with better survival in a small number of subjects, there was no difference in the number of cancers, the number of late-stage cancers, the number of resectable cancers, or the number of cancer deaths between the two groups. The same study done at Johns Hopkins produced what were essentially the same results (10).

A Czech study enrolled 6364 men and evaluated the screening group with chest X-ray and sputum cytology every 6 mo for 3 yr. The control group had an initial prevalence screen, followed by a chest X-ray 3 yr later. Subsequently, each group had a yearly chest X-ray for an additional 3 yr. In the initial screening, 36 cancers were found in the screening group, 25% resectable, with a 25% 5-yr survival. In the control group, 19 cancers were found, 15% resectable, with no 3-yr survival. Over the entire 6-yr period, however, there were 85 deaths with 108 cancers in the screened group and 67 deaths with 82 cancers in the control group. The differences were not statistically significant. Like the Mayo Clinic Project study, the screened group showed advantages in stage distribution, resectability, and survival in early-detected tumors but not an improvement in overall survival (11).

CURRENT PRACTICE BY PRIMARY CARE PHYSICIANS

Interestingly, a recent survey (1996) revealed that 25% of Australian family physicians recommend an annual chest X-ray as a screening test for lung cancer in asymptomatic heavy smokers. Although this is fewer than the 44% reported in surveys by the American Cancer Society in 1984 and 1989, it still represents a significant departure from recommendations related to the Mayo Clinic Project and other studies noted earlier (12). Older physicians who responded were more likely to believe in the value of annual screening for lung cancer. It is not clear from the available data whether they are ignorant of or simply reject the recommendation not to screen.

CURRENT STATUS OF POTENTIAL SCREENING METHODS

Chest X-Ray

Of studies potentially useful in the detection of early-stage lung cancer, the chest X-ray is the most frequently employed. Unfortunately, it has been reported that a radiologist working under standard conditions has about a 50% likelihood of failing to identify a pulmonary nodule 5 mm or smaller. Nonetheless, screened groups continue to show detection of smaller Stage I tumors, higher resectability rates, and higher survival for patients whose tumors are detected early.

A 1993 retrospective study in Japan reviewed the X-rays of all patients with lung cancer arising in a >40-yr-old population undergoing mass screening *(13)*. No attempt was made to identify highest-risk patients and both smokers and nonsmokers were screened.The sensitivity of cancer detection was greatest for adenocarcinoma (85%), consistent with the understanding that adenocarcinomas have a mean duration from Stage I to advanced disease of at least 4 yr. Detection at quite a small size would appear to be crucial, as 58% of adenocarcinomas larger than 2.0 cm had already metastasized at the time of detection. Small lesions were difficult to see as judged by their frequent visibility in retrospect. Squamous-cell tumors were more likely to progress from invisible (even in retrospect) to larger than 2.0 cm within 1 yr, reducing the sensitivity for squamous-cell tumors to 52% and making the utility of yearly chest X-ray screening questionable. Overall, only 103 Stage I lung carcinomas were detected in over 300,000 cases. It is clear from these data that highest-risk patients should be targeted in any reasonable screening effort.

Salomaa in 1998 reported finding 93 cancers out of 33,743 screened with a single X-ray in a cancer prevention study *(14)*. Screen-detected tumors were diagnosed at an earlier stage, had higher resectability rates, and better survival than a comparable unscreened group whose chest X-rays were done related to "ordinary health care."

Although interest in chest X-ray screening persists, it is becoming eclipsed by the prospect of low-dose helical computed tomogrpahy (CT) scanning, as the time commitment and cost per scan have diminished and would likely be further reduced in any higher-volume screening campaign.

Low-Dose Helical CT Scan

Multiple studies have now documented that CT scanning is more sensitive than conventional chest X-ray for detection of small lung cancers. Low-dose CT scanning does not require dye injection, can be

Chapter 12 / Screening for Lung Cancer

accomplished in about 20 s of scanning time, and does not expose the patient to a large radiation dose (a dose comparable to that provided with mammography), making it a potentially suitable screening technique. Low-dose helical CT scanning has shown a higher detection rate of lung cancer than conventional chest X-ray (0.48% compared with 0.04%) with a mean lesion size of 17 mm in diameter (15), comparable to another study that confirmed a lung cancer detection rate of 0.37% with most cancers found at Stage I with a mean tumor diameter of 15 mm and a 3-yr survival rate of 83%. In one Japanese study of elderly heavy smokers (mean age 60.7 yr), lung cancer was found in 22 of 1443 subjects screened with low-dose helical CT and sputum analysis (16). CT scanning has been found to be sensitive with a dose setting not less than 6 Ma (17). However, there are still limited data available to assess the overall survival impact of such early detection related to CT scanning. Furthermore, there are only early data looking at the morbidity or mortality related to lung nodules small enough and nonspecific enough to require invasive biopsy or excision for diagnosis. The positive predictive value of CT scanning in the diagnosis of lung cancer has been estimated to be about 8.5%, based on an incidence of 19 cancers in 223 suspicious CT lesions recently reported (15). As most of the early detection of lung cancers by CT has been reported with prevalence studies, there is little information in the literature about the frequency of CT scanning that would be optimal in a regular screening program.

The Early Lung Cancer Action Project (ELCAP), begun in 1992, may answer questions about the utility of low-dose CT scanning by screening 1000 high-risk patients aged 60 and over for lung cancer (18). Not surprisingly, a preliminary report has confirmed the capability of CT scanning at baseline to detect small, noncalcified lung nodules in 23%, compared with 7% detected by chest X-ray. Malignant disease was detected in 2.7% by CT (23 of 27 at Stage I) and 0.7% by chest X-ray. Even the Stage I tumors detected by CT were smaller than those detected by chest X-ray. Documentation that noncalcified nodules are detectable at three times the rate with chest X-ray, malignant tumors at four times the rate, and Stage I tumors at six times the rate of chest X-ray raises serious questions as to whether chest X-rays can be effective as a screening strategy. Twenty-six of 27 malignancies were resectable. Of the 233 noncalcified nodules, only 28 were biopsied, one of which was benign.

A schedule of CT follow-up scans has been used for small nodules judged to be of low risk for malignancy based on their radiological appearance, limiting the morbidity and costs associated with large numbers of biopsies. The investigators report no cases of malignancy thus far in lesions so followed. This begins to address a long-standing con-

202 Part VI / Screening for Respiratory Cancers

cern about avoiding unnecessary thoracotomy for the evaluation of detected nodules that are found to be benign. New technologies may be helpful in this area, including less debilitating video-assisted thoracoscopic surgery (VATS).

Positron emission tomography (PET) complements other radiological assessment and FDG-PET (F-2-deoxy-D-glucose labeled scanning) shows a high specificity for malignant nodules in the elderly population. Increasingly, it should become unnecessary to resort to invasive procedures for management of nodules detected by low-dose CT scanning.

The ELCAP study has not matured enough to report survival data or such epidemiological data as cost per estimated year of life saved. Nonetheless, estimates of survival rates of 80% would be expected for small Stage I tumors, consistent with other screening studies' data. With awareness that only about 20% of all new lung cancers are diagnosed in Stage I or II and with confirmation already that CT scanning can detect 80% of lung cancers in Stage I, it is clear that lung cancer screening by low-dose helical CT scan may benefit the high-risk patient.

SPUTUM CYTOLOGY ANALYSIS

The examination of sputum smears for malignant cells, introduced in the mid-1930s, has been a valuable tool in the diagnosis of lung cancers suspected from clinical illness or radiological abnormality. Accuracy of analysis requires skilled interpretation and can be labor intensive, with increased efficiency provided using thin-smear and cell block techniques. The sensitivity of conventional sputum cytology has been found to be only 64.5%, albeit with a 97.9% specificity. Unfortunately, in general, the sensitivity of conventional sputum cytology is greatest with central, more advanced-stage lung cancers, which are less likely to result in improved survival after early detection.

Despite discouraging results over the last 20 yr with conventional sputum cytology as a screening measure, there is continued interest in technologic modifications that might increase sensitivity. In 1997, Payne et al. subjected 73 archived sputum specimens from the Mayo Clinic Project to repeat analysis for "malignancy-associated changes" with quantitative microscopy, looking for subvisual nuclear changes that may be found associated with tumors in visually normal nuclei *(19)*. They looked at negative specimens from the Mayo study and compared the results for those who did not develop lung cancer during the years of follow-up with those who did. A higher sensitivity for tumor cell detection could be developed (83%) but with a positive predictive value of only 50%. Tockman et al. used monoclonal antibodies for early lung cancer detection and reported a sensitivity of 64% *(20)*. Subsequent

Chapter 12 / Screening for Lung Cancer 203

reports have indicated even higher sensitivity and specificity. It may be that combinations of such approaches in sputum analysis will enhance sensitivity enough to make screening more productive, although the detection of small peripheral tumors is likely to remain elusive because of the absence of tumor or tumor-affected cells in expectorated specimens. Monoclonal antibodies used in immuno-staining sputum to recognize difucosylated Lewis X and a 31-kDa protein have shown a correlation between positive staining and later development of lung cancer *(21)*.

Sputum screening of patients with significant smoking histories and chronic airway obstructive disease has identified carcinoma or severe dysplasia in 2.5% and moderate dysplasia in 25% *(22)*. Such screening may identify a subset of patients who would benefit from standard or autofluorescent bronchoscopic examination of the central airways for tumor detection.

STRATEGY FOR PRIMARY CARE PHYSICIANS

Pending additional studies that should clarify the utility of various screening modalities in terms of their sensitivity, specificity, risk, survival benefit, and cost, what should be the approach by the primary physician to the patient at risk for lung cancer?

Prevention

The primary objective for the primary physician should be to prevent exposure of any patient to the carcinogens in cigaret smoke. This would obviate the need for screening, which surely would be inappropriate to apply to nonsmokers (even individuals with asbestos, second-hand tobacco smoke, or radon exposure) whose relative risk of lung cancer is insufficient to justify screening. Part of the physician's role in prevention, in addition to general health promotion and individual counseling of young patients not to begin smoking, is to advocate elimination of tobacco smoke exposure in public environments. Focused radon and asbestos detection and abatement should also be advocated.

Risk Recognition

The primary care physician should recognize the patient at high risk for lung cancer. A comprehensive history will determine the duration and intensity of cigaret smoking. It should include a thorough occupational and environmental history sufficient to detect asbestos or other carcinogenic exposures so as to allow for risk stratification. Patients over 50 yr old with a heavy smoking history (>30 pack-years), and especially those with chronic airflow obstruction (FEV1 <70% of predicted) and/or asbestos exposure, carry the highest risk. It is important to evaluate heavy smokers for the presence of chronic airway obstruction (in general, a simple flow-volume loop is sufficient), which develops in about 15% of smokers, as it establishes an additional Algorithm 1).

Risk Reduction

Smoking cessation is effective in reducing the chronic smoker's risk of lung cancer, with gradual diminution of risk of mortality ratios from at least 10:1 to 2:1 over 15–20 yr. Adjunctive supports to smoking cessation such as nicotine replacement and psychotropic medications such as buproprion have been shown to enhance the effectiveness of strong physician counseling.

Screening

Although routine interval chest X-ray screening for lung cancer is currently not recommended, there is room for individualization of approach by the primary care physician. In high-risk patients, one could consider obtaining a yearly chest X-ray or lowering one's threshold for obtaining a chest ray for acute or persistent respiratory symptoms not likely to be related to cancer. In the Mayo Clinic Project study, many early-stage lung cancers were found with X-rays done for other purposes.

Data from prevalence screening with low-dose CT scanning are already favorable and reproducible enough to suggest a benefit from screening of high-risk patients. The primary care physician who wishes to consider individualizing such screening for high-risk patients will need to confirm the availability of appropriate scanning technique, the interpretive expertise of the consulting radiologist, and the willingness of the patient to accept surgical intervention for a positive finding. Insurance reimbursement could be a problem unless and until a consensus favoring such screening is reached.

At present, the role of sputum analysis as a screening device for lung cancer is ill defined, although new technology may make it an attractive adjunct to radiological study in the future. It remains a reasonably sensitive test for central airway tumors, particularly squamous-cell cancers.

Literature Surveillance and Awareness

A number of studies underway, including ELCAP, are beginning to result in a change in attitude and likely in recommendations about screening for lung cancer. If recommendations for screening are developed, attention needs to be paid to the lower limit of age appropriate for screening, as risk of lung cancer is heavily influenced by advancing age as well as smoking history. Additionally, there is likely to be controversy about the

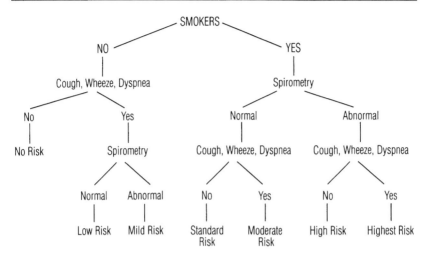

Algorithm 1. Algorithm to assist in the determination of lung cancer risk level in smokers vs nonsmokers. (From Petty TL. [1998] Where to catch a fish: a commentary on the early diagnosis of lung cancer. *Curr Clin Trials Thoracic Oncol* 2(1):7. Used with permission.)

optimal frequency of screening. The primary care physician will need to remain vigilant and begin to apply new strategies such as low-dose CT scanning on an individual basis after discussion with high-risk patients or on a wider scale if a consensus develops that it is beneficial and cost-efficient. Such a consensus would, of course, be widely reported in the media, as it would represent a major divergence from the practice of the past 20 yr.

Specialist Referral

Risk stratification for lung cancer is dependent on a careful history related to respiratory symptoms, tobacco use, occupational and other environmental carcinogenic exposures, family history, and detection of airflow obstruction. None of these issues falls outside of the expertise of the primary physician. Health promotion, with smoking prevention and smoking cessation, is also part of the daily practice of the primary physician. However, as in any area of medicine, there are difficult patients who may require additional opinion, reinforcement, and motivation to adhere to a prescribed regimen, making specialty consultation appropriate. The detection of a lung nodule by chest X-ray or CT scan is a frequent impetus to the review of a case by a pulmonary specialist, who likely has more experience in dealing with the differential diagnoses and probabilities. Primary physician–pulmonologist–radiologist collaboration is likely to be essential when decisions need to be made about whether and how to approach asymptomatic lesions, no matter how they came to be imaged.

SUMMARY

- The persistence of an epidemic of lung cancer, associated with an unyielding high mortality related to symptomatic disease, continues to cry out for a successful screening strategy.
- A recommendation in place for over more than a decade not to employ widespread screening, based on available survival data, remains controversial.
- Newer technologies are likely to make screening for lung cancer a viable option, with low-dose helical CT scanning the most attractive option at present.
- We have the information needed to stratify risk and thereby determine who is at most need of screening.
- We need additional data regarding appropriate screening methods, impact on disease survival, optimal frequency of screening interventions, and cost-efficiency.
- As is the case with other screening, such as mammography, prostatic-specific antigen, stool for occult blood, if lung cancer screening is recommended, the primary care physician will be its coordinator.

REFERENCES

1. Fontana RS, Sanderson DR, Taylor WF, et al. (1984) Early lung cancer detection: results of the initial (prevalence) radiologic and cytologic screening in the Mayo Clinic Study. *Am Rev Resp Dis* 130:561–565.
2. Muhm JR, Miller WE, Fontana RS, Sanderson DR, Uhlenhopp MA. (1983) Lung cancer detected during a screening program using four-month chest radiographs. *Radiology* 148:609–615.
3. U. S. Preventive Services Task Force. (1990) Screening for lung cancer. *Chest* 41:1763–1766.
4. Flehinger BJ, Kimmel M, Polyak T, Melamed MR. (1993) Screening for lung cancer. *Cancer* 72:1573–1580.
5. Strauss GM. (1997) Measuring effectiveness of lung cancer screening. *Chest* 112:216S–28S.
6. Wolpaw DR. (1996) Early detection in lung cancer. *Med Clin N Am* 80(1):63–82.
7. Strauss GM, Gleason RE, Sugarbaker DJ. (1995) Chest x-ray screening improves outcome in lung cancer. *Chest* 107:270S–279S.
8. Epstein DM. (1990) The role of radiologic screening in lung cancer. *Rad Clin NA* 28:489–495.
9. Melamed MR, Flehniger BJ, Zaman MB, et al. (1984) Screening for early lung cancer. *Chest* 86:44–53.
10. Frost JK, Ball WC, Levin ML, et al. (1984) Early lung cancer detection: results of the initial (prevalence) radiologic and cytologic screening in the Johns Hopkins Study. *Am Rev Resp Dis* 130:549–554.
11. Kubik A, Polak J. (1986) Lung cancer detection. *Cancer* 57:2427–2437.
12. Sladden MJ, Ward JE. (1999) Do Australian family physicians screen smokers for lung cancer? *Chest* 115:725–728.
13. Soda H, Tomita H, Kohno S, Oka M. (1993) Limitation of annual screening chest radiography for the diagnosis of lung cancer. *Cancer* 72(8):2341–2346.

Chapter 12 / Screening for Lung Cancer 207

14. Salomaa E, Liippo K, Taylor P, et al. (1998) Prognosis of patients with lung cancer found in a single chest radiograph screening. *Chest* 114:1514–1518.
15. Sone S, Takashima S, Feng L, et al. (1998) Mass screening for lung cancer with mobile spiral computed tomography scanner. *Lancer* 351:1242–1245.
16. Kaneko M, Eguchi K, Ohmatsua H, et al. (1996) Peripheral lung cancer screening and detection with low-dose spiral CT vs. radiography. *Radiology* 201:796–802.
17. Nitta N, Takahashi M, Murata K, Morita R. (1998) Ultra low-dose helical CT of the chest. *Am J Roentgen* 171:383–385.
18. Henschke CI, McCauley DI, Yankelevitz DF, et al. (1999) Early Lung Cancer Action Project: overall design and findings from baseline screening. *Lancet* 354:99–105.
19. Payne PW, Sebo TJ, Doudkine A, et al. (1997) Sputum screening by quantitative microscopy: a reexamination of a portion of the National Cancer Institute Cooperative Early Lung Cancer Study. *Mayo Clin Proc* 72:697–704.
20. Tockman MS, Gupta PK, Myers JD, et al. (1988) Sensitive and specific monoclonal antibody recognition of human lung cancer antigen on preserved sputum cells: a new approach to early lung cancer detection. *J Clin Oncol* 6:1685–693.
21. Mulshine JL, Scott F. (1995) Molecular markers in early cancer detection. *Chest* 107:280S–286S.
22. Kennedy TC, Proudfoot SP, Franklin WA, et al. (1996) Cytopathological analysis of sputum in patients with airflow obstruction and significant smoking histories. *Cancer Res* 56:4673–4678.

VII
SCREENING FOR CANCER IN HIGH-RISK GROUPS

13 Screening for Esophageal Cancer in High-Risk Groups

Barrett's Esophagus

Elisabeth I. Heath, MD
and Marcia I. F. Canto, MD

KEY PRINCIPLES

- Adenocarcinoma of the esophagus is rising in incidence and carries a significant morbidity and mortality.
- Barrett's esophagus is the major risk factor for developing adenocarcinoma of the esophagus.
- Endoscopic surveillance of Barrett's esophagus using a rigorous biopsy protocol is a cost-effective method of screening.
- Warning signs such as heartburn, regurgitation, long-standing reflux symptoms, dysphagia, odynophagia, family history of Barrett's esophagus or esophageal cancer, or prior history of Barrett's esophagus indicate a referral to a subspecialist for further workup.
- Treatment of Barrett's esophagus includes therapy for gastroesophageal reflux disease (using H-2 blockers, proton-pump inhibitors, or prokinetic agents), or surgical therapy.
- Mucosal ablation is an endoscopic therapy that is currently under evaluation for eradication of Barrett's esophagus and dysplasia.

INTRODUCTION

Esophageal cancer is a disease of high mortality and morbidity. Despite major advances in the field of oncology, the age-adjusted mor-

From: *Cancer Screening: A Practical Guide for Physicians*
Edited by: K. Aziz and G. Y. Wu © Humana Press Inc., Totowa, NJ

tality for this cancer remains almost similar to the incidence, indicating the high mortality rate for this cancer. The survival statistics have not changed significantly within the past 30 yr *(1)*. One of the major factors for the poor survival rate is the advanced stage of the disease at the time of diagnosis. In a symptomatic patient, the 5-yr survival is less than 10% *(2)*. The prognosis is considerably improved when patients are diagnosed at an early stage of esophageal cancer. Thus, strategies for identifying high-risk patients, implementation of an early detection and surveillance program, and the design of primary and secondary preventive measures are critical in improving the rate of survival.

EPIDEMIOLOGY OF ESOPHAGEAL CANCER

Cancer of the esophagus has one of the highest variations in geographic distribution and sex ratios of any solid malignancy. There is a 17-fold difference in the mortality between the high- and the low-incidence areas. The reason for this extreme variation in the incidence is unclear, but it is probably related to nutritional and environmental factors *(3)*. Squamous-cell carcinoma (SCC) and adenocarcinoma (AC) account for more than 95% of all esophageal tumors. The estimated number of new cases of squamous cell carcinoma and adenocarcinoma of the esophagus in the United States is 12,300 and the estimated number of deaths is 11,900 *(4)*. Historically, SCC has been considered synonymous with esophageal carcinoma in the United States. In a study of 1312 esophageal carcinomas diagnosed between 1946 and 1963, only 3.3% were adenocarcinomas, however, within the last three decades, the incidence of AC has increased significantly and recent data suggest that AC accounts for almost 60% of newly diagnosed esophageal cancers, an increase of more than 350% *(5–7)*. The incidence of SCC, on the other hand, has not changed significantly during the same time period *(8)*. The incidence of AC has not only increased in the United States, but also in Scandinavia and areas of Western Europe. However, in Asian countries, such as Japan and China, the incidence has not changed significantly. SCC is the prevalent type of esophageal cancer in these countries.

In the United States, there are racial differences with regard to the histologic type of cancer. In white males over the age of 65 yr, the age-adjusted rates for developing esophageal adenocarcinoma has increased three- to fourfold *(9)*. In contrast, SCC of the esophagus is six times more likely to occur in African-American males compared to white males *(10)*.

The reasons for the rising incidence of esophageal adenocarcinoma are unclear. However, two major risk factors have been identified. These

Chapter 13 / Screening for Esophageal Cancer 213

include Barrett's esophagus (BE) and chronic gastroesophageal reflux disease (GERD). Patients with Barrett's esophagus have a 30–125 times increased risk of developing AC as compared to the age-matched population, with a yearly cancer risk of 1.37% *(11,12)*. GERD and other acid peptic disorders are also significant risk factors for developing esophageal cancer. Recently, a large case-control population-based study suggests that the esophageal AC is strongly associated with GERD, even in the absence of Barrett's esophagus. Lagergren et al. reported recurrent symptoms of reflux are associated with a 7.7-fold (95% confidence interval [CI] = 5.3–11.4) increased risk of developing adenocarcinoma of the esophagus. GERD has not been shown to increase the risk of SCC of the esophagus *(13)*.

The high mortality and the lack of efficacy of chemotherapy and radiation therapy provide the rationale for promoting surveillance endoscopy in patients with chronic GERD symptoms, particularly those with known Barrett's metaplasia. This chapter will describe the epidemiology, risk factors, and screening recommendations for Barrett's esophagus.

RISK FACTORS FOR BARRETT'S ESOPHAGUS

Barrett's esophagus occurs when metaplastic columnar epithelium (specialized columnar epithelium defined by the presence of goblet cells) replaces normal stratified squamous epithelium of the distal esophagus *(14)*. The estimated prevalence of Barrett's esophagus is 700,000, however, this is probably an underestimation because of the high number of undiagnosed asymptomatic patients *(15)*. The risk factor for the development of Barrett's esophagus is primarily GERD. GERD results in chronic inflammation involving the mucosa and submucosa, which is manifested as reflux esophagitis. It is thought that this, in turn, leads to a change in the epithelial cells, perhaps from some progenitor cells, to columnar epithelium *(16,17)*. The origin of the progenitor cells is unknown but currently thought to be from either the esophageal basal epithelial cells, esophageal glands, gastric rests in the distal esophagus, fundic mucosa in the stomach, or duodenal or gastric cells in the refluxate. Approximately 12–18% of patients with GERD will develop Barrett's esophagus *(18)*. Although not well understood, it is thought that certain genetic changes occur in the metaplastic tissue that eventually lead to neoplastic progression.

Barrett's metaplasia occurs in patients of all ages. The average age at diagnosis of Barrett's esophagus varies from 55 to 63 yr *(19)*. Barrett's esophagus, however, is not solely a disease of the elderly. Several series of pediatric patients with Barrett's esophagus have been reported *(20)*.

214 Part VII / Screening for Cancers in High-Risk Groups

The prevalence of Barrett's esophagus increases with age until a plateau is reached in the 60s *(21)*. The age-specific prevalence ranged from 0.147% in 10–19 yr olds, to 0.257% in 30–39 yr olds, to 0.920% in 70–79 yr olds. About one-quarter of the final prevalence was reached by age 30 and one-half by age 40 *(22–24)*.

For reasons that remain unclear, men are at a greater risk for developing adenocarcinoma of the esophagus. In several large series, nearly 80% of patients with Barrett's esophagus were men *(25–27)*. This difference in risk occurs despite the fact that reflux has similar prevalence in males and females across various age groups *(28)*.

RISK OF ADENOCARCINOMA IN BARRETT'S ESOPHAGUS

The estimated annual risk for adenocarcinoma ranges from 0.2 to 2% in patients with Barrett's esophagus. Tumor progression occurs when metaplastic columnar tissue leads to dysplastic tissue, which, in turn, leads to adenocarcinoma. Dysplasia is defined as precancerous tissue because the basement membrane is intact. It is currently classified as absent, low grade, indefinite, or high grade. High-grade dysplasia, which was previously called carcinoma *in situ*, has the highest potential for developing malignancy. Data on 285 patients from four centers that have performed prospective studies showed 34% patients with high-grade dysplasia developed AC during a follow-up period of 0.2–4.5 yr, 18% with low-grade dysplasia developed AC during a follow-up period of 1.5–4.3 yr, and 3% without dysplasia developed AC over an interval of 3.4–10 yr *(29–32)*.

The diagnostic pathology criteria for dysplasia in Barrett's esophagus are difficult and even expert pathologists often have discrepancy in their diagnosis, particularly with low-grade and indefinite dysplasia. However, there is a higher concordance with high-grade dysplasia and carcinoma (85 vs 72%) *(33)*. With high-grade dysplasia, it is important to obtain an adequate sample, so that invasive adenocarcinoma is not overlooked. Hence, once high-grade dysplasia is diagnosed by biopsy, immediate confirmation is required by repeat endoscopy and biopsy.

The length of Barrett's esophagus (short-segment vs long-segment Barrett's esophagus) and the risk of developing AC has been a subject of controversy for a long time. Association between AC and long-segment Barrett's esophagus is well known. In recent years, several studies have emphasized the premalignant potential of short-segment Barrett's esophagus. Data from three large studies suggests that the risk of AC for short-segment Barrett's esophagus (<3 cm) is less than long-segment Barrett's esophagus (>3 cm). The rate of dysplasia was 15.4% for the

Chapter 13 / Screening for Esophageal Cancer

long-segment Barrett's esophagus and 8% for the short-segment Barrett's esophagus *(34–36)*.

THE MOLECULAR BASIS FOR CARCINOGENESIS IN BARRETT'S ESOPHAGUS

Barrett's mucosa has been studied intensively for histologic and molecular changes that may predispose it to malignancy. Several abnormalities have been demonstrated in the Barrett's mucosa histologically and by flow cytometry. These include chromosomal abnormalities detected in short-term cultures of Barrett's mucosa, with chromosomal rearrangement, and clonal proliferation of karyotypically abnormal cells *(37)*.

Ornithine decarboxylase (ODC) activity in Barrett's mucosa is elevated compared with that in the adjacent gastric or small intestinal epithelium, which suggests that the regulation of polyamine metabolism by this enzyme may be altered in this premalignant tissue. In 15 patients with Barrett's mucosa, high-grade dysplasia had more ODC activity than low-grade dysplasia *(38)*.

P53 mutations were identified in four of seven samples of Barrett's epithelium that had little or no dysplasia but were located adjacent to esophageal adenocarcinomas. This finding suggests that p53 mutations may be a marker for premalignant changes in Barrett's mucosa. These findings were confirmed by Schneider and co-workers *(39)* in a prospective evaluation of patients with Barrett's epithelium or Barrett's epithelium and carcinoma. Mutations of p53 were involved in the pathogenesis of Barrett's cancer for a subset of patients (46%) with cancer. In patients with Barrett's epithelium and no- or low-grade dysplasia, mutations were not found; however, in one of three patients with high-grade dysplasia, p53 mutations were found. These findings support the hypothesis that p53 mutations may be a useful marker for patients at increased risk for the development of invasive cancer.

METHODS OF SCREENING

Screening Endoscopy for Chronic GERD and Suspected Barrett's Esophagus

Screening patients who are at high risk for developing esophageal adenocarcinoma requires identification of the appropriate patient population. Patients with recurrent symptoms of GERD and/or suspected Barrett's esophagus should be referred for upper endoscopy. Currently, the American College of Gastroenterology (ACG) recommends upper endoscopy for individuals over the age of 50 who have had symptomatic

GERD for at least 5–10 yr *(40)*. Endoscopy is the gold standard in evaluating the upper alimentary tract. It allows for direct visualization of the target organ. At the time of endoscopy, the presence of columnar-type epithelium, hiatal hernia, and any lesions such as nodules, polyps, ulcers, strictures, or esophagitis are noted. The location of the gastroesophageal junction and squamo-columnar junction are also recorded. The latter is the most proximal level of the gastric folds with minimal air insufflation. The estimated length of Barrett's esophagus is also clinically relevant; this is equal to the distance of the gastroesophageal junction (or proximal level of the gastric folds) from the gums minus that of the squamo-columnar junction. Biopsies from columnar-type epithelium should be obtained and the location of the biopsies (distance from the gums) recorded. Care should be taken not to biopsy from within the hiatal hernia because intestinal metaplasia at the gastric cardia has been shown to be a common finding (prevalence 19–22%) and may not necessarily confer the same risk of esophageal cancer as Barrett's esophagus *(34)*. The presence of distinctive Barrett's epithelium is necessary because there are patients who have only gastric cardia or fundic-type metaplasia in the distal esophagus or intestinal metaplasia in the gastric cardia.

Surveillance Endoscopy for Established Barrett's Esophagus

Patients with biopsy-proven Barrett's esophagus should undergo periodic endoscopic surveillance, depending on the individual patient risk–benefit ratio. Surveillance is only appropriate for patients who are fit for therapy.

The technique for optimal screening or surveillance for cancer in Barrett's esophagus has not been established nor definitively proven to be of benefit by any randomized trial. A systematic biopsy protocol has been generally recommended. This technique obtains biopsy specimens from each quadrant of the esophagus every 1–2 cm from the gastroesophageal junction to 1 cm above the squamo-columnar line *(27)*. The "Seattle" protocol was originally described in patients with high-grade dysplasia, in whom the risk of cancer is between 33 and 45%. The group from the University of Washington in Seattle showed that all incidental cancers that develop in Barrett's esophagus could be diagnosed using their rigid biopsy protocol *(27)*. However, others have criticized this technique because of the number of biopsies required, particularly for long segments of Barrett's esophagus, and the associated costs and time required.

There is no accepted optimal method for tissue sampling. Although the large ("jumbo") biopsy forceps is often used in the research setting, this is clearly not routinely used in practice *(40)*. Indeed, only 15% of

Chapter 13 / Screening for Esophageal Cancer   217

gastroenterologists in the United States take jumbo biopsies for Barrett's esophagus surveillance *(40)*. The reason for this is not clear, but it could be related to the need for an endoscope with a large "therapeutic" channel in order to pass the jumbo forceps. Whereas the American College of Gastroentrology does not specifically recommend the Seattle protocol, it describes a biopsy technique that involves obtaining multiple biopsies from normal-appearing and abnormal BE (ulcer, nodule, stricture) *(41)*. The American Society of Gastrointestinal Endoscopy (ASGE) describes "one acceptable method" for surveillance biopsy as four-quadrant biopsies with jumbo biopsies taken at 2-cm intervals starting 1 cm below the esophagogastric junction and extending 1 cm above the squamo-columnar junction *(42)*. This is a modification of the original Seattle technique that samples from four-quadrants at 1-cm intervals. Unfortunately, this modified Seattle biopsy technique may still miss unsuspected adenocarcinomas in BE, with only high-grade dysplasia identified in endoscopic biopsies *(40)*.

Transnasal Balloon Cell Sampling

There has been some attempt to study a nonendoscopic method for screening patients for Barrett's esophagus, dysplasia, and cancer using a transnasal balloon for sampling cells for cytological examination *(43,44)*. This balloon has soft cones to enhance cell collection and is 9 mm wide when deflated and 3 cm wide when inflated. In a study of 63 patients with established BE, cytological specimens were obtained from the esophagus using the Brandt esophageal cytology balloon (Wilson-Cook Medical, Winston-Salem, NC) followed by EGD with biopsy and brush cytology *(43)*. Only 83% of patients with established BE had adequate sampling of columnar epithelium. Furthermore, the sensitivity of balloon cytology for high-grade dysplasia or adenocarcinoma was 80% but only 25% for low-grade dysplasia. In another study, investigators were unable to find specialized columnar epithelium in any of the patients with established BE using the same balloon cytology technique, however, the number of patients enrolled in this study was small *(44)*. Although the potential cost savings is great for diagnosis and surveillance of BE, this nonendoscopic method does not appear to be sufficiently sensitive for use in clinical practice.

Special Techniques: Chromoendoscopy

During endoscopy, staining the mucosa with Lugol's solution or methylene blue may enhance the diagnosis of Barrett's esophagus, dysplasia, and esophageal cancer. Lugol's solution contains iodine and potassium iodide. Within a few minutes of spraying this solution on the mucosal surface, the normal epithelium changes to a dark brown/greenish brown color. However, dysplastic or malignant tissue will not stain. This technique has been evaluated in China and Japan for increasing the detection of SCC of the esophagus *(45)*. This technique has also been used in Barrett's esophagus *(46)*. A second technique uses toluidine blue, in which cellular nuclei are stained. This method has a high sensitivity and specificity, but it cannot differentiate between gastric and intestinal metaplasia *(47)*. Another endoscopic staining method uses methylene blue (chromoendoscopy) to help detect Barrett's esophagus tissue. Methylene blue is a stain that is taken up by tissue such as small-intestine and colonic epithelia and allows for the differentiation between gastric and intestinal metaplasia. Canto et al. have studied methylene blue staining in 47 patients *(48)*. All patients with high-grade dysplasia did not take up the stain, as predicted. In another study of 43 patients evaluated in a randomized, sequential fashion, dysplasia and/or cancer was diagnosed in more patients with methylene blue-directed biopsy than random, four-quadrant jumbo biopsy (44 vs 28%, $p = 0.03$) *(49)*.

A noninvasive approach to detect Barrett's esophagus or esophageal cancer utilizes barium esophagrams. This screening technique has been studied in patients with SCC of the esophagus *(50)*. For detecting carcinoma limited to the submucosal layer, routine esophagram done every 12 mo was found to be adequate. However, this study was not successful in detecting carcinoma *in situ*. To date, there have been no studies using barium esophagram in the screening for Barrett's esophagus.

Endoscopic Ultrasound

The role of endoscopic ultrasound (EUS) in Barrett's esophagus is limited. EUS is not generally recommended as part of screening or surveillance procedures. However, investigators have shown that the appearance of Barrett's esophagus is so distinctive with high-frequency catheter ultrasonography that it can be reliably distinguished from reflux esophagitis *(51)*. Furthermore, studies published and presented only in abstract form suggest that there may be a future role for EUS in certain high-risk patients with Barrett's esophagus. Two preliminary reports suggest that EUS has the potential for detecting cancer in patients with BE when endoscopy does not, particularly when performed in carefully selected patients with dysphagia, focal nodule, or stricture with only high-grade dysplasia in biopsies *(51,52)*. However, a normal EUS may or may not accurately exclude the presence of an intramucosal cancer *(53)*. When superficial cancer is present, it may appear as focal thickening located in the first two (T1 mucosal) or three (T1submucosal) layers. It is therefore reasonable to perform EUS

Chapter 13 / Screening for Esophageal Cancer 219

in patients with high-grade dysplasia because of the risk for adenocarcinoma, which, in turn, can be detected and staged at the same procedure.

SURVEILLANCE RECOMMENDATIONS FOR BARRETT'S ESOPHAGUS

The challenge in proposing standard of care screening guidelines lies not only in the difficulty of the biopsy protocol but also in determining the adequate frequency of surveillance endoscopy (*see* Algorithm 1). The intervals for surveillance are currently controversial. A set of guidelines suggested at the International Conference on Ablation Therapy for Barrett's Mucosa is as follows: (1) Patients without dysplasia should have follow-up endoscopy yearly. After two negative consecutive examinations, then it may be changed to every 3 yr. (2) Patients with low-grade dysplasia should have follow-up endoscopy every 6 mo. After two negative consecutive examinations, it may be changed to every year. (3) Patients with high-grade dysplasia should have an expert confirmation of their diagnosis and then should undergo surgical resection of the esophagus if high-grade dysplasia is confirmed *(54)*.

The ASGE recommends surveillance endoscopy every 1–3 yr if there is no dysplasia. If the highest grade of dysplasia is low grade, then endoscopy and biopsy every 6–12 mo is recommended. However, the ACG recently published recommendations on the management of Barrett's esophagus, which increased the surveillance intervals for patients with no and low-grade dysplasia *(41)*. Specifically, patients with no dysplasia should have follow-up endoscopy every 2–3 yr using a systematic biopsy protocol. For patients with low-grade dysplasia, the surveillance interval is 6 mo. If two consecutive sets of biopsies show no dysplasia, then the surveillance interval can increase to 12 mo. Although these recommendations are fully endorsed by the ASGE and the American Gastroenterological Association, they are not supported by any data and are based only on expert opinion. Hence, the practicing physician is forced to make clinical decisions based on recommendations that have not been substantiated or proven by any randomized clinical trial, such as the National Polyp Study.

The 1990 Barrett's Esophagus Working Party of the World Congress in Gastroenterology and the ACG are essentially the same *(55)*. However, one difference is in the management of high-grade dysplasia patients. These latter guidelines suggest continuing follow-up endoscopy every 3 mo until there is a firmer indication for surgical extirpation of the esophagus. There have been multiple clinical trials supporting endoscopic surveillance of patients with Barrett's esophagus, especially patients with dysplasia *(56,57)*.

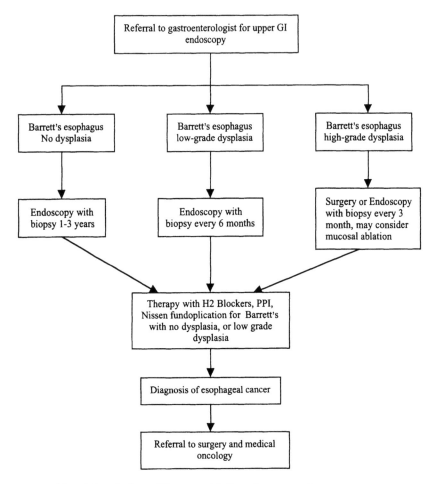

Algorithm 1. Surveillance guidelines for Barrett's esophagus.

COST-EFFECTIVENESS OF SCREENING

In the age of rising health care costs, a natural question to ask is whether endoscopic surveillance of Barrett's esophagus is cost-effective. Upper endoscopy is not inexpensive, and although the incidence of esophageal adenocarcinoma is rising, this type of cancer is relatively uncommon when compared to breast cancer. Streitz et al. studied this very question and were able to conclude that surveillance endoscopy is as cost-effective as surveillance mammography (12).

In this study, endoscopic surveillance was performed in 149 patients with benign Barrett's esophagus. Of the 149 patients screened, 13

Chapter 13 / Screening for Esophageal Cancer 221

patients were discovered to have esophageal adenocarcinoma. The rest of the patients were followed on average for 17 mo and seven cancers were detected. Of the 12,537 mammograms performed, 50 occult breast cancer cases were detected. The costs of detecting both types of cancers were comparable: $37,928 for Barrett's esophagus and $54,513 for occult breast cancer. The costs for treatment of the cancers were $83,340 and $83,292, respectively. Certainly when applying mammography as a breast cancer screen, more lives will be saved because of the larger number of women at risk for developing breast cancer. However, the comparable costs of detection and treatment for esophageal cancer support continuing surveillance endoscopy.

Other studies have reported different cost values for the detection and treatment of esophageal cancer. Clearly, the costs will be dependent on the standard of care in a particular geographic area and other factors such as the cost of endoscopy. The cost-effectiveness of screening is dependent on selecting the patient population of highest risk. Intuitively, mass screening or screening the average-risk person will not be cost-effective. Although esophageal cancer is a much less common disease, the high morbidity and mortality rate, as well as the comparable detection and treatment costs, justifies continuing endoscopic surveillance in patients with Barrett's esophagus.

TREATMENT AND PREVENTION OF BARRETT'S ESOPHAGUS

One approach to medically treating Barrett's esophagus is treating GERD, because this condition is one of the most common risk factors for Barrett's esophagus and esophageal adenocarcinoma. To reduce the gastric acid, H-2 blockers and proton-pump inhibitors are used. These medications have contributed significantly to reducing the acid level and improving symptoms of GERD. However, controlling acid exposure does not appear to aid in the regression of Barrett's esophagus. The challenge in determining the efficacy of these medications is the difficulty in accurately measuring the affected surface area and precisely repeating the biopsy from the same affected area at every follow-up endoscopy. Nonetheless, specific guidelines for therapy (on package insert) are dependent on which medication is prescribed.

A more aggressive approach is to perform surgery. In patients with Barrett's esophagus with no evidence of dysplasia, an esophagectomy can hardly be justified. However, a Nissen fundoplication procedure (antireflux surgery) will anatomically reduce or eliminate acid reflux of the stomach or duodenum. Two studies reported rare incidence of developing esophageal adenocarcinoma after this surgical procedure *(58,59)*. Therefore, this type of surgical procedure may be offered as a treatment for gastroesophageal reflux disease, but there is no evidence that it will definitely prevent Barrett's esophagus or esophageal adenocarcinoma. Surgical treatment is frequently recommended for patients with high-grade dysplasia. In surgically fit candidates, this would be the current standard of care. In expert hands, esophagectomy carries a reasonably low morbidity and mortality rate. However, this difficult procedure will still be performed in patients without cancer. Therefore, recommendations to wait until invasive early cancer is detected by close surveillance are also valid. An aggressive biopsy protocol should be followed to increase the likelihood that carcinoma will be diagnosed in patients with severe dysplasia *(41)*.

Another treatment modality for Barrett's esophagus is to perform mucosal ablation. Examples of mucosal ablation are laser ablation, monopolar/bipolar electrosurgery, and photodynamic therapy. Photodynamic therapy (PDT) utilizes a photosensitizing compound (such as porfimer sodium or Photofrin), which, when activated, produces a toxin to kill dysplastic or tumor cells. Overholt et al. performed PDT on patients with Barrett's esophagus *(60)*. Disappearance of Barrett's mucosa was documented in 43 patients and dysplasia was eliminated in 78 patients. These results are encouraging, but PDT is still under evaluation. Side effects, such as photosensitivity and stricture formation, impact negatively on the quality of life. Also, there have been reports that the mucosal ablation is superficial, and underneath the "normal" epithelium there can be columnar epithelium, with or without dysplasia. Hence, until the results of ongoing randomized Phase 3 trials are available, PDT remains a potential therapy for Barrett's esophagus.

In terms of the prevention of Barrett's esophagus and cancer, the trials conducted have primarily focused on secondary prevention. For primary prevention to succeed, definitive risk factors such as diet and nutrition, environmental hazards, and tobacco and alcohol need to be identified. Certainly recommendations can be made to change these particular risk factors, but the impact on the prevention of Barrett's esophagus is unknown. Secondary prevention focuses on detecting and treating disease at an early stage. At present, there are no medications to prevent Barrett's esophagus, dysplasia, or cancer, but epidemiologic and other data support drugs such as NSAIDs (aspirin, sulindac, celecoxib) and selenium as potential chemopreventive agents. Cyclooxygenase-2 is over expressed in Barrett's esophagus and esophageal cancer. Hence, a selective cyclooxygenase-2 inhibitor such as celecoxib will soon be tested a potential chemopreventive agent in a

Chapter 13 / Screening for Esophageal Cancer 223

Phase 2 trial. Another compound called DFMO is an inhibitor of ornithine decarboxylase. Preclinical data have shown decreased incidence of esophageal tumors in rodents treated with DFMO. Currently, a trial evaluating the role of DFMO in Barrett's esophagus is also ongoing.

INDICATIONS FOR CONSULTING THE SUBSPECIALIST

The identification of warning signs that place patients in the high-risk category for esophageal adenocarcinoma is of utmost importance. Such signs include (1) heartburn, regurgitation, or both at least once a week, (2) heartburn, regurgitation, or both at least once a week at night, (3) long-standing reflux symptoms (>20 yr), (4) dysphagia or odynophagia, (5) weight loss, (6) tobacco and alcohol use, (7) family history of Barrett's esophagus or esophageal adenocarcinoma, and (8) prior history of Barrett's esophagus or esophageal adenocarcinoma. Gastrointestinal bleeding or heme-positive stools are also possibly associated with occult Barrett's esophagus (severe esophagitis) or early cancer with an ulcer. With these signs and symptoms, a referral to a gastroenterologist is indicated.

SUMMARY

Barrett's esophagus, once considered a medical curiosity without any clinical significance, is now known to be a major complication of gastroesophageal reflux disease and the single most important risk factor for AC of the esophagus. The incidence of AC is rising faster than any other cancer in the body. Dysplasia is considered the prerequisite intermediate step from metaplasia to carcinoma in Barrett's esophagus. There is no effective therapy for the primary prevention of Barrett's esophagus and the management includes aggressive treatment of GERD and periodic surveillance endoscopies with biopsy to detect dysplasia or early cancer.

REFERENCES

1. Pope, CE II. (1973) Tumlors. In: Sleisenger MH, Fordtran JS, eds., *Gastrointestinal Disease*. Philadelphia: WB Sanders, p. 455.
2. Cedarquist C, Nielsen J, Berthelsen A, et al. (1971) Cancer of the esophagus. II. Therapy and outcome. *Chir Scand* 144:233–240.
3. Craddock VW. (1992) Aetiology of oesophageal cancer: some operative factors. *Eur J Cancer Prev* 1:89–103.
4. Landis SH, Murray T, Bolden S, et al. (1998) Cancer statistics. *CA Cancer J Clin* 48:6–29.
5. Raphael HA, Ellis FH Jr, Dockerty MB. (1996) Primary adenocarcinoma of the esophagus: 18-year review and review of the literature. *Ann Surg* 64(5):785–796.
6. Conio M, Cameron AJ. (1999) Barrett's esophagus and adenocarcinoma: prevalence and incidence in Olmsted County. *Gastroenterology* 116(G1):682.

224   **Part VII / Screening for Cancers in High-Risk Groups**

7. Devesa S, Blot WJ, Fraumeni J. (1998) Changing patterns in the incidence of esophageal and gastric carcinoma in the United States. *Cancer* 83:2049–2053.
8. Kim R, Rose S, Shar AO, et al. (1997) Extent of Barrett's metaplasia: a prospective study of the serial change in area of Barrett's measured by quantitative endoscopic imaging 1996. *Gasrointest Endosc* 45:456–462.
9. Devesa SS, Blot WJ, Fraumeni JF. (1998) Changing patterns in the incidence of esophageal and gastric carcinoma in the United States. *Cancer* 83:2049–2053.
10. Chalasani N, Wo JM, Waring JP. (1998) Racial differences in the histology, location, and risk factors of esophageal cancer. *J Clin Gastroenterol* 26:11–13.
11. Provenzale D, Kemp JA, Arora S, et al. (1994) A guide for surveillance of patients with Barrett's esophagus. *Am J Gastroenterol* 89:670–680.
12. Streitz JM, Ellis FH, Tilden RL, et al. (1998) Endoscopic surveillance of Barrett's esophagus: a cost-effectiveness comparison with mammographic surveillance for breast cancer. *Am J Gastroenterol* 93:911–915.
13. Lagergren J, Bergstrom R, Lindgren A, et al. (1999) Symptomatic gastroesophageal reflux as a risk factor for esophageal adenocarcinoma. *N Engl J Med* 340:825–831.
14. Spechler SJ, Goyal RK. (1986) Barrett's esophagus. *N Engl J Med* 315:362–371.
15. Champion G, Richter JE, Vaezi MF, et al. (1994) Duodenogastroesophageal reflux: relationship to pH and importance in Barrett's esophagus. *Gastroenterology* 107:747–754.
16. Armstrong D, Blum AL, Savary M. (1982) Reflux disease and Barrett's esophagus. *Endoscopy* 1972;24:9.
17. Monnier PH, Ollyo J-B, Fontolliet CH, et al. (1995) Epidemiology and natural history of reflux esophagitis. *Sem Laparosc Surg* 2:2–9.
18. Winters JR, Sparling TJ, Chobanian SJ, et al. (1987) Barrett's esophagus: a prevalent, occult complication of gastroesophageal disease. *Gastroenterology* 92:118–124.
19. Menke-Pluymers MB, Hop WC, Dees J, van Blankenstein M, Tilanus, HW. (1993) Risk factors for the development of an adenocarcinoma in columnar-lined (Barrett's) esophagus: the Rotterdam Esophageal Tumor Study Group. *Cancer* 72:1155–1158.
20. Hassall E, Weinstein WM, Ament ME. (1985) Barrett's esophagus in childhood. *Gastroenterology* 89:1331–1337.
21. Cameron AJ, Lomboy CI. (1992) Barrett's esophagus: age, prevalence, and extent of columelium. *Gastroenterology* 103:1241–1245.
22. Brown LM, Silvennan DT, Pottern LM, et al. (1994) Adenocarcinoma of the esophagus and esophagogastric junction in white men in the United States: alcohol, tobacco, and socioeconomic factors. *Cancer Causes Control* 5:333–340.
23. Brown LM, Swanson CA, Gridley C, et al. (1995) Adenocarcinoma of the esophagus: role of obesity and diet. *J Natl Cancer Inst* 87:104–109.
24. Katzka BA, Reynolds JC, Saul Sll, et al. (1987) Barrett's metaplasia and adenocarcinoma of the esophagus in scleroderma. *Am J Med* 82:46–52.
25. Garidou A, Tzonou A, Lipworth L, et al. (1996) Life-style factors and medical conditions in relation to esophageal cancer by histologic type in a low-risk population. *Intl Cancer* 68:295–299.
26. Harle IA, Finley RJ Belsheim M, et al. (1985) Management of adenocarcinoma in columnar-lined esophagus. *Ann Thorac Surg* 40:330–336.
27. Levine DS, Haggitt RC, Blunt PL, et al. (1993) An endoscopic biopsy protocol on differentiate high-grade dysplasia from early adenocarcinoma in Barrett's esophagus. *Gastroenterology* 105:40–50.
28. Locke CR III, Talley NJ, Fett SL, et al. (1998) Prevalence and clinical spectrum of gastroesophageal reflux: a population-based study in Olmsted County, Minnesota. *Gastroenterology* 112:1448.

Chapter 13 / Screening for Esophageal Cancer 225

29. Robertson CS, Mayberry IF, Nicholson DA, et al. (1988) Value of endoscopic surveillance in the detection of neoplastic changes in Barrett's esophagus. *Br J Surg* 75:760–773.

30. Hammeeteman W, Tytgat IN, Houthoff HI, et al. (1989) Barrett's esophagus: development of dysplasia and adenocarcinoma. *Gastroenterology* 69:1249–1256.

31. Miros M,Kerlin P, Walker N. (1991) Only patients with dysplasia progress to adenocarcinoma in Barrett's esophagus. *Gut* 32:1441–1446.

32. Reid BJ, Blount PL, Rubin CE, et al. (1992) Flow cytometric and histological progression to malignancy in Barrett's esophagus: prospective endoscopic surveillance of a cohort. *Gastroenterology* 102:1212–1219.

33. Reid BJ, Haggitt R C, Rubin CE, et al. (1988) Observer variations in the diagnosis of dysplasia in Barrett's esophagus. *Human Pathol* 19:166–178.

34. Hirota W K, Loughney T M, Lazas DJ, et al. (1999) Specialized intestinal metaplasia, dysplasia, and cancer of esophagus and esophagogasric junction: prevalence and clinical data. *Gastroenterology* 116:277–285.

35. Sharma P, Morales T G, Bhattacharyya A, et al. (1997) Dysplasia in short-segment Barrett's esophagus: a prospective 3 year follow up. *Am J Gastroentrol* 92:2012–2016.

36. Weston A P, Krmpotich P T, Cherian R, et al. (1997) Prospective long term endoscopic and histologic follow-up of short segment Barrett's esophagus: comparison with traditional long segment Barrett's esophagus. *Am J Gastroenterol* 92:407–413.

37. Garewal HS, Sampliner R, Liu Y, Trent JM. (1989) Chromosomal rearrangement in Barrett's esophagus: a pre-malignant lesion of esophageal adenocarcinoma. *Cancer Genet Cyto-genet* 42:281.

38. Grawal HS, Sampliner R, Gerner E, et al. (1988) Ornithine decarboxylase activity in Barrett's esophagus: a potential marker for dysplasia. *Gastroentrology* 94:819.

39. Schneider PM, Casson AG, Levin B, et al. (1996) Mutations of p53 in Barrett's esophagus and Barrett's cancer: a prospective study of ninety eighty cases. *J Thorac Cardiovasc Surg* 111:323.

40. Falk GW, Rice TW, Goldblum JR, Richter JE. (1999) Jumbo biopsy forceps protocol still misses unsuspected cancer in Barrett's esophagus with high-grade dysplasia. *Gastrointest Endosc* 49(2):170–176.

41. Sampliner RE. (1998) Practice guidelines on the diagnosis, surveillance, and therapy of Barrett's esophagus. The Practice Parameters Committee of the American College of Gastroenterology. *Am J Gastroenterol* 93(7):1028–1032.

42. ASGE. (1998) The role of endoscopy in the surveillance of premalignant conditions of the upper gastrointestinal tract. *Gastrointest Endosc* 48(6):663–668.

43. Falk GW, Chittajallu R, Goldblum JR, et al. (1997) Surveillance of patients with Barrett's esophagus for dysplasia and cancer with balloon cytology [see comments]. *Gastroenterology* 112(6):1787–1797.

44. Fennerty MB, DiTomasso J, Morales TG, et al. (1995) Screening for Barrett's esophagus by balloon cytology. *Am J Gastroenterol* 90(8):1230–1232.

45. Sugimachi K, Kitamura K, Baba K, et al. (1992) Endoscopic diagnosis of early carcinoma using Lugol's solution. *Gastrointest Endosc* 38:657–661.

46. Woolf GM, Riddell RH, Irvine EJ, et al. (1989) A study to examine agreement between endoscopy and histology for the diagnosis of columnar lined (Barrett's) esophagus. *Gastrointest Endosc* 35:541–544.

47. Chobanian SJ, Catau EL, Winters C, et al. (1987) In vivo staining with toluidine blue as an adjunct to the endoscopic detection of Barrett's esophagus. *Gastrointest Endosc* 33:99–101.

48. Canto MI, Setrakian S, Petras RE, et al. (2001) Methylene blue staining of dysplastic and nondysplastic Barrett's esophagus. An in vivo and ex vivo study. *Gastrointest Endosc,* in press.

226 Part VII / Screening for Cancers in High-Risk Groups

49. Canto MI, Setrakian S, Willis J, et al. (2000) Methylene blue-directed biopsy for improved detection of intestinal metaplasia and dysplasia in Barrett's esophagus: a controlled sequential trial. *Gastrointest Endosc* 51(5):560–568.
50. Ohno S, Kabashima A, Tomoda M, et al. (1997) Significance of routine annual esophagram for early detection of carcinoma of the esophagus. *Hepato-Gastroenterology* 44:539–545.
51. Adrain AL, Ter HC, Cassidy MJ, et al. (1997) High-resolution endoluminal sonography is a sensitive modality for the identification of Barrett's metaplasia. *Gastrointest Endosc* 46(2):147–151.
52. Stotland B, Kochman M, Smith D, et al. (1997) Endosonography is indicated for selected patients with Barrett's esophagus. *Gastrointest Endosc* 45(4):AB181.
53. Parent J, Levine D, Haggitt R, et al. (1997) Role of endoscopic ultrasound in patients with Barrett's esophagus and high grade dysplasia. *Gastrointest Endosc* 45(4):AB76.
54. Bremner CG, Deemester TR. (1997) Proceedings from an international conference on ablation therapy for Barrett's mucosa. *Dis Esophagus* 11:1–27.
55. Dent J. (1991) Working party report to the world congresses of gastronenterology, Sydney 1990: Barrett's oesophagus. *J Gastroenterol Hepatol* 6:1–22.
56. Sandick JW, Lanschot JJ, Kuiken BW, et al. (1998) Impact of endoscopic biopsy surveillance of Barrett's oesophagus on pathological stage and clinical outcome of Barrett's carcinoma. *Gut* 43:216–222.
57. Peters JH, Clark GW, Ireland AP, et al. (1994) Outcome of adenocarcinoma arising in Barrett's esophagus in endoscopically surveyed and nonsurveyed patients. *J Thorac Cardiovasc Surg* 05:813–821.
58. McCallum RW, Polpalle S, Davenport K, et al. (1991) Role of anti-reflux surgery against dysplasia in Barrett's esophagus. *Gastroenterology* 100:100–106.
59. McDonald MI, Trastek VF, Allen MS, et al. (1996) Barrett's esophagus: does an antireflux procedure reduce the need for endoscopic surveillance? *J Thorac Cardiovasc Surg* 111:1135–1138.
60. Overholt B, Panjehpour M, Haydek J. (1999) Photodynamic therapy for Barrett's esophagus: follow-up in 100 patients. *Gastrointest Endosc* 49:1–7.

14 Screening for Esophageal Cancer in China

You-Lin Qiao, MD, PhD
and Guoqing Wang, MD

KEY PRINCIPLES

- China has one of the highest incidences of esophageal carcinoma in the world.
- Marked variations exist in the incidence of esophageal cancer in neighboring areas in China, suggesting an important role played by the environmental and dietary factors in the pathogenesis of esophageal cancer in China.
- Many simple and inexpensive techniques are used for mass screening for esophageal cancer in China. Abrasive balloon cytology is the most commonly used and is highly effective with significant reduction in the mortality in the screened population.

INTRODUCTION

Esophageal cancer (EC) has been endemic in China for generations. It was first recorded in China in 300 BC, when it was referred to as *Ye Ge*, meaning dysphagia and belching, or *Ge Shi Ging*, difficult to swallow, with blockage of the gullet and vomiting after eating *(1)*. The existence of *Houwang Miao* (the throat god temple) reflects the profound fear and high prevalence of this disease in the ancient Chinese. Even today, the efficacy of the most modern treatment for advanced EC is similar to praying to the throat god.

The world's highest incidence and mortality of esophageal cancer occurs in the north central parts of the People's Republic of China,

From: *Cancer Screening: A Practical Guide for Physicians*
Edited by: K. Aziz and G. Y. Wu © Humana Press Inc., Totowa, NJ

particularly in the Taihang Mountain area, which is the border of the Henan, Hebei, and Shanxi provinces. The highest rates of esophageal cancer mortality within China are found in Linxian, a rural county in the north central part of the country, where the cumulative death rates to age 75 for esophageal cancer exceed 20% in both sexes *(2,3)*.

In the United States the 5-yr survival for esophageal carcinoma is approximately 10%, and there has been no significant change in the mortality in the last 50 yr. In contrast in China, the 5-yr survival is 90% in the screened population and the mortality has changed remarkably within the last 50 yr *(4,5)*.

EPIDEMIOLOGY

The global incidence of EC is one of the highest of all cancers *(6)*. Combined with cancers of the mouth and pharynx, which often have a similar etiology, the incidence of these upper digestive tract cancers is the highest of any form of cancer. Worldwide, EC was responsible for 316,000 new cases and 286,000 deaths in 1990 *(7)*. The area with the highest incidence is the notorious "cancer belt," stretching from Iran to China, certain regions in South Africa, and the Normandy district of France *(8)*. In China, EC constitutes 15% of all cancers and is the fourth site characterized by very poor survival, together with the liver, pancreas, and lung *(9)*. The age-adjusted mortality of esophageal cancer in China in 1992 was 27.7 per 100,000 men and 13.6 per 100,000 women *(10)*.

There are striking geographic variations in the incidence of esophageal cancer. These variations are seen not only in the various regions of the world but also between the neighboring areas within China. The incidence of esophageal carcinoma in the Taihang Mountains in the northern part of China is 139.80/100,000, and 1.43/100,000 in the neighboring Hunyuan county. The ratio between high- and low-risk areas is approximately 100:1 *(11)*. In the United States, the annual incidence is 0.4/100,000, which is the lowest in the world. In north China, the ratio of male to female patients with EC is 1.6:1, ranging from 1.44:1 to 2.63:1. The ratio is lower in areas with higher mortality rates and higher in areas with lower mortality rates. EC is not common among children and young adults. In Linxian, the incidence rate for those 25 yr old is below 5/100,000. Above this age, the incidence gradually increases. At age 60, it is about 800/100,000. The highest mortality rate of EC is in the 60- to 69-yr age group, accounting for 37–39% of the total deaths from EC. For those 50–59 yr old and for those over 70, the values are 23 and 28%, respectively *(11)*.

Chapter 14 / Screening for Esophageal Cancer in China 229

ETIOLOGY

The dramatic epidemiological differences in the incidence of EC in various regions of the world and within China and the fact that gullet cancer in chickens is also observed in the high-incidence areas led to the hope that the causes of the EC would be relatively easy to identify. However, in spite of extensive surveys, no single predominating cause has been detected. It is probable that several risk factors are involved *(12,13)*.

With regard to EC, nations can be divided into three groups. In group 1, the cancer rate is very high, as in China and Iran. The predominant factor in this group is related to the diet, including micronutrient deficiencies, low levels of the protective factors that occur in fresh fruit and vegetables, and consumption of food containing high levels of initiating carcinogens (i.e., nitrosamines). In group 2 countries, including most of Europe and the United States, the cancer rate is very low and the major cause is smoking and excessive consumption of alcohol. Group 3 countries, such as Japan and South Africa, have intermediate cancer rates. Several causes are important, including alcohol, cigaret smoking, and dietary deficiencies. Additional factors in Japan include consumption of very hot tea gruel and toxic plants (e.g., bracken), whereas in South Africa, certain unusual procedures practiced during pipe smoking seem to be important. Thus, the position of a country on the EC scale depends mainly on the environmental factors, and no race or religious group has been shown to be especially vulnerable *(14)*. A number of factors have been identified, which may be contributing to the high risk of EC in China. These are discussed in the following subsections.

Nitrosomine Compounds

Of all the groups of known chemical carcinogens, the *N*-nitroso compounds possess characteristics that make them the most likely agents in the induction of human cancer. A significant amount of volatile and nonvolatile nitrosamines, several of which are carcinogenic for the esophagus, have been found and assayed in a variety of foods. Moldy meat, salted or smoked fish, and cheese are especially suspect. The areas with high consumption of these food items have the highest incidence of EC *(15)*.

The local diet consumed in Linxian County has been extensively studied because of the highest incidence of squamous-cell carcinoma in this region. The diet is severely restricted, comprised mainly of gruel and pickled vegetables. A previously unknown compound, Roussin red methyl ester, was isolated from pickled vegetables. This is thought to be derived, in part, from the metal jars used for storage. The chronic administration of Roussin red methyl ester to rats and mice induced papillomas in the forestomach, suggesting that this compound could be carcinogenic for the esophagus. In addition, Roussin red can react with benzylamine to form NMBzA, a potent esophageal carcinogen *(16)*.

The water supply in Linxian County is often inadequate, and water is collected from wells containing high levels of nitrates and nitrites. In addition, water is stored in earthenware jars for a considerable period, during which time bacterial reduction of nitrate to nitrite takes place. The vegetables, mainly turnips and sweet potato leaves, are fermented in water, without the addition of salt or vinegar. During the storage period, nitrate formed by bacteria from nitrate in the water or in the vegetables can react with amines in the plant material to form nitrosamines.

In addition, molds grow on the surface of the pickles and these fungi produce not only mycotoxins but also reduced nitrate to nitrite and methylated primary amines to form asymmetric secondary amines. In addition, the previously unknown nitrosamine, *N*-3-methyl-*n*-butyl-*N*-1-methylacetonylnitrosamine (NMAMBA) has been found in corn bread that had been inoculated with *F. moniliforme* and incubated with a low concentration of nitrite *(17)*. Similarly, *N*-2-methyl-*n*-propyl-*N*-methyacetonylnitrosamine was detected in millet and wheat flour that had been treated in the same way. NMAMBA induced tumors in the forestomach, an organ often regarded as an extension of the esophagus, in rats and mice.

Another high-risk area for esophageal cancer in which the diet has been examined for its nitrosamine content is the Kashmir region in India. Kashmiris have a unique diet, which differs from that of surrounding areas where there is a lower incidence of esophageal cancer. The long, severe winters in Kashmir necessitate the storage of food, which is often kept for more than 2 yr. Plant foods are sun-dried or pickled and fish is sun-dried or smoked. With similar food items to north central China, fungi and bacteria have the opportunity to convert nitrate to nitrite, which then reacts with amines in the food to form nitrosamines *(18–20)*.

Dietary and Micronutrient Deficiencies

Although the total caloric intake in the areas with high incidence of EC in China is adequate, there is a low intake of vitamins A and C, riboflavin, animal protein, fat, fresh vegetables, and fruits *(21)*. The dietary and micronutrient deficiencies are markedly severe during the winter months. Riboflavin, molybdenum, copper, zinc, and manganese deficiencies are associated with esophageal cancer in experi-

Chapter 14 / Screening for Esophageal Cancer in China 231

mental animals. In a study of 29,584 adults in Linxian, there was a 42% reduction in the prevalence of esophageal cancer among those who received supplementation of β-carotene, vitamin E, and selenium. A population-based case-control study in Shanghai showed that after adjustment for cigaret smoking, alcohol consumption, and other risk factors, increasing consumption of fruits, dark orange vegetables, and beef or mutton was associated with a statistically significant decreasing trend in the risk of development of esophageal cancer *(22)*.

Fungal and Other Microorganism Invasion

In the high-incidence areas of EC, invasion of the esophagus with various microorganisms is common. These include fungi and the human papilloma virus. In one study, the presence of fungus, as determined by cytosmear, correlated with the degree of dysplasia. For example, fungus was found in the esophagi of 31% of normal and mild dysplasia subjects, 72% of those with severe dysplasia, and 90% of those with carcinoma of the esophagus *(23)*. Fungal invasion of the esophagus was also studied in biopsies and resected specimens *(24)*. Among 185 samples, the incidence of fungal invasion was 30% in the hyperplastic epithelium of noncancerous patients, 50% in the hyperplastic epithelium of early EC, 15% in the cancerous tissue of early EC, and 3.1% in normal epithelium.

Electron microscopy showed that the fungi invade between the esophageal epithelial cells as well as inside the cytoplasm of the cells. The epithelial cells adjacent to the invading fungi showed various degrees of change, ranging from simple hyperplasia to mild and severe dysplasia, and to early malignant change. The average age of patients with the infection is about 7 yr younger than that for the EC patients *(23)*.

Candida species is the most common invader, and a pure culture of *Candida albicans* has been isolated from the hyperplastic epithelium and carcinoma *in situ* of the esophagus. *Candida tropicalis, C. krusei, C. parapsilosis, Torulopsis glabrata,* and *T. tomata* have also been isolated from oral and esophageal samples *(25)*. Human papilloma virus DNA was also noted in almost 50% of squamous-cell carcinoma in several studies. The role of these microorganisms in the malignant change of the esophagus is under active investigation. They may act indirectly on the esophageal epithelium either by forming carcinogens or other products to enhance or attenuate carcinogenesis or by directly affecting the esophagus itself.

Temperature of Drinks and Food Consumed

In one survey in 1965, it was found that 77% of the inhabitants in Linxian habitually ate food with temperatures of 60–70°C *(26)*. Some even ingested food at 80°C. In experimental animals, severe coagulation necrosis and acute interstitial necrosis were noted 12 h after forcefully feeding the animals water at 80°C. Within 1–3 d, severe ulceration and epithelial regeneration was observed. These symptoms disappeared after 1 wk, but hyperplasia and mild dysplasia could be observed in some animals. With water at 75°C, the damage was less, but hyperplasia was seen in some of the animals. Damage, however, was not observed with water at 60–70°C. DNA damage in the esophagus is repaired only slowly and repeated thermal trauma to the esophagus may induce restorative hyperplasia and dysplasia, thereby acting as a potent initiating or promoting factor in esophageal carcinogenesis *(27)*.

Miscellaneous Factors

Several factors are important and specific to certain areas and contribute to the higher incidence of esophageal cancer in these areas. These include occupational exposure to silica, drinking mutagenic water, coal cooking, and consumption of certain herbal beverages at a very high temperature *(28–30)*.

BIOLOGY OF ESOPHAGEAL CANCER

Squamous-cell carcinoma is the predominant cancer of the esophagus in China. According to the research data of endoscopic examination, clinical pathology, and epidemiology, there is a parallel incidence of dysplastic changes in the esophagus and esophageal cancer in different areas of China *(31,32)*. The epithelial cells undergo hyperplasia, followed by increasing grades of dysplasia and ultimately cancerous lesions. In a prospective study, patients with hyperplasia, mild dysplasia, moderate dysplasia, and severe dysplasia of the basal cells on endoscopic biopsy were followed for up to 3.5 yr. The rate of development of carcinoma was 5, 5.3, 26.7, and 65.2%, respectively *(33)*. In another study of 105 patients with mild dysplasia, 15.2% progressed to severe dysplasia. Forty percent remained unchanged and 44.8% returned to normal over a 4-yr period. Of 79 patients with severe dysplasia, 26.6% progressed to cancer, 32.9% stayed about the same, and 40.5% regressed to mild dysplasia or normal histology *(34)*.

In an endoscopic study, the rate of progression of severe dysplasia to carcinoma was evaluated. In this study, 327 patients with severe dysplasia were followed for 1–2 yr: 7.9% progressed to cancer. In 142 patients followed for 2–5 yr, 20.5% progressed to cancer. Of 44 cases followed for 5–9 yr, 34% progressed to cancer, and in a small group of 17 patients followed for 9–12 yr, 53% progressed to cancer. Severe dysplasia was

Chapter 14 / Screening for Esophageal Cancer in China 233

thus seen as a high-risk marker for the development of esophageal cancer, the risk increasing with time *(32,35)*.

The time-course for the progression of early esophageal carcinoma to advanced disease was estimated by a study of 91 patients with early esophageal cancer who did not undergo surgery for various reasons. The patients were followed endoscopically for 19–24 mo. Eight of the 91 patients developed advanced disease during this period, but 83 cancers remained superficial. The authors concluded that early esophageal cancer in most cases progressed in a relatively slow manner, estimating that it usually takes about 3–4 yr, to develop advanced cancer from *in situ* disease *(36)*. In another small study of 23 patients with early EC, 12 patients remained unchanged, 11 progressed to advanced cancer in a follow-up period of 4–6 yr, and 78% were alive at 5 yr.

The apparently rather slow progression from normal histology through dysplasia to early carcinoma over a period of years, followed by another relatively long period before the disease becomes advanced, is encouraging, and periodic screening every 1–2 yr will allow detection of most cases in early stage. The finding of dysplasia, particularly severe dysplasia, on cytology or biopsy would seem to indicate a high risk for cancer and the need for a more frequent surveillance interval *(37)*.

SCREENING FOR ESOPHAGEAL CANCER IN CHINA

In the high-risk areas of the world, several inexpensive, simple, and innovative techniques have been used to obtain cytological material from the esophagus to identify asymptomatic individuals who harbor malignant or premalignant cells (*see* Algorithm 1). In Iran and Italy, a standard endoscopic brush is passed via a nasogastric tube; in Japan, sponge cytology with an expandable sponge in a dissolvable capsule retrieved by a string is used; in South Africa, a suction abrasive tube is used; in China, several methods have been developed and used for screening, the most common method being abrasive balloon cytology.

Chinese Balloon Cytology

One of the most outstanding works on EC in China is the mass screening using the technique of *lawang*, meaning to pull a (fish) net. It consists of a single- or double-lumen rubber balloon covered with a mesh net (Fig. 1). The balloon is swallowed by the patient and once the balloon is in the stomach, it is inflated and gradually pulled out. The cancer cells are easier to exfoliate than the normal cells and stick to the mesh. The balloon is smeared onto the glass slides uniformly and then washed off with 15 cm^3 of normal saline, which is centrifuged, and cells are examined under the microscope.

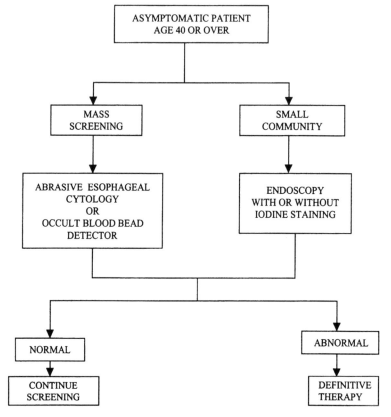

Algorithm 1. Screening for esophageal carcinoma in China.

Shu has recently reviewed the experience in China using this basic technique. From 1959 to 1979, some 500,000 people in China had abrasive balloon cytology of the esophagus. Those found to have malignant cells or premalignant dysplastic changes were sent for further testing with barium esophagrams and endoscopy and biopsy. The accuracy for cancer detection was about 80% in the mass-screening projects, approaching 90% in outpatient clinics (37). Of particular note was that 75% of the cancers detected in mass screenings were early lesions, carcinoma in situ, or minimally invasive with negative regional lymph nodes. The surgical cure rate was 90% in the patients with these early cancer (37).

Japanese Sponge Cytology

Although the balloon technique is simple and efficacious, it is associated with considerable discomfort to patients and has a lower acceptance rate. The Japanese sponge technique is less painful with better patient compliance rate. In this technique, an encapsulated sponge is

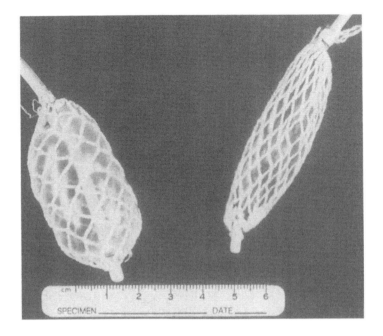

Fig. 1. Chinese cytology balloon.

swallowed by the patient with water and left in the stomach for 3–5 min to allow the capsule to dissolve and the sponge to expand. The sponge is then pulled out and rolled on a slide and washed with normal saline in a fashion similar to that described for the balloon technique. In a study of 439 patients with histologically proven dysplasia or carcinoma, the Japanese sponge technique had lower sensitivity and specificity as compared to balloon cytology (sensitivity 24 vs 47% and specificity 81 vs 92% for dysplasia and squamous-cell carcinoma, respectively) *(38)*.

Occult Blood Bead Detector

In the early stages, the majority of the upper digestive tract cancers bleed because 95% of these lesions cause erosion, ulceration, or inflammation. Only 5% are located beneath the mucous membrane and have a normal mucosal surface. A small bead designed by Qin has shown promising results and is able to detect blood in the upper digestive tract. It is a simple, inexpensive, and effective method that can be repeated periodically. The occult blood bead is less than 1 cm in diameter with an attached thread (Fig. 2). On an empty stomach, the bead is swallowed with 50 cm^3 of cold water. After 3 min, it is pulled out and the color observed; light blue, blue, and dark blue color are designed weakly

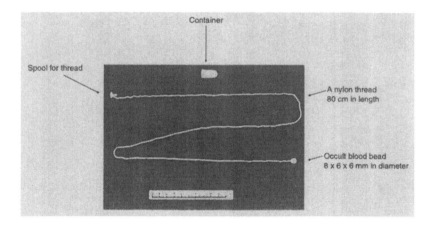

Fig. 2. Occult blood bead detector.

positive (+), positive (++), and strongly positive (+++), respectively. In 11 provinces in China, 233,825 subjects (age range: 30–70 yr) were screened. A positive occult blood test result was found in 28,557 subjects (12%). Of these, 16,918 underwent a gastroscopy, resulting in the detection of 581 cancers that were located in similar frequencies in the esophagus, gastric cardia, and gastric body; 70% of the lesions were in early or moderately advanced stage. Among 119 patients with early-stage cancer, the 3-yr survival rate was 98.3% *(39)*. The occult blood bead detector costs approx 30 cents and may be practical for large-scale screening of cancer of the upper digestive tract in developing areas. In a pilot study of 34 patients with known gastric or esophageal cancer, the occult blood bead test was positive in all patients with gastric cancer, but false-negative in 19% of patients with esophageal cancer *(40)*. Further studies are required to assess the sensitivity and specificity of this test in EC.

Endoscopy

Endoscopy is the best method for screening and diagnosis of early esophageal cancer in the high-risk areas. Standard endoscopic biopsies and brush cytology are complementary to endoscopy with a diagnostic accuracy of approx 90–95%. The diagnostic accuracy can be further improved by staining esophageal mucosa with Lugol's iodine. The iodine stains normal squamous epithelial cells brown as a result of the presence of glycogen. Dysplastic and neoplastic cells are devoid of glycogen and are not stained. These areas become apparent even in the absence of a discrete lesion on endoscopy *(41)*. However, endoscopy is

Chapter 14 / Screening for Esophageal Cancer in China   237

expensive as an initial test for mass screening and is not universally available in all parts of China. It is usually recommended in patients who have abnormal balloon cytology.

CHINESE EXPERIENCE AND RECOMMENDATIONS

The Chinese oncologists are faced with two problems: to reduce the mortality rate and increase the survival rate of esophageal cancer. For this purpose, an intensive public-education campaign was undertaken by the Chinese government, in which groups of young children trained in choral and dance performance related to the cancer campaign traveled to the high-risk areas. They emphasized the warning signs of EC and importance of the "three earlies": early discovery, early diagnosis, and early treatment for the masses. However, despite these public-education campaigns, very few asymptomatic patients with early esophageal cancer sought medical advice. On the other hand, those who already had difficulty in swallowing with or without accompanying pain usually suffered from a moderate or advanced lesion. The results of treatment of these patients were inevitably poor. At present, periodic public screening, using exfoliative cytology or gastric occult blood bead tests in the high-risk population to discover early lesions, is the only means of identifying the favorable cases. Following this, endoscopic verification and localization would establish the diagnosis beyond doubt.

Since 1974, Wang and his associates, working in the Taihang mountains, have initiated and organized the public screening in adults over 35 yr of age by balloon cytology and gastric occult blood bead tests to screen for the early detection of cancer. A total of 150,000 subjects were screened 12 times during this period and 16,500 fiber-optic endoscopies were performed, leading to the detection of early esophageal carcinoma in 620 cases and early cancer of gastric cardia in 420. As these early patients were free from symptoms, most of them refused an operation. Among the 1040 patients, only 200 were operated on and some were treated by radiation therapy. The rest opted to follow-up until they developed obvious clinical symptoms. The 5-yr survival in the screened patients who underwent definitive therapy was over 90% *(42)*.

In the last 26 yr (1973–1999), 160 million participants have been screened in China. Balloon cytology or occult blood bead detector is recommended as the initial procedure of choice for mass screening in the high-risk areas. This reduces the high-risk population to 10–20% of the large sample. The screening is recommended in all the patients over the age of 40 in these areas. The optimal screening interval is not well defined. Most mass-screening surveys are performed every 5 yr. As

238 Part VII / Screening for Cancers in High-Risk Groups

there is slow progression from hyperplasia to the development of carcinoma, which takes several years, screening every 1–2 yr seems adequate. Endoscopic examination is recommended if dysplasia or cancer is suspected on balloon cytology for definitive diagnosis. The patients with dysplasia on endoscopic biopsies will merit more frequent screening. However, for smaller communities, endoscopy with or without iodine staining is suggested as the primary screening procedure of choice *(43)*.

An important phenomenon worth mentioning is the presence of a second concomitant primary tumor, the "double primaries." It is not uncommon to see a second primary tumor, usually in the gastric cardia, oropharynx, or lung in this high-risk population. The prognosis obviously depends on the treatment of both primary ones.

COST-EFFECTIVENESS

There are no studies on the cost-effectiveness of esophageal cancer screening in China. However, several facts have emerged after various mass-screening surveys.

Screening has shown to improve the prognosis. The 5-yr survival rate has increased from 8–10% to over 90% in the screened population. Some of the early cancers have been treated with local therapy (e.g., electroheating, argon plasma coagulation, or endoscopic mucosal resection), thus reducing the need, mortality, and morbidity associated with extensive surgery.

In the high-risk group, the estimated cost to screen one case of cancer or precancer is approx 800 yuan (approx US $78). Therefore, the methods used for screening EC in China are inexpensive, simple, and effective and may be applicable to other high incidence areas in the world.

SUMMARY

Esophageal cancer is one of the most unpleasant forms of cancer, and one with an exceptionally poor prognosis. In China, EC is ranked second after gastric carcinoma as the leading cause of cancer death. Several innovative and highly effective techniques for mass screening have been developed and applied. These techniques along with an intense public-education campaign have resulted in the marked reduction in the mortality and morbidity from this inevitably lethal disease.

REFERENCES

1. Huang GJ, Wu YK. (eds.) (1984) *Carcinoma of the Esophagus and Gastric Cardia.* New York: Springer-Verlag.

Chapter 14 / Screening for Esophageal Cancer in China   239

2. National Cancer Control Office. (1980) *Atlas of Cancer Mortality in the People's Republic of China*. Shanghai: China Map Press.
3. National Cancer Control Office. (1980) *Data of Cancer Mortality in China*. Beiging: Ministry of Public Health.
4. Shu YJ. (1983) Cytopathology of the esophagus. An overview of esophageal cytopathology in China. *Acta Cytol* 27:7–16.
5. Ries LAG, Miller BA, Hankey BF. (1994) *SEER Cancer Statistic Review, 1973–1991: Tables and Graphs*. Bethesda, MD: National Cancer Institute.
6. Parkin DM, Laara E, Muir CS. (1988) Estimates of worldwide frequency of sixteen major cancers in 1980. *Int J Cancer* 41:184–197.
7. Parkin DM, Pisani P, Ferlay, J. (1999) Global cancer statistics. *CA Cancer J Clin* 49(1):33–64.
8. Sales D, Levin B. (1985) Incidence, epidemiology and predisposing factors. In: DeMeester TR, Levin B, eds., *Cancer of the Esophagus*. Grune and Stratton, Orlando, FL, pp. 1–19.
9. Li LD, Lu FZ, Zhang SW, et al. (1996) Analysis of cancer mortality rates and distribution in China: 1990–92. *Chin J Oncol* 18(6):403–407.
10. Day NE, Munoz N, Ghadiria P. (1982) Epidemiology of cancer of the digestive tract. In: Correa P, Haenszel W, eds, *Epidemiology of Esophageal Cancer: A Review*. The Hague Martinus, Boston, MA.
11. Coordinating Group for Research on Etiology of Esophageal Cancer in North China. (1975) The epidemiology and etiology of esophageal cancer in North China: a prelimnary report. *Chin Med J* 1:167–177.
12. Munoz N, Day NE. (1996) Esophageal Cancer. In: Schottenfeld D, Fraumeni JF Jr. eds., *Cancer Epidemiology and Prevention*. Philadelphia: Saunders, pp. 681–706.
13. Brown LM, Hoover RN, Greenberg RS, et al. (1994) Are racial differences in squamous cell esophageal cancer explained by alcohol and tobacco use? *J Natl Cancer Inst* 86: 5.
14. Craddock VW. (1993) Cancer of the Esophagus. Approaches to the etiology (ed). Cambridge University.
15. Tricker AR, Perkins MJ, Massey RC, et al. (1984) The incidence of some non-volatile N-nitroso compounds in cured meat. *Food Addit Contam* 1:245–252.
16. Liu JG, Li MH. (1989) Roussin red methyl ester, a tumor promoter isolated from pickled vegetables. *Carcinogenesis* 10:617–620.
17. Li M, Ji C, Cheng S. (1986) Occurrence of nitroso compound in fungi-contaminated foods: a review. *Nutr Cancer* 8:63–69.
18. Siddiqi M, Tricker AR, Preussmann R. (1988) The occurrence of preformed N-nitroso compounds in food samples from a risk area of esophageal cancer in Kashmir, India. *Cancer Lett* 39:37–43.
19. Siddiqi M, Tricker AR, Preussmann R. (1988) Formation of N-nitroso compounds under simulated gastric conditions from Kashmir foodstuffs. *Cancer Lett* 39:259–265.
20. Siddiqi M, Preussmann R. (1989) Esophageal cancer in Kashmir: an assessment. *J Cancer Res Clin Oncol* 115:111–117.
21. Li M, Li P, Li B. (1980) Recent progress in research on esophageal carcinoma in China. *Adv Cancer Res* 33:173–249.
22. Gao YT, McLaughlin JK, Gridley G, et al. (1994) Risk factors for esophageal cancer in Shanghai, China. II. Role of diet and nutrients. *Int J Cancer* 58(2):197–202.
23. Cancer Institute (Hospital) of the Chinese Academy of Medical Sciences. (1978) Annual Report [in English]. Beijing, pp. 855–860.
24. Xia Qj, Zhao Y. (1978) Fungal invasion in esophageal tissue and its possible relation to esophageal carcinoma. *Chin. Med.* Cancer Institute and Ritan Hospital of the

240 **Part VII / Screening for Cancers in High-Risk Groups**

Chinese Academy of Medical Sciences. Collection of Papers for the Twentieth Anniversary of the Cancer and Ritarr Hospital, Beijing.

25. TPTRGHP. (1978) Isolation of fungi from the oral cavity and esophagus of esophageal cancer patients. *Med Ref* 7:13–19.
26. Yang J, Chen ML, Hu GG, Jin Y, Wang SH. (1980) Preliminary studies on the etiology and conditions of carcinogenesis of the esophagus in Linxian. In: Yang J, Gao J, eds., *Experimental Research on Esophageal Cancer.* Beijing: Renmin Weisheng, p. 82.
27. Craddock VM, Henderson AR. (1986) Effect of N-nitrosamine carcinogenic for oesophagus on O^6-alkyl-guanine-DNA-methyl transferase in rat oesophagus and liver. *J Cancer Res Clin Oncol* 111:229–236.
28. Mumford JL, Lee X, Lewtas J, Young TL, Santella RM. (1993) DNA adducts as biomarkers for assessing exposure to polycyclic aromatic hydrocarbons in tissues from Xuan Wei women with high exposure to coal combustion emissions and high lung cancer mortality. *Environ Health Perspect* 99:83–87.
29. Pan G, Takahashi K, Feng Y, et al. (1999) Nested case control study of esophageal cancer in relation to occupational exposure to silica and other dusts. *Am J Ind Med* 35(2):272–280.
30. Tao X, Zhu H, Matanoski GM. (1999) Mutagenic drinking water and risk of male esophgeal cancer. A population based case control study. *Am J Epidemiol* 150(5):443–452.
31. Jass JR, Morson BC. (1983) Epithelial dysplasia in the gastrointestinal tract. In: Sherlock P, George B, Glass J, eds.), *Progress in Gastroenterology,* Vol. 4. New York: Grune & Stratton, pp. 345–371.
32. Shu YJ, Yang 56, Gin SP. (1980) Further studies on the relationship between epithelial dysplasia and carcinoma of the esophagus. *Natl Med J China* 60:39–41.
33. Wang ZY, Wang GQ, Liu FS, et al. (1998) Comparison of the findings detected by x-ray, esophagoscope and histopathology on early esophageal cancers. *Chin Med J* 88(12):693–695.
34. Nabeya K. (1983) Markers of cancer risk in the esophagus and surveillance of high risk groups. In: Sherlock P, Morson BC, Barbara L, et al., eds., *Precancerous Lesions of the Gastrointestinal Tract.* New York: Raven, pp. 71–86.
35. Yang CS. (1980) Research on esophageal cancer in China. A review. *Cancer Res* 40:2633–2644.
36. Guanrei Y, He H, Sungliang Q, et al. (1982) Endoscopic diagnosis of 115 cases of early esophageal carcinoma. *Endoscopy* 14:157–161.
37. Shu YJ. (1983) Cytopathology of the esophagus. An overview of esophageal cytopathology in China. *Acta Cytol* 27:7–16.
38. Roth MJ, Liu SF, Dawsey SM, et al. (1997) Cytologic detection of esophageal squamous cell carcinoma and precursor lesions using balloon and sponge samplers in asymptomatic adults in Linxian, China. *Cancer* 80:2047–2059.
39. Qin DX, Wang GQ, Zuo JH, et al. (1992) Experiences on primary screening of esophageal and gastric cancers with occult-blood bead detector. *Chin J Oncol* 14:77.
40. Qin DX, Wang GQ, Yuan FL. (1988) Screening for upper digestive cancer with an occult blood bead detector. *Cancer* 62:1030–1034.
41. Dawsey SM, Fleischer DE, Wang GQ, et al. (1998) Mucosal iodine staining improves endoscopic visualization of squamous dysplasia and squamous cell carcinoma of the esophagus in Linxian, China. *Cancer* 83:220–231.
42. Dawsey SM, Shen Q, Nieberg RK, et al. (1997) Studies of esophageal balloon cytology in Linxian, China. *Cancer Epidemiol Biomarkers Prev* 6:121–130.
43. Wang GQ. (1989) Data analysis of gastroscopic screening among 2,000 population. *Chin J Oncol* 11(3):201–203.

15 Screening for Liver Cancer in China

Boheng Zhang, MD and Binghui Yang, MD

KEY PRINCIPLES

- Men beginning at age 45 and women at 55 with serological evidence of hepatitis B virus and cirrhosis secondary to hepatitis C virus infection and other forms of chronic hepatitis have increased risk for primary liver cancer and require screening for liver cancer.
- α-Fetoprotein and ultrasonography should be offered every 6 mo to all the patients who are at an increased risk for primary liver cancer.
- Further diagnostic evaluation is recommended in patients with a positive screening test.
- Health care providers who perform the tests should have appropriate proficiency and the tests should be performed correctly.

EPIDEMIOLOGY AND BIOLOGY OF PRIMARY LIVER CANCER IN CHINA

Incidence and Prevalence

In 1990, an estimated 541,000 new cases of primary liver cancer (PLC) were diagnosed and 501,000 people died from liver cancer worldwide, among them, 318,000 (58.8%) new cases and 293,000 (58.5%) deaths occurred in China *(1)*. Since 1990, liver cancer has become the second most common cancer killer in China, accounting for 18.74% of all cancer deaths *(2)*. There are marked geographic variations in the incidence of liver cancer in China. The high-incidence areas include

From: *Cancer Screening: A Practical Guide for Physicians*
Edited by: K. Aziz and G. Y. Wu © Humana Press Inc., Totowa, NJ

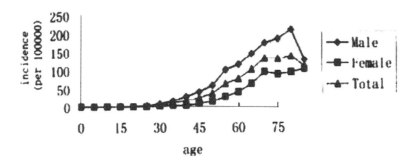

Fig. 1. Incidence of primary liver cancer in Shanghai in 1987–1989.

Jiangsu, Fujian, Guangdong, and Guangxi provinces and other southeast coast areas. The highest incidence occurs in Qidong County, Haimen City, and Fusui County, where the incidence rate is over 50/100,000.

As shown in Fig. 1, the incidence of PLC increases with age; the male-to-female ratio is about 3:1. Factors, including differences in the stage of the disease at the time of diagnosis and aggressiveness of the therapy, have been postulated as contributing to the observed disparity in the survival. However, none of these factors completely explains this observed incongruity.

RISK FACTORS FOR LIVER CANCER IN CHINA

More than 90% of all new cases of PLC occur in people with a background of hepatitis B virus (HBV) infection or chronic hepatitis in China. Incidence increases with age, beginning at 45 yr in men and 55 yr in women (Fig. 1). The risk factors for PLC in China include: (1) chronic viral hepatitis, (2) aflatoxin, and (3) contamination of drinking water.

Chronic Viral Hepatitis

Chronic hepatitis B and C are well recognized as the major risk factors for PLC. Hepatitis B is more predominant compared to hepatitis C in China. The risk of the liver cancer is even greater when a person is infected with both hepatitis B and hepatitis C. A classic study conducted in Taiwan by Beasley *(3)* found that the relative risk of developing hepatocellular carcinoma (HCC) in the HBsAg carriers is 98% compared to the non-HBsAg carriers. Meta-analyses were conducted to summarize the relation between HBV, hepatitis C virus (HCV), infection, and liver cancer in China *(4–6)*. HBsAg positive patients had a

Chapter 15 / Screening for Liver Cancer in China

relative risk of 8.06 (95% confidence interval [CI]: 3.99–16.27) for developing PLC from six cohort studies and an odds ratio of 11.6 (95% CI: 6.37–21.44) from 16 case-control studies. Anti-HCV positive patients had an odds ratio of 5.49 (95% CI: 2.8–10.60) from nine case-control studies. The odds ratio increased to 29.92 (95% CI: 15.41–58.08) if the patient was infected with both HBV and HCV.

Aflatoxin

A mycotoxin formed by *Aspergillus flavus* is a frequent contaminant of improperly stored grains and nuts. Aflatoxin B1 is the most potent and naturally occurring hepatocarcinogen and is active in all animal species. In the endemic areas of PLC in China, the high incidence of PLC may be related to ingestion of foods contaminated with aflatoxin. However, this association is blurred by the frequent coexistence of hepatitis B infection in this population. Results from a nested case-control study conducted in Shanghai suggested the relative risk of PLC in a population exposed to aflatoxin was 2.4. There was a strong interaction between serological markers of chronic hepatitis B infection and aflatoxin exposure in liver cancer risk: The relative risk increased up to 60 *(7)*.

Contaminated Water

Evidence from epidemiological studies shows people drinking pond water have increased risk of developing PLC in the rural area in China. The odds ratio from a meta-analysis for 10 case-control studies was 1.41 (95% CI: 1.10–1.81). Recently, studies found that toxin from blue-green algae, a strong promoter for hepatocarcinogenesis, may play an important role in cancer development *(8)*.

CLINICAL FEATURES

Symptoms and signs of PLC may include abdominal pain, hepatomegaly, and an abdominal mass. Clinical stages of PLC have been arbitrarily defined as Stage I (subclinical; without obvious liver cancer symptoms or signs), Stage II (moderate; between criteria for Stages I and III), and Stage III (late; with cachexia, jaundice, ascites, or distant metastases). Survival from PLC is closely related to the clinical and pathological stages of the disease at diagnosis (*see* Table 1) *(9)*.

NATURAL HISTORY OF PRIMARY LIVER CANCER

The natural history of PLC can be arbitrarily classified into four stages. The total time to develop clinically apparent liver cancer is estimated to be at least 2 yr *(10)*.

Table 1
Treatment and Prognosis in Different Stages

Stage	Resection rate	5-yr survival
I	60.0%	72.9%
II	24.7%	16.1%
III	0	0

- The early subclinical Stage I is from the onset of disease to the diagnosis of subclinical PLC, the median period being around 10 mo, which is also the time needed for a tumor to grow to 4.0 cm.
- The subclinical Stage I is from the diagnosis of subclinical PLC to the occurrence of symptoms, lasting 8–9 mo. PLC can be detected by mass screening using α-fetoprotein (AFP) for an average of 7.9 mo before symptoms occur.
- The moderate Stage II is from the appearance of symptoms and signs to that of jaundice, ascites, or distant metastasis, and lasts about 4 mo. During this period, diagnosis is not difficult.
- The late Stage III is from the appearance of jaundice, ascites, or distant metastasis to death, and lasts 2 mo. No means can effectively prolong survival.

RATIONALE AND STRENGTH OF EVIDENCE FOR SCREENING

Although the importance of primary prevention of PLC was universally acknowledged, the HBV vaccination in newborn babies seems limited as a global strategy to prevent PLC, because HCV may also be involved in the development of PLC. Even in endemic areas of HBV, evaluation of the effects of HBV vaccination as an effective means of preventing PLC may not be possible until after at least 30 yr. The secondary prevention of PLC is another important approach in reducing PLC mortality in the short term.

Primary liver cancer fulfills all of the criteria for justification. First, it causes substantial morbidity and mortality and is the second leading cause of death from cancer in China. Treatment of patients with advanced PLC is largely unsuccessful. Second, screening tests have been shown to achieve accurate detection of early-stage cancers. Third, evidence from controlled trials and uncontrolled studies suggest, with various degrees of persuasiveness, that detecting early-stage cancer reduces mortality from this disease. Finally, cost-effectiveness analysis shows that screening benefits outweigh its harms.

Chapter 15 / Screening for Liver Cancer in China

The natural history of PLC also suggests that screening can be effective. Contrary to the previous concept of relatively short survival time in patients with PLC, the natural history of PLC suggests that patient survival is probably over 2 yr *(10)*. Although not as long as other cancers, PLC still provides a window of opportunity for detecting early-stage cancers. Thus, screening strategies can be directed toward detecting cancers at an early stage to reduce mortality.

Although great advances have been made in the management of symptomatic liver cancer, there has been little overall reduction in mortality from liver cancer during the past 30 yr. Surgical resection offers the reasonable chance of cure for patients at an early stage. Unfortunately, by the time most of these tumors cause symptoms that bring patients to their doctors, most tumors have already spread and the chance of surgical cure is less than 5%.

BRIEF HISTORY OF SCREENING FOR LIVER CANCER IN CHINA

α-Fetoprotein has been used for liver cancer screening since 1971 in China. During 1971–1973, agar gel diffusion (AGD) assay for AFP was used for screening, which had a relatively low sensitivity. The screening was conducted in 343,999 normal people with AGD assay, 147 asymptomatic patients were found to be positive for AFP and 88.4% of these patients were subsequently proven to have HCC during a 2- to 10-mo follow-up period *(11)*. During the period from 1971 to 1976, 1,967,511 patients were screened for serum AFP in Shanghai. Of the 300 HCC patients detected, 134 (44.7%) were diagnosed as subclinical HCC, and the 3-yr survival rate after resection was 57.1% *(12)*. In Qidong City, an endemic area of PLC in China 1,223,912 subjects were screened using serum AFP during the period 1974–1977. Of these, 35.2% patients had subclinical PLC and the 2-yr survival rate after resection for these patients was 69.0% *(13)*.

In the early 1980s, little progress was made in screening for PLC. Because the sensitivity and specificity of AFP as a screening tool was poor, a combination of AFP and ultrasonography was recommended for PLC screening. A randomized controlled trial (RCT) for PLC was carried out among male HBsAg carriers aged 30–69 yr during 1992 to 1995 *(14)*. In this trial, 5581 carriers were randomly assigned to a screening group (3712) with 1869 as a control group. Two hundred fifty-seven PLCs were detected with an incidence of 1341.65 per 100,000 and a mortality rate of 1138.06 per 100,000 in the screening group, whereas in the control group, 117 PLCs were diagnosed, with an incidence of

1195.64 per 100,000 and mortality rate of 1113.89 per 100,000. There was no statistically significant difference in the mortality rates between the two groups. From 1993 to 1997, a well-organized trial was conducted in urban Shanghai by the present authors *(15)*. In this trial, 19,200 people aged 35–59 yr with serum evidence of HBV or a history of chronic hepatitis were randomly allocated to screening (9757) or no screening (control, 9443) group. Screening-group participants were invited to have a serum AFP test and a screening ultrasound every 6 mo. The compliance rate for the screening was 58.2%. When the screening group was compared with the control, the number of patients with PLC was 86 vs 67, 52 patients in the screened group had subclinical PLC versus 0 in the control groups, 40 patients (46.5%) in the screening group had resection versus 5 (5.7%) in the control group, and 1-, 3-, and 5-yr survival rates were 65.9, 52.6, and 46.4% vs 31.2, 7.2, and 0%, respectively. The mortality rate from PLC was significantly lower in the screened group than in the control group: 83.2 per 100,000 and 131.5 per 100,000, respectively, with a mortality ratio of 0.63 (95% CI: 0.41–0.98) *(see* Table 2). The results from these two trials were controversial; the main reason for this difference may be attributed to different strategy of treatment. Only 25% (25 of 100) subclinical PLCs received curative treatment in Qidong *(16)*, whereas 75% subclinical PLCs received curative treatment in the authors' study.

Rationale for the Techniques Used

The most commonly used screening tests are serum AFP testing and ultrasonography scanning. Application of AFP as a screening tool is based on the direct evidence discussed in this chapter and on indirect evidence from clinical practice. The specificity of AFP for screening is not satisfactory, especially in the patients with chronic hepatitis, as it may increase with the flare up of active hepatitis, but the latter can often be differentiated easily by alanine transaminase (ALT) testing. Ultrasonography alone is not helpful as screening tool particularly if the patient has advanced cirrhosis and if the tumor size is too small. The combination of both these tests is complementary and corrects some of the limitations of each test and has been shown to be more effective than either test alone *(18,19)*. As these two tests have small effects on overall inconvenience and cost, they could be applied frequently. The major disadvantage is the decline in the sensitivity and specificity as the tumor size decreases because the objective of the screening is to find early-stage cancer. Overall, these tests are acceptable both to the patients and the clinicians with a reasonable accuracy, simplicity, cost, and safety.

Table 2

Selective Screening Programs for PLC Conducted in China

	Population screened	Screening tools	No. of PLCs detected	Incidence per 100,000	Subclinical PLC
Natural population					
Shanghai (1971–1976)	1,967,511	AFP	300	15.3	134 (44.7%)
Qidong (1974–1980)	1,310,871	AFP	499	38.1	177 (35.5%)
With liver disease					
Shanghai and Qidong	76,660	AFP	253	330.0	NA[a]
Qidong	4,875	AFP	48	948.6	NA
Shanghai	2,997	AFP	15	500.5	5 (33.3%)
Qidong[b] (1992–1995)	19,155 (male)	AFP	257	1342.0	76 (29.6%)
Shanghai[b] (1993–1997)	38,444	AFP + US[a]	86	233.7	52 (60.5%)

[a]US: ultrasonography scanning; NA: not available.
[b]Randomized control trial.
Source: Adapted from ref. 17 with permission.

METHODS OF SCREENING

High-Risk Population

The high-risk population for liver cancer is defined as patients who have background chronic hepatic disease (chronic hepatitis, serological evidence of infection with HBV or HCV, and liver cirrhosis) and are over 40 yr of age. It is clear that the incidence of PLC in this group is increased. In a randomized controlled trial in Shanghai, the incidence of PLC in those 35–59 yr of age with positive HBsAg was 310 per 100,000 for men (12 times higher than normal population) and 76.4 per 100,000 for women (8.5 times higher than the normal population in Shanghai) *(15)*. In Qidong County, the incidence of PLC among male HBsAg carriers age 30–69 yr was 1292.3/100,000 *(14)*. Patients with Child C liver disease are usually excluded from screening, as the prognosis is universally poor and transplantation is not widely available.

Screening Tools

α-Fetoprotein

α-Fetoprotein is produced by the fetal liver and the yolk sac and teratoma of gonads. In some patients, AFP can increase with a flare-up of active hepatitis. The detection of AFP in the serum of patients with PLC has provided a new clue for the early detection and diagnosis of PLC. About 70% patients with PLC have positive AFP. Generally, the concentration of AFP increases with the size of tumor. Patients with the positive results must undergo further diagnostic evaluation, consisting of ALT, ultrasound, or computed tomography (CT). Elevated AFP in active hepatitis is always accompanied with elevated ALT, whereas in PLC, there is usually a normal ALT.

Several methods are used to measure the AFP concentration; these methods include AGD, countercurrent immunoelectrophoresis (CIEP), hemagglutination (RPH), enzyme-linked immunosorbent assay (ELISA), and radioimmunoassay (RIA). The sensitivity and specificity of AFP for PLC screening reported in different studies varied considerably. This variation may be the result of several factors: the different types of test used in the studies; different populations (with or without HBV infection) tested; and whether the test is used for a prevalence screen or an incidence screen. Also, the sensitivity of a test at one point in time is less than if several values are obtained over several years. The performance of characteristics of AFP differs when used for screening or diagnosis.

If the cutoff point of the AFP level for PLC is increased, the sensitivity will decrease while the specificity increases. The usual cutoff point of AFP for screening is 20 mg/L in our institution. Two randomized

Chapter 15 / Screening for Liver Cancer in China

controlled trials of screening using a serial measurement of AFP reported sensitivity and specificity of 80.0%, 80.9% and 68.6%, 95.0%, respectively. The results are significantly superior to obtaining a single value *(14,18)*.

COMBINED AFP AND ULTRASONOGRAPHY

As a screening method, ultrasonography allows clinicians to visualize the liver directly. The unsatisfactory performance of AFP alone led to the use of ultrasonography in addition to or in place of AFP. However, there is no reported program using ultrasonography alone as a screening test in China. There are theoretical reasons for combining AFP testing with ultrasound scanning. Ultrasonography offsets the performance of AFP. In the cirrhotic liver, AFP provides a clue for detecting small cancers. In a randomized controlled trial, when AFP and ultrasonography were used in parallel, the sensitivity and specificity were 92 and 92.5%, respectively *(18)*. Compared with AFP testing alone, the sensitivity was greatly increased without significant loss of specificity.

Screening Interval

There are no studies that directly address the question of how frequently the screening should be performed. Reported screening intervals vary from 3 to 12 mo. However, reasons for choosing these intervals are often not reported. The rationale for performing a screening every 6 mo is based on the indirect evidence reflecting current knowledge of the natural history of the disease and existing data on the performance and relative cost and safety of the procedures. It is generally accepted that the subclinical stage, from the diagnosis of subclinical PLC to the occurrence of symptoms, is approx 8–9 mo *(10)*. It means that most cancers will be detected at subclinical stage if screening is performed every 6 mo. In asymptomatic PLC less than 5 cm in size, the median tumor doubling time was 117 d. *(20)*. The most rapid growing tumors take 5 mo to increase in size from 1 to 3 cm. Therefore, 6-mo screening is a reasonable interval to detect tumors growing from undetectable to detectable size.

Algorithm for PLC Screening and Diagnosis

There is no literature to guide decision-making on the most appropriate way to deal with abnormal screening test results. Empirically, the diagnostic procedure is presented in Algorithm 1.

COST-EFFECTIVENESS

Given effective surveillance, a program still faces challenges to its eventual success. Among them, the challenge of cost-effectiveness has been the most important.

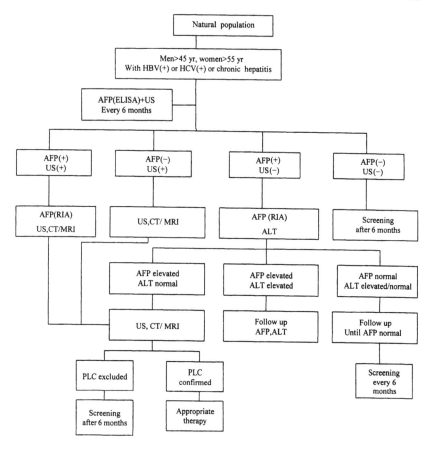

Algorithm 1. PLC screening and diagnosis.

Cost-Effectiveness of Screening Tests

There are limited analyses of the cost of screening for PLC. A cost-analysis study by the present author detected 51 PLCs on screening 20,294 HBV carriers. Further analysis showed that when AFP and ultrasound were used in combination, 36 small PLCs (less than 5 cm) were detected, the cost for each PLC detected was $3639. Using ultrasound alone, 32 small PLCs were detected; the cost for each small PLC was $1982. Using AFP alone, 25 small PLCs were detected, the cost for each small PLC was $3029 *(18)*.

Cost-Effectiveness for Program

The detection of small PLC is consistent with effectiveness but is fallible. So we analyzed the cost-effectiveness of the program. Assuming a population of 100,000 subjects aged 35–59 yr with history of

Chapter 15 / Screening for Liver Cancer in China 251

chronic hepatitis or HBsAg carrier, performing screening for PLC for 1 yr with compliance to screening 58.2% (as reported previously). The results indicated that the cost for each participant in screening group would be $15, and $14 for each individual without screening. The screening group would gain 508 yr of life per 100,000 participants screened compared with no screening. The cost per year of life gain is $213. Using sensitivity analyses, we found that screening will be more cost-effective if the incidence of PLC is higher. If the incidence exceeds 273/100,000, screening would be effective as well as cost saving. It also means that screening in women aged 35–59 might be not so cost-effective. The change of compliance may improve the effectiveness greatly, but improve little on the cost-effectiveness ratio *(21)*.

INDICATIONS FOR CONSULTING THE SUBSPECIALIST

Patients with evidence of HBV or cirrhosis should be informed about the risk of liver cancer. Prompt referral to a subspecialist is warranted if a patient at risk for HCC has a high AFP or abnormal US. Abrupt deterioration in the general condition in a cirrhotic or patient with HBV may indicate development of HCC even in the absence of an abnormal screening test and should be evaluated by a subspecialist.

CONTROVERSIAL AREAS

Screening for PLC has become accepted practice by hepatologists worldwide in patients with a background of HBV and cirrhosis because of HCV or other causes. Cancers can certainly be detected earlier through screening, with a better outcome. Given the effectiveness of screening, many questions should be answered before the program is advocated. One of the major issues is the age at which the screening should be instituted in patients with chronic HBV infection and the cost-effectiveness of screening women because the incidence is much lower in women and they tend to develop PLC at a later age than men. Furthermore, it is unclear if more aggressive screening should be offered to patients with a family history of PLC. It has been shown that HBV-induced PLC may be familial. In a study conducted in Haimen City *(22)*, another endemic area of PLC in China, 40.29% of 278 families had more than two HCC patients. Complex segregation analysis of 490 extended families showed that a recessive allele with a population frequency of approx 0.25 yielded a lifetime risk of PLC of 0.84 for males and 0.46 for females in the presence of both HBV infection and genetic susceptibility. In the absence of genetic susceptibility, the lifetime risk of PLC is 0.09 for HBV-infected males and 0.01 for HBV-infected females, regardless of the genotype. It is virtually zero for uninfected persons. The results provide

252 Part VII / Screening for Cancers in High-Risk Groups

evidence for the interaction of genotype HBV infection in determining the occurrence of PLC.

SUMMARY

Hepatocellular carcinoma ranks as one of the most common neoplasms worldwide and China has the highest incidence of HCC in the world. Almost 60% of all the liver cancers in the world occur in China. The high incidence of HCC in China is a reflection of the very high number of HBV carriers in this country. The peak age of incidence and mortality in China is 10 yr earlier than in the United States and other countries, where the incidence is low. Screening using AFP and ultrasonography for HCC is widely available in China and has shown to detect malignant lesions at an early and potentially treatable stage. However, compliance for the screening is low and massive public education along with the primary preventative measures with HB vaccinations are needed to reduce the mortality of HCC in this country.

REFERENCES

1. Murray CJ, Lopez AD (eds.) (1996) *Global Health Statistics.* Geneva: WHO/ Harvard School of Public Health, World Bank, pp. 551,552.
2. Li L, Zhang S, Lu F, et al. (1997) Research on characteristics of mortality spectrum and type composition of malignant tumors in China. *Chin J Oncol* 19:323–328.
3. Beasley RP. (1988) Hepatitis B virus. The major etiology of hepatocellular carcinoma. *Cancer* 61:1942–1956.
4. Zhao N, Yu SZ. (1994) A meta-analysis of prospective studies for the relationship between Hepatitis B, aflatoxin and liver cancer. *Tumor* 14:225–227.
5. Zhao N, Yu SZ. (1994) A meta-analysis of risk factors for liver cancer; 16 case-control studies. *Chin Prey Control Chronic Dis* 2:10–12.
6. Yu SZ. (1999) Epidemiology and prevention of primary liver cancer. In: Tang ZY, Yu YQ, eds., *Primary Liver Cancer.* 2nd edition. Shanghai: Shanghai and Technology Press, pp. 86–112.
7. Ross RK, Yuan JM, Yu MC, et al. (1992) Urinary aflatoxin biomarkers and risk of hepatocellular carcinoma. *Lancet* 339:943–946.
8. Yu SZ, Chen G. (1994) Blue-green algae toxins and liver cancer. *Chin J Cancer Res* 6:9–12.
9. Tang ZY. (1989) Efforts in the past decades to improve the ultimate outcome of primary liver cancer. In: Tang ZY, Wu MC, Xia SS, eds., *Primary Liver Cancer.* Berlin: Springer-Verlag, pp. 469–481.
10. Tang ZY. (1981) A new concept on the natural course of hepatocellular carcinoma. *Chin Med J* 94:585–588.
11. The Coordinating Group for Research on Liver Cancer, China. (1974) Alpha-fetoprotein assay in primary hepatocellular carcinoma mass survey and follow-up studies. *Tumor Prevent Treat Study* 2:277–286.
12. Tang ZY, Yu EX, Wu CE, et al. (1974) Diagnosis and treatment of primary hepatocellular carcinoma in early stage report of 134 cases. *Chin J Med* 92:801–806.

Chapter 15 / Screening for Liver Cancer in China 253

13. Zhu YR. (1981) AFP serosurvey and early diagnosis of liver cell cancer in the Qidong area. *Chin J Oncol* 3:35–37.
14. Chen JG, Lu JH, Chen QG, et al. (1997) Study on effect of screening on mortality of primary cancer of liver. *Chin J Public Health* 16:341–343.
15. Yang B, Zhang B, Tang Z. (1999) Randomized controlled prospective study of secondary prevention for primary liver cancer. *Natl Med J China* 79:887–889.
16. Zhang BC, Wang MR, Chen JG, et al. (1994) Analysis of patients with primary liver cancer detected (I) at mass screening and (II) during follow-up period in a high risk population. *Chin J Clin Oncol* 2(1):489–491.
17. Tang ZY, Yang BH. (1995) Secondary prevention of hepatocellular carcinoma. *J Gastroenterol Hepatol* 10:683–690.
18. Zhang B, Yang B. (1999) Combined α-fetoprotein testing and ultrasonography as a screening test for primary liver cancer. *J Med Screen* 6:108–110.
19. Yang B, Tang Z. (1989) The value of ultrasound in mass screening for primary liver cancer. *Tumor* 9:118–120.
20. Sheu JC, Sung JL, Chen DS, et al. (1984) Growth rates of asymptomatic hepatocellular carcinoma and its clinical implications. *Gastroenterology* 86:1404–1409.
21. Zhang B, Yang B. (1999) Cost-effectivenss analysis of screening for primary hepatic cancer. *Clin Med J Chin* 6:106–108.
22. Shen FM, Lee MK, Gong HM, et al. (1991) Complex segregation analysis of primary hepatocellular carcinoma in Chinese families: interaction of inherited susceptibility and hepatitis B viral infection. *Am J Hum Genet* 49:88–93.

16 Screening for Gastric Cancer in Japan

Masao Ichinose, MD, Naohisa Yahagi, MD, Masashi Oka, MD, Hitoshi Ikeda, MD, Kaumasa Miki, MD, and Masao Omata, MD

KEY PRINCIPLES

- Japan has one of the highest incidences of stomach cancer in the world.
- Several risk factors for stomach cancer have been identified, including salt, nitrates, and low intake of fresh fruits and vegetables; however, *Heliobacter pylori* infection and atrophic gastritis are strongly related to gastric cancer. The prevalence of *H. pylori* and atrophic gastritis in Japan is markedly higher than other industrialized nations of the world.
- In Japan, gastric cancer mass screening has been conducted since 1960, with a significant reduction in mortality and morbidity.
- Traditionally, barium X-rays have been used for gastric cancer screening. Recently, the addition of serum pepsinogen to the barium X-ray has been shown to improve the detection rate of gastric cancer.

INTRODUCTION

Stomach cancer remains one of the leading causes of cancer-related death worldwide. The highest rate of stomach cancer is in Chile and Japan; one of the lowest rates is in the United States. In Japan, a gastric cancer screening program was introduced in the 1960s as a public health

From: *Cancer Screening: A Practical Guide for Physicians*
Edited by: K. Aziz and G. Y. Wu © Humana Press Inc., Totowa, NJ

service that has gradually been extended to include the whole nation. Currently, screening is performed throughout the country and more than 6 million people annually undergo screening provided by either a community service or the workplace. As a result, thousands of stomach cancer cases are detected each year, and cancer screening has greatly contributed to the reduction in the stomach cancer mortality rates. Screening most frequently includes the use of double-contrast barium X-rays or panendoscopy. Serum pepsinogen tests were recently introduced for mass screening to identify individuals at high risk for stomach cancer. Individuals testing positive for extensive atrophic gastritis based on their serum pepsinogen levels undergo endoscopic examination or a high-quality barium X-ray to test for the presence of stomach cancer. The results of the serum screening tests are comparable and, in some respect superior to, those of traditional screening. The objective of this chapter is to describe the current status of the screening for stomach cancer in Japan.

EPIDEMIOLOGY

Despite a consistent decline in incidence throughout the world, stomach cancer is still one of the leading causes of cancer-related death in Japan. The stomach is the most common site for cancer; in 1993, the estimated incidence was 63,404 among males and 33,478 among females (1). The age-adjusted mortality rate per 100,000 was 45.4 for males and 18.5 for females (2). The worldwide decline in stomach cancer is an unexpected phenomenon that cannot be explained simply by advances in medical diagnosis and treatment. Rather, changes in diet and attention to environmental factors that contribute to carcinogenesis are considered largely responsible (3,4). The decline in the incidence of gastric cancer in Japan may be partly the result of the westernization of the Japanese diet in the last three or four decades. Although there are several risk factors for stomach cancer, such as salt, nitrates, and low intake of fresh fruits and vegetables, the accumulated pathologic and epidemiological evidence suggests that atrophic gastritis together with intestinal metaplasia is a precursor of stomach cancer (4–6). Areas of the world with high rates of stomach cancer also have a high prevalence of atrophic gastritis, and follow-up studies indicate that almost all stomach cancer occurs in patients with atrophic gastritis (7–10). Therefore, individuals with atrophic gastritis are populations at high risk for cancer. The high incidence of *Helicobacter pylori* in both symptomatic and asymptomatic persons with gastritis indicates a contributory role for *H. pylori* in initiating the mucosal injury and subsequent development of

Chapter 16 / Screening for Gastric Cancer in Japan

atrophic gastritis. An association between *H. pylori* and stomach cancer was recently reported in several prospective and cross-sectional studies *(11–19)*, and has received widespread attention among epidemiologists and gastroenterologists. Atrophic gastritis is now considered a risk factor for stomach carcinogenesis. The prevalence of *H. pylori* infection and atrophic gastritis is markedly higher in Japan than in other industrialized countries, although the reason for the high prevalence is not fully understood. Several studies indicate a recent trend toward a reduction in the prevalence of *H. pylori* infection and atrophic gastritis *(20,21)*, which appears to be related to the recent decline in the incidence of stomach cancer in Japan. The relatively high incidence of *H. pylori* infection in the noncancerous population, however, indicates that most people with *H. pylori* do not develop stomach cancer and that other contributing factors are important in the pathogenesis *(16,22)*.

As it is unclear when atrophic gastritis begins in any individual case, it is difficult to predict the resulting incidence of the cancer. Various studies, however, indicate that a relatively small proportion, approx 10%, of subjects with gastritis will develop stomach cancer and a relatively long period of time (10–20 yr) is required for the development of the cancer *(7–10,23)*.

PATHOLOGY AND BIOLOGY OF STOMACH CANCER

Adenocarcinoma is the major type of malignant stomach neoplasm, representing approx 95% of the total cases. The remaining 5% include lymphomas, sarcomas, and other less common types, such as squamous-cell carcinoma, adenoacanthoma, carcinoid, and so forth. The term *stomach cancer* usually refers to adenocarcinoma of the stomach. According to the Lauren classification system, adenocarcinoma is classified into two histologically distinct groups: the intestinal type and the diffuse type *(24)*. This classification, based on tumor histology, effectively characterizes two types of stomach cancer that manifest distinctively different pathological, epidemiological, and biological characteristics. The intestinal type of the cancer typically arises within intestinal metaplasia, a highly frequent lesion of the gastric antrum, whereas the diffuse type is less frequently associated with intestinal metaplasia and typically arises in the corpus *(24)*.

The intestinal type is characterized by epithelial cells that form discrete glands and is more likely to present as a protruding polypoid lesion. In contrast, sheets of epithelial cells characterize the diffuse type of cancer or cells scattered in the stromal matrix without evidence of gland formation. The diffuse type of adenocarcinoma tends to be cytologically less differentiated and has a predilection for extensive submucosal spread and early metastasis. Therefore, this pathologic type is associated with a poorer prognosis than the intestinal type. The incidence of intestinal-type, but not diffuse-type, stomach cancer varies widely depending on geographic regions *(25,26)*. The incidence of the intestinal type of cancer has been declining over the past several decades. In contrast, there has been little, if any, decrease in the incidence of the diffuse type *(27)*. These facts strongly suggest that the mechanisms involved in carcinogenesis are different between the two types of cancer and that the intestinal type is more dependent on environmental factors. The current model of the histological changes that precede intestinal-type cancer begins with gastritis, proceeds to extensive atrophic gastritis together with intestinal metaplasia, and then to dysplasia *(28)*. Although the association between atrophic gastritis together with intestinal metaplasia and intestinal-type cancer is very strong, as suggested by various pathologic, clinical, and epidemiological evidence, there is only a weak association, if any, between atrophic gastritis and diffuse-type cancer *(29,30)*.

DIAGNOSIS OF STOMACH CANCER

Symptoms of stomach cancer are vague and nonspecific and do not occur until advanced stages. Because the cancer is a highly curable disease following adequate resection when detected at an early stage, the importance of early detection is repeatedly stressed in Japan, where, in the 1970s and early 1980s, mortality rates were the highest in the world. The medical establishment in Japan has historically concentrated on early detection and treatment of stomach cancer. The low cost of health care allowed for the widespread use of double-contrast barium X-ray and endoscopy, which has led to dramatic progress in the diagnosis of early stomach cancer. Currently, high-resolution video image endoscopy is widespread. High-resolution video image endoscopy, together with dye-spraying methods, allows for visualization of minute lesions (<5 mm in size), and the detection of minute cancers is not rare. The proportion of early cancers in the surgically resected cases now exceeds 50% in our hospital *(31)*. Early stomach cancers are defined as carcinoma confined to the mucosa or submucosa irrespective of lymph node involvement *(32)*. Because the depth of the cancer invasion is closely correlated with lymph node metastasis (mucosal cancer, 3%; submucosal cancer, 20%) *(33)*, it strongly influences the prognosis of the cancer and the survival rates decrease dramatically with the progression of the stage; relative 5-yr survival rates are as follows, for Stage

Chapter 16 / Screening for Gastric Cancer in Japan 259

Ib 75.9 %; Stage II, 68.4%; Stage III, 28.3%; and Stage IV, 3.0% (data from the First Department of Surgery, University of Tokyo Hospital). Although aggressive radical gastrectomy with extensive lymph-node dissection is used to treat advanced cancer, the possibilities for endoscopic treatment without laparotomy or gastrectomy with minimal node dissection for small early-stage stomach cancers, patients at high operative risk, or elderly patients are being debated. Thus, the detection of the depth of cancer invasion is becoming more important, not only for making the prognosis but also for selection of the treatment strategy. Algorithm 1 shows the regular process in the diagnosis of stomach cancer in Japan. Following detection and confirmation of the histology of the cancer, the extent of cancer invasion and metastasis is evaluated. The accuracy of endoscopic diagnosis based on pathomorphological criteria decreases as the depth of the cancer invasion increases; therefore, endoscopic ultrasonography has been used in recent years for the assessment of the depth of invasion and for the detection of regional lymph node metastasis. If a small intestinal-type cancer (<2 cm in diameter) is diagnosed as mucosal cancer, the patient can avoid laparotomy when the lesion is resected completely by endoscopic surgery. Until now, Japanese physicians have adopted an aggressive approach toward early and precise diagnosis of the cancer to reduce the alarming mortality rate of stomach cancer. In Japan, the current 5-yr survival rate for stomach cancer is estimated to be approx 60% on average *(34)*. This high survival rate can also be attributed to nationwide gastric mass screening.

STOMACH CANCER SCREENING IN JAPAN

As described in the previous sections, stomach cancer is a serious public health problem in Japan. Therefore, a screening program for stomach cancer detection was introduced over a quarter of a century ago, and continues to be extensively conducted as a nationwide public service. The Health and Medical Services Law for the Aged was established in 1983. The aim of the screening program, based on the law, was to screen 30% of the population aged 40 and over (approx 12 million people each year) *(35)*. Currently, more than 6 million people of cancer-prone age are screened annually, and the screening often includes the use of double-contrast barium X-rays or endoscopy.

Barium X-Rays

In the mass screening, a double-contrast barium X-ray is the traditional first screening step, after which those suspected of having cancer (approx 12% of the screened subjects) are further investigated using a

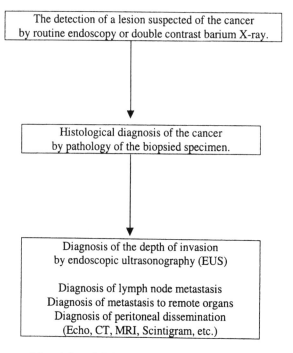

Algorithm 1. Diagnosis of stomach cancer.

higher-quality barium X-ray using photofluorography with six standard views or by endoscopy. The cost is relatively low (about 3500 yen per capita); thus, more than 80% of the screening throughout Japan uses the barium X-ray *(36)*. The remaining 20% of the subjects are screened directly using high-quality barium X-ray, and less than 1% are screened using endoscopy. In 1997, 6,446,917 people underwent stomach cancer screening, and, as a result, 6891 persons were diagnosed with stomach cancers (a detection rate of 0.107%) *(36)*. Among them, 3,266,613 persons were screened by local community health services and 2,940,276 screened by the workplace (Table 1). The detection rate of the cancer is approximately three times higher through the community health services than through the workplace, partly because the proportion of people younger than 40 yr of age is higher in the workplace (2.9 vs 20.5%), but mainly because nearly half of the subjects positive in the first screening are not further screened. With the introduction of screening, the proportion of cancers detected in the early stages has increased progressively; currently two-thirds of surgically operated cancers detected in the screening are in the early stage (Tables 2 and 3) *(36)*. Of these cancers, 15.5% were less than 1 cm in diameter, and approx 10% of the cancers were resected endoscopically. These screenings, together with endoscopies

Chapter 16 / Screening for Gastric Cancer in Japan

Table 1

The Results of Japanese Conventional Stomach Mass Screening in 1997

	By Community Health Service	By workplace	Total
No. of subjects	3,266,613	2,940,276	6,206,889
No. of positive subjects by barium X-ray	411,200	333,234	744,434
Incidence of the above	12.6%	11.3%	12.0%
No. of positive subjects to undergo the second step of screening	344,195	188,450	532,645
Incidence of the above	83.7%	56.6%	71.6%
No. of stomach cancers detected	5153	1524	6677
Detection rate	0.16%	0.05%	0.11%

Table 2

Stomach Cancers Detected by Mass Screening in 1997: Surgically Resected Stomach Cancers According to Their Histological Stages

Total no. of cases	m	sm	mp	ss	s	m + sm	mp + ss +
5151 (100.0%)	2058 (40.0%)	1433 (27.8%)	538 (10.4%)	562 (10.9%)	560 (10.9%)	3491 (67.8%)	1660 (32.2%)

Note: m, cancer invasion of mucosa; sm, submucosa; mp, muscularis propria; ss, subserosa; serosa.

Table 3

Treatment of the Cancers Detected by Mass Screening in 1997

Total no. of cases	5449
Surgical operation	4700
Laproscopic surgery	40
Endoscopic surgery	543
Chemotherapy	47
No treatment	76
Others	43

performed on symptomatic patients, have increased 5-yr survival rates to more than 95% for early stomach cancer (37). Therefore, Japanese physicians are reasonably convinced that an aggressive approach toward early detection of stomach cancer has led to a substantial reduction in mortality rates from stomach cancer. In fact, the rate of death from stomach cancer has declined, even as the population is rapidly aging. In addition, when different areas of Japan are compared, the decline in the rate is closely correlated with the intensity of the mass screening *(38)*. Because the screening program has been introduced as a public health service and is widely available, it is difficult to make randomized clinical trials for any formal evaluation of the efficacy of the cancer screening. Several retrospective studies reveal a substantial reduction in mortality rates from stomach cancers as a result of screening *(39–41)*. Fukao et al. examined medical records in the Miyagi prefecture during the period from 1960 to 1991 and estimated that there was an approximately 60% reduction in mortality rates for individuals over the age of 50 screened by the mass survey at least once in the past 5 yr *(40,41)*. Nationwide stomach cancer screening has been an unparalleled success; however, the number of people screened has not increased, attaining only 50% of the level intended by the Health and Medical Services Law for the aged. The cancer screening covers only 7.25% of the cancer-prone-age population throughout Japan. Furthermore, the sensitivity of the barium X-ray is not very high (sensitivity for early stage cancer is 39% and that for advanced cancer is 92%) *(42)*. Also, because of its low resolution, the barium X-ray is usually only indicative of abnormalities in the stomach mucosa; therefore, more than half of the early cancer cases are not diagnosed. The recent addition of pepsinogen in the screening strategy has significantly increased the detection rate of gastric cancer.

Serum Pepsinogen

As described in the previous section, chronic atrophic gastritis together with intestinal metaplasia is a well-known precancerous lesion, pepsinogen gastritis *(43–45)*. It is classified into two biochemically and immunologically distinct types, namely, PGI and PGII (PGI is also called PGA, and PGII is also called PGC). PGI is produced by chief and mucous neck cells in the fundic glands, while PGII is produced by these cells and also by the cells in the pyloric glands and Brunner's glands *(43)*. It is widely accepted that serum pepsinogen levels reflect the functional and morphologic status of stomach mucosa. As the fundic gland mucosa reduces, PGI levels gradually decrease, whereas PGII levels remain fairly constant *(46)*. As a result, a stepwise reduction of the PGI/ II ratio is closely correlated with the progression from normal gastric mucosa to extensive atrophic gastritis with a sensitivity of 93.3% and specificity of 87.7% *(46)*.

Chapter 16 / Screening for Gastric Cancer in Japan

The single use of pepsinogen tests is by no means sufficient for stomach cancer screening; however, it provides a valuable measure for selecting population that needs further screening with either barium X-rays or endoscopy *(46,47)*. Serum pepsinogen was introduced for cancer screening to identify individuals with extensive atrophic gastritis *(48,49)*. Individuals testing positive for extensive atrophic gastritis by serum pepsinogen levels (PGI<70 ng/mL, a I/II ratio<3.0) undergo endoscopic examination or high-quality barium X-ray to test for the presence of stomach cancer. It has shown a sensitivity of 80%, specificity of 70%, cancer detection rate of 0.44%, and a positive predictive value of 1.5% *(50)*. In the past 8 yr, a considerable number of screening services provided by workplaces and also by community health services have adopted the serum tests as a primary screening tool *(48–50)*. Results of these screenings demonstrate that the cancer detection rate of the screening with the serum tests is superior and more cost-effective as compared to the conventional barium X-ray mass screening (Table 4). Furthermore, the percentage of early cancers detected by the new serum test screening is higher than conventional screening and a considerable number of patients have been treated by endoscopic surgery. Because the tests detect extensive atrophic gastritis coexisting with cancer, it is possible that the diffuse type of cancer will not be detected by the serum tests. The results of the mass screenings clearly indicate that this is not true, although the serum test screening is especially useful in detecting small asymptomatic cancers, nonulcerated morphology type, and differentiated histology type. Small asymptomatic cancers of this type are relatively difficult to detect using barium X-rays, whereas conventional screening is good for detecting cancers with an ulcerated morphology type and an undifferentiated histology type, which are frequently symptomatic. Because the cancers detected by the two screening methods are different, the combination of the two methods has greatly improved the screening efficacy and is more cost-effective. Algorithm 2 shows some of the examples of cancer screenings performed in Japan using a combination of the two methods.

SUMMARY

Mortality from gastric cancer in Japan has been decreasing; however, it is still the leading cause of cancer deaths in Japan. Mass screening for stomach cancer in high-incidence areas has resulted in a steady decline in the number of late-stage cancers diagnosed and a corresponding increase in the earlier-stage tumors. Mass screening for gastric cancer is not applicable to the US population because of the very low incidence; however, in

Table 4

Comparison of Cost-Effectiveness Among the Stomach Cancer Screening Methods in Japan

Screening method	No. of screens	Total net cost (10,000 yen)	No. of stomach cancers (%) (early cancer)	Detection rate (%) (early cancer)	Net cost for detection of one gastric cancer (early-stage cancer)
Serum pepsinogen tests[a]	16,596	5864	38 (29)	0.23 (0.17)	154 (202)
Indirect barium X-ray[b]	5808	3180	10 (5)	0.17 (0.09)	318 (636)
High-quality barium X-ray[c]	1379	2004	4 (4)	0.29 (0.29)	501 (501)
Barium X-ray in total	7187	5183	15 (9)	0.21 (0.13)	346 (576)

[a]2000 yen/capita.
[b]4,116 yen/capita.
[c]11,311 yen/capita.
Note: Encoscopy for the second step of screening: 13,000 yen/capita.

Chapter 16 / Screening for Gastric Cancer in Japan

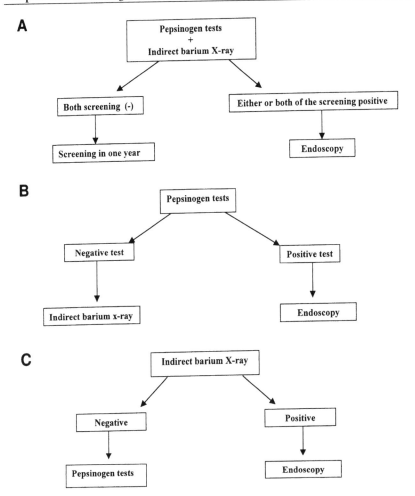

Algorithm 2. Stomach cancer screening with combination of the two methods: pepsinogen tests and conventional barium X-ray.

areas of high incidence such as western Pacific, Central and South America, and northern Europe, it can reduce mortality and there is a need to develop a cancer control program in these areas.

REFERENCES

1. The Research Group for Population-Based Cancer Registration in Japan (1999) In: Tominaga S, Oshima A, eds., *Cancer Mortality and Statistics*, Tokyo: Japan Scientific Societies Press, pp. 83–143.
2. Kuroishi T, Hirose K, Tajima K, Tominag, S. (1999) Cancer mortality in Japan, In: Tominaga S, Oshima A, eds., *Cancer Mortality and Statistics*, Tokyo: Japan Scientific Societies Press, pp. 1–82.
3. Correa P. (1991) The epidemiology of gastric cancer. *World J Surg* 15:228–234.

266 Part VII / Screening for Cancers in High-Risk Groups

4. Kono S, Hirohata T. (1994) A review on the epidemiology of stomach cancer. *J. Epidemiol* 4:1–11.
5. Kurtz RC, Sherlock P. (1985) The diagnosis of gastric cancer. *Sem Oncol* 12:11–18.
6. Boeing H. (1991) Epidemiological research in stomach cancer. Progress over the last ten years. *J Cancer Res Clin Oncol* 117:133–143.
7. Imai T, Kubo T, Watanabe H. (1971) Chronic gastritis in Japanese with reference to high incidence of gastric carcinoma. *J Natl Cancer Inst* 47:179–195.
8. Siurala M, Vuorinen Y. (1963) Follow-up studies of patients with superficial gastritis and patients with a normal gastric mucosa. *Acta Med Scand* 173:45–52.
9. Munoz N, Matko I. (1972) Histological types of gastric cancer and its relationship with intestinal metaplasia. *Recent Results Cancer Res* 39:99–105.
10. Cheli R, Santi L, Ciancamerla SG, Canciani GA. (1973) A clinical and statistical follow-up study of atrophic gastritis. *Am J Dig Dis* 18:1061–1065.
11. Correa P, Fox J, Fontham E. (1990) Helicobacter pylori and gastric carcinoma. Serum antibody prevalence in populations with contrasting cancer risks. *Cancer* 66:2569–2574.
12. Forman D, Sitas F, Newell DG. (1990) Geographic association of Helicobacter pylori antibody prevalence and gastric cancer mortality in rural China. *Int J Cancer* 46:608–611.
13. Nomura A, Stemmermann GN, Chyou PH, et al. (1991) Helicobacter pylori infection and gastric carcinoma among Japanese Americans in Hawaii. *N Engl J Med* 325:1132–1136.
14. Parsonnet J, Friedman G D, Vandersteen DP. (1991) Helicobacter pylori infection and infection and the risk of gastric carcinoma. *N Engl J Med* 325:1127–1131.
15. Sipponen P, Kosunen TU, Valle J, Riihela M, Seppala K. (1992) Helicobacter pylori infection and chronic gastritis in gastric cancer. *J Clin Pathol* 45:319–23.
16. The Eurogast Study Group. (1993) An international association between Helicobacter pylori infection and gastric cancer. *Lancet* 341:1359–1362.
17. Blaser MJ, Perez-Perez GI, Kleanthous H, et al. (1995) Infection with Helicobacter pylori strains possessing cagA is associated with an increased risk of developing adenocarcinoma of the stomach. *Cancer Res* 55:2111–2115.
18. Huang, JQ, Sridhar S, Chen Y, Hunt RH. (1998) Meta-analysis of the relationship between Helicobacter pylori seropositivity and gastric cancer. *Gastroenterology* 114:1169–1179.
19. Eslick GD, Lim LL, Byles JE, Xia HH, Talley NJ. (1999) Association of Helicobacter pylori infection with gastric carcinoma: a meta-analysis. *Am J Gastroenterol* 94:2373–2379.
20. Youn HS, Baik SC, Cho YK, et al. (1998) Comparison of Helicobacter pylori infection between Fukuoka, Japan and Chinju, Korea. *Helicobacter* 3:9–14.
21. Haruma K, Okamoto S, Kawaguchi H, et al. (1997) Reduced incidence of Helicobacter pylori infection in young Japanese persons between the 1970s and 1990s. *J Clin Gastroent* 25:583–586.
22. Megraud F, Brassens-Rabbe MP, Denis F, Belbouri A, Hoa DQ. (1989) Seroepidemoiology of Campylobacter pylori infection in various populations. *J Clin Microbiol* 27:1870–1873.
23. Findley JW, Kirsner JB, Palmer L. (1950) Atrophic gastritis: a follow-up study of 100 patients. *Gastroenterology* 16:347–355.
24. Lauren P. (1965) The two histological main types of gastric carcioma: diffuse and so-called interstiitial type carcinoma. *Acta Pathol Microbial Scand* 64:31–49.
25. Munoz N, Correa P. Cuello C, Duque E. (1968) Histologic types of gastric carcinoma in high- and low-risk areas. *Int J Cancer* 3:809–818.

Chapter 16 / Screening for Gastric Cancer in Japan 267

26. Correa P, Sasano N, Stemmermann GN, Haenszel W. (1973) Pathology of gastric carcinoma in Japanese populations comparisons between Miyagi prefecture, Japan and Hawaii. *J Natl Cancer Inst* 51:1449–1459.
27. Fujimoto I, Hanai, A. (1987) Trends of cancer incidence by site and histological types in Osaka, Japan, 1963-1983. *Gann Monogr Cancer Res* 33:25–31.
28. Correa P. (1988) A human model of gastric carcinogenesis. *Cancer Res* 48:3554–3560.
29. Ngayo T. (1977) Precursors of human gastric cancer. Their frequencies and histological characteristics. In: Farber E, ed., *Pathophysiology of Carcinogenesis in the Digestive Organs*. Baltimore: University Park Press, pp. 151–160.
30. Correa P. (1984) Chronic gastritis and gastiric cancer. In: Ming SC, ed., *Precursors of Gastric Cancer*. New York: Praeger Publishers, pp. 105–116.
31. Sano T, Kobori O, Muto T. (1992) Lymph node metastasis from early gastric cancer: endoscopic resection of tumor. *Br J Surg* 79:241–244.
32. Kajitani T. (1981) The general rules for the gastric cancer study in surgery and pathology. Part I: clinical classification. *Jpn J Surg* 11:127–139.
33. Hioki K, Nakane Y, Yamamoto M. (1990) Surgical strategy for early gastric cancer. *Br J Surg* 77:1330–1334.
34. Inokuchi K. (1991) Prolonged survival of stomach cancer patients after extensive surgery and adjuvant treatment: an overview of the Japanese experience. *Semin Surg Oncol* 7:333–338.
35. Oshima A. (1988) Screening for stomach cancer: the Japanese program. In: Chamberlain J, Miller AB, eds., *Screening for Gastrointestinal Cancer*. Toronto: Hans Huber (for UICC), pp. 65–70.
36. Annual report on gastrointestinal mass survey [in Japanese]. In: *Statistic Committee of Japanese Association of Gastrointestinal Mass Survey*, pp. 196–207.
37. Yamazaki H. (1995) On the prognosis of stomach cancer of the aged detected by mass screening [in Japanese]. *J Gastroenterol Mass Survey* 33:445–455.
38. Kuroishi T, Hirose K, Nakagawa N, Tominaga S. (1983) Comparison of time trends of stomach cancer death rates between the model area of the screening program and the control are [in Japanese]. *J Gastroenterol Mass Survey* 58:45–52.
39. Oshima A, Hirata N, Ubukata T, Umeda K, Fujimoto I. (1986) Evaluation of a mass screening program for stomach cancer with a case-control study design. *Int J Cancer* 38:82,933.
40. Abe Y, Mitsushima T, Nagatani K, Ikuma H, Minamihara, Y. (1995) Epidemiological evaluation of the protective effect for dying of stomach cancer by screening programme for stomach cancer with applying a method of case-control: a study of efficient screening programme for stomach cancer [in Japanese]. *Jpn J Gastroent* 92:836–845.
41. Fukao A, Tsubono Y, Tsuji I, et al. (1995) The evaluation of screening for gastric cancer in Miyagi prefecture, Japan: a population-based case-control study. *Int J Cancer* 60:45–48.
42. Nishizawa M. (1993) Present status and prospect for cancer screening [in Japanese]. *J Gastroenterol Mass Survey* 78:100–103.
43. Samloff IM. (1982) Pepsinogens I and II: purification from gastric mucosa and radioimmunoassay in serum. *Gastroenterology* 82:26–33.
44. Samloff IM, Secrist DM, Passaro E. (1975) A study of the relationship between serum group I pepsinogen levels and gastric acid secretion. *Gastroenterology* 69:1196–2000.
45. Ichinose M, Miki K, Furihata C, et al. (1982) Radioimmunoassay of serum group I and group II pepsinogens in normal controls and patients with various disorders. *Clin Chim Acta* 126:183–191.

46. Miki K, Ichinose M, Shimizu A. (1987) Serum pepsinogens as a screening test of extensive chronic gastritis. *Gastroenterol Jpn* 22:133–141.
47. Miki K, Ichinose M, Kawamura N. (1989) The significance of low serum pepsinogen levels to detect stomach cancer associated with extensive chronic gastritis in Japanese subjects. *Jpn J Cancer Res* 80:111–114.
48. Miki K, Ichinose M, Ishikawa K, et al. (1993) The clinical application of the serum pepsinogen I and II levels as a mass screening method to detect stomach cancer. *Jpn Cancer Res* 84:1086–1090.
49. Kodoi A, Yoshihara M, Sumii K, Haruma K, Kajiyama G. (1995) Serum pepsinogen in screening for gastric cancer. *J Gastroenterol* 30:452–460.
50. Miki K. (1999) New Gastric cancer screening with serum pepsinogen. *Front Gastroenterol* 4:139–150.

VIII

FUTURE PROSPECTS IN CANCER SCREENING

17 Advanced Imaging Technology for Future Cancer Screening

Jeff L. Fidler, MD

KEY PRINCIPLES

- Recent advances in the field of radiology have revolutionized CT and MRI technology.
- There has been significant improvement not only in the speed of acquisition of images but also in the clarity and quality of images obtained.
- The newer techniques have shown promising results in the screening of several cancers, however, they are not currently utilized because of their high cost.
- The cost-effectiveness of these techniques need to be addressed before their implementation in the cancer screening.

TECHNICAL CONSIDERATIONS

Within the past several years, there has been a significant improvement in computer technology, which has translated into rapid advancement in computed tomography (CT) and magnetic resonance imaging (MRI) technology. These improvements have allowed CT and MRI to expand their clinical roles to include oncologic applications. In this section, we will discuss and describe these advancements.

CT

The major changes in CT technology have been in the geometry of image acquisition and postprocessing techniques. In the early 1990s helical or spiral CT scanners were introduced that allowed several

From: *Cancer Screening: A Practical Guide for Physicians*
Edited by: K. Aziz and G. Y. Wu © Humana Press Inc., Totowa, NJ

advantages over the previously available incremental technique. Incremental scanning acquired images by rotating the radiation source around the patient. The individual slices were acquired at a preselected thickness or collimation. Following this image acquisition, the table moves the patient to the next location and the process is repeated. This process required approx 2 s for the rotation and a 6-s delay to position the table into the next location.

Spiral CT revolutionized the way CT was performed. Spiral or helical CT acquires images by continually rotating the radiation source around the patient during continual table movement through the radiation source. This produces a "spiral" or "corkscrew" appearance of the acquisition. A single image can now be obtained in 1 s. This improvement in speed leads to improved sensitivity and specificity, as images can be acquired during the time of optimal organ enhancement with improved conspicuity of pathology. Also, several passes or phases can be performed through pathology, allowing dynamic information to be obtained. Because helical data are a continuous acquisition, this creates a large volume set that can undergo several computer manipulations. Images can be reconstructed so that they overlap each other, leading to improved resolution. Also, data can be reconstructed in three-dimensional views. These techniques lead to a decrease in partial voluming artifacts (reduced false-positive results). The three-dimensional views can also allow a better perspective of the relationship of pathology to normal tissues.

A further increase in speed by performing incomplete rotations of the radiation source led to the development of CT fluoroscopy. Several images can be obtained per second and allow real-time visualization of interventional equipment. However, this speed comes at a trade-off in resolution.

The most recent breakthrough in CT is multislice or multidetector scanners. A conventional helical CT has one row of detectors in the ring around the scanners. Multidetectors have several rows of detectors that can be utilized in a single rotation of the radiation source, thus creating more images per rotation. This technology further increases the speed of the exam. For example, 5-mm-thick images can be obtained through the entire chest, abdomen, and pelvis in a total time of less than 20 s. A multislice detector is currently undergoing investigation to determine the further improvements in sensitivity and specificity allowed with this technique. As the CT speed increases, two scenarios can occur. Thinner slices with improved resolution can be obtained and multiple phases or passes through regions of interest can be performed. This leads to the creation of hundreds of images per examination. In order to manipulate

Chapter 17 / Advanced Imaging Technology 273

this amount of data, computer postprocessing techniques and networking technology have had to improve. The time for the computer to reconstruct the images is much faster today. Three-dimensional models can be reconstructed relatively quickly. Today, interpretation of these studies are often performed on workstations, as filming of all of the images acquired would be prohibitive. It is likely that in the future, data will be reviewed and displayed three-dimensionally instead of the current axial projections.

MRI

Advances in MRI technology can be discussed in one of several categories, including the magnet, coils, pulse sequences, and contrast agents. Magnet design has improved in several areas. Magnets are now not as confining and most vendors have open MRI scanners. These magnets allow improved patient tolerance with a decrease in the number of inadequate or suboptimal exams because of claustrophobia. Magnet strength is stronger, which allows a higher resolution and faster scans. Some vendors now have magnets that are dedicated for certain applications, including neurology, cardiac, and musculoskeletal.

Coils are very important in obtaining high-resolution images. Many dedicated coils are currently available that allow the coil to be placed near the region of interest. Examples include the breast, torso, endoluminal, and a variety of musculoskeletal coils.

Parameters that are utilized in MRI to obtain images, referred to as pulse sequences, have also improved. The majority of these improvements have been to decrease examination times. Decreased scan time improves the examination in several areas. Motion artifacts, which lower the sensitivity and specificity especially in the upper abdomen, have nearly resolved. Many scans can be performed while the patient is holding his breath (1). The faster scans allow improved resolution and also decrease the amount of time the patient is required to stay within the magnet. New pulse sequences allow further improvement in tissue contrast. One area that has an expanded clinical role has been in MR hydrography. Heavily T2-weighted images, which turn fluid bright and surrounding structures relatively dark, can be obtained in seconds. This allows an evaluation of the bile and pancreatic ducts (MR cholangiopancreatography), urinary tract (MR urography), and the fluid-filled bowel. MRCP techniques have been the most extensively evaluated with excellent results (2). Extremely rapid images can be obtained using echoplanar imaging and spiral pulse sequence. As with CT, there are trade-offs for increased speed, such as a decrease in tissue contrast.

One area in which these sequences have allowed new information to be obtained is in perfusion, diffusion, and functional imaging. Perfusion

274 Part VIII / Future Prospects in Cancer Screening

allows information regarding blood flow to tumors; diffusion assesses the Brownian motion of molecules, which is important in the characterization of pathology *(3)*. Functional imaging allows assessment of the relationship of pathology to areas in the brain of specific function. All of these will likely play increasing roles in the evaluation of oncologic patients in the future.

Although the aforementioned advances have lead to better sensitivity and specificity, there can still be significant improvement. Organ-specific contrast agents are currently being investigated to further improve results. The main two areas of contrast development have been in liver imaging with the development of furomoxide and manganese agents and vascular-contrast agents. As CT and MRI continue to advance, several issues will need to be addressed. For CT, radiation exposure will need to be carefully monitored as the number of slices and phases obtained per examination increases. Newer and faster postprocessing software will need to be developed that will allow the routine clinical use of various three-dimensional displays.

In MRI, magnetic strength will continue to be pushed to the limits, as this will decrease the scan time and improve resolution. For MRI to play an increasing role in screening for malignancies, several issues will need to be addressed, including the cost-effectiveness, availability, and accuracy of the competing modalities such as CT.

SCREENING OF MALIGNANCIES

General Comments

Computed tomography and MRI are not currently utilized in widespread oncologic screening programs, primarily because of their cost. A CT of certain body parts is generally over $500 and an MRI slightly less than $1000. Because of this, these modalities are primarily used in patients suspected of having an underlying malignancy, staging of malignancies, or as a problem-solving technique. As these techniques have improved, they are clearly the imaging procedure of choice for the detection of certain malignancies. To become incorporated into a widespread screening algorithm, the cost-effectiveness issues must be addressed.

Faster technology is now allowing scans to be performed more rapidly and many institutions are offering reduced charges for these exams, thus making them more cost competitive. In the following subsection we will discuss the role of CT and MRI in screening for various malignancies, advantages and limitations of the modalities over currently utilized techniques, and the future of these techniques.

Chapter 17 / Advanced Imaging Technology

Breast Cancer

In the past few years, there has been an increasing interest in using MRI to evaluate breast cancer. This interest has grown because of the inherent advantages of superior tissue contrast with MRI and the relative limitations of mammographys less-than-perfect sensitivity, difficulty in the evaluation of dense breast tissue, and radiation exposure.

Specific technical developments that have allowed the performance of breast MR include dedicated breast coils, which allow extremely high resolution images to be obtained. Faster imaging sequences have been developed that now allow three-dimensional examinations to be performed during the dynamic injection of contrast. Several repetitive sequences can be performed that allow sequential evaluation of the enhancement characteristics of breast masses. Postprocessing subtraction techniques are available that can display areas of enhancement and help improve lesion conspicuity.

On MRI, malignancies appear as areas of enhancement (Fig. 1). The sensitivity of MRI has exceeded that of mammography. One of the major limitations of MRI has been its poor specificity (37–97%), as other abnormalities such as fibroadenomas, ductal hyperplasia, lobular neoplasia, inflammatory disease, scar less than 6 mo old in nonradiated breast, scar less than 18 mo old in radiated breast, fibrocystic disease, and normal tissue in different phases of the menstrual cycle can also enhance *(4,5)*. Therefore, other features have been assessed to improve the specificity. These include the degree of contrast uptake and washout in these lesions *(6)*. Also, morphologic appearances have been helpful, including a peripheral rim of enhancement in malignancies, linear areas of enhancement in DCIS, internal septations of fibroadenomas, tiny cysts of fibrocystic disease, absence of enhancement in benign processes, and irregular or spiculated borders in malignancies *(7)*. Using these features, some studies have demonstrated improvements in specificity to 70–80%. Another limitation to MR is the cost of the examination, as discussed previously.

The current role of breast MR is still under investigation. Current uses have been mainly as a problem-solving technique. Potential indications include differentiating a benign from a malignant mass, detecting cancer when the clinical exam or conventional imaging is negative or equivocal, evaluating for cancer recurrence after breast conservation therapy, staging newly diagnosed cancer, and detecting occult cancer in patients presenting with axillary lymph-node metastases *(8–10)*.

In the future, several issues will need to be addressed before MRI will have widespread clinical usage. The specificity will need further

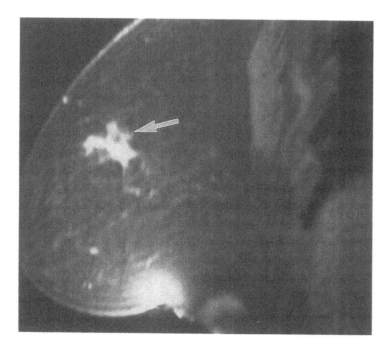

Fig. 1. Breast cancer. Contrast-enhanced MRI shows an irregular enhancing breast mass (arrow).

improvement. Research will need to be performed evaluating the cost-effectiveness of MRI. Coils and hardware are now being developed that will allow MRI-guided biopsies and localizations to be performed *(11)*. This will be necessary to allow differentiation of true positive from false-positive enhancing areas.

Lung Cancer

Computed tomography is clearly the imaging study of choice in the screening of lung cancer. The resolution with CT has significantly improved with the development of spiral CT and multislice detectors. This allows very thin-collimation, high-resolution images of the lungs to be obtained in a single breath-hold, avoiding misregistration because of breathing. Early cancers (tiny nodules) can be missed and are usually related to misinterpretation as blood vessels. The ability of the radiologist to scroll through the lungs in a movie fashion has improved the differentiation of nodules from vessels.

One of the major limitations of CT has been the specificity. Tiny nodules are often visualized, however, they are nonspecific and can also represent noncalcified granulomas, small intrapulmonary lymph nodes,

Chapter 17 / Advanced Imaging Technology

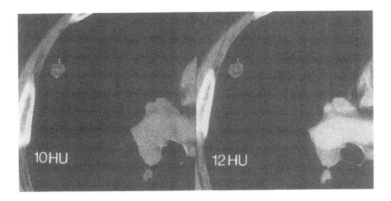

Fig. 2. Granuloma. Precontrast enhanced (**A**) and postcontrast enhanced (**B**) CT show the lack of enhancement of a pulmonary nodule.

hamartomas, and so forth. CT is currently used to screen patients with possible lung cancer. Several issues must be addressed and are currently being investigated that may allow CT to be utilized in widespread screening programs for high-risk patients. Studies are currently ongoing, evaluating the sensitivity of low-dose scans to determine the lowest possible exposure that can be utilized *(12)*.

If CT is to be implemented into widespread screening programs, it must be cost-effective and have high specificity in assessing the multiple tiny nodules it detects. Poor specificity will lead to expensive follow-up and many unnecessary surgeries. Therefore, studies are ongoing to improve the specificity. One of these includes the evaluation of nodule enhancement. The lack of enhancement of nodules suggests a benign process *(13)* (Fig. 2). Other characteristics such as growth rate are also being evaluated.

Hepatocellular Carcinoma

Hepatocellular carcinoma (HCC) has been one of the most difficult tumors to identify by imaging techniques because of the associated altered background of cirrhosis. Several modalities are available, including ultrasound, CT, MR, CT with angiography, and lipiodol-CT. There is no agreement on an appropriate algorithm. Preferences will vary and be based on institutional or regional biases, equipment, and expertise available *(14,15)*. A reasonable cost-effective screening algorithm includes the use of α-fetoprotein levels and ultrasound, reserving CT and/or MRI for problematic cases (those with high clinical suspicion) or for preoperative staging. Advances in CT and MRI have improved the detection rates of HCC. The ability to perform faster scans

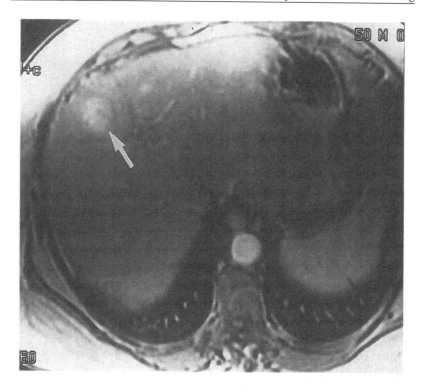

Fig. 3. Hepatocellular cancer. Arterial phase MR image shows a hyperenhancing mass (arrow).

allows multiple phases to be performed. Because HCC has arterial blood supply, obtaining images during early arterial enhancement can detect additional HCC nodules. This technique can be utilized with both CT and MRI *(16–20)* (Fig. 3).

New liver MR contrast agents have been useful as well. Hepatoselective agents such as furomoxides and mangafodipir trisodium (Mn-DPDP) are taken up in hepatocytes, increasing the conspicuity of neoplasms. However, certain tumors with hepatocytes, including well-differentiated HCC, can also show uptake *(21)*. Characterization of the nodular carcinogenic spectrum that occurs in the setting of cirrhosis has been reported; however, it appears that there is overlap and differentiation may not be possible *(16)*.

In the future, new contrast agents will continue to be developed and refined to help improve detection rates. Faster scans will allow a reduced cost of examination. There will need to be an ongoing assessment of these techniques compared to the others available, to determine the most cost-effective algorithm for screening.

Chapter 17 / Advanced Imaging Technology

Pancreas

Unfortunately, there are no good data to show the sensitivity of CT or MRI in screening for or detecting early pancreatic adenocarcinoma. Most patients that present to imaging have advanced disease; therefore, most of the data available have assessed the accuracy of staging the malignancy.

New technology has allowed us to detect smaller tumors and at an earlier stage. Helical and, more recently, multislice CT allows us to image the pancreas with a very high resolution and during several phases of enhancement improving tumor conspicuity *(22)*. MR technology also is allowing higher-resolution scans to be obtained. Gadolinium agents administered dynamically and Mn-DPDP, a manganese agent taken up in the liver and pancreas may allow further improvement in detection.

Computed tomography is still the most widely used modality and most cost-effective with good sensitivities. CT has a high positive predictive value for determining nonresectability; however, there are still a large number of cases (up to 30%) that are felt to be resectable by CT and found to be nonresectable at surgery.

Recent results with MRI show that MRI may be even more accurate than some CT techniques, especially for smaller tumors *(23,24)*. Future studies will need to compare the high-resolution, multiphase techniques of CT and MRI to other imaging techniques such as endoscopic ultrasound in the detection of small tumors *(25,26)*.

Colon Cancer

Colon cancer is the second leading cause of death in the United States. Colon cancer screening is unique to other cancer screening in that it detects the precursor, which can be removed before the cancer develops, thus curing the patient. Several screening techniques are available and various combinations have been incorporated into different screening algorithms. These include fecal occult blood testing, flexible sigmoidoscopy, colonoscopy, and barium enema.

A new technique, CT colonography (CTC), has the potential to be incorporated rapidly into colon cancer screening algorithms. CTC has many advantages. It can be performed rapidly, is well tolerated by patients, is noninvasive, and has good sensitivity. The technique for CTC is continuing to be refined; however, currently it is generally being performed very similarly at the leading institutions. The patient is required to have bowel prep prior to the examination. To perform CTC, air is inflated into the colon. Carbon dioxide appears to be better tolerated than room air. Glucagon can be administered; however, it has not

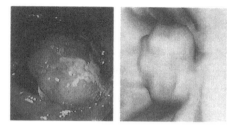

Fig. 4. Colon cancer. Polypoid mass as seen by (A) colonoscopy, (B) two-dimensional, and (C) three-dimensional images from CT colonography.

yet been shown to improve results. Images are acquired with thin slices, usually 5 mm thick, and then reconstructed to create overlapping imaging, thus, providing higher resolution. Many investigators are using both supine and prone images to assure adequate distension of all portions of the colon and to help in the differentiation of stool from polyps.

When CTC was first being investigated, the total interpretation time was very lengthy. Following the acquisition of the CT, three-dimensional fly-through movies were being created, which appeared similar to those views that could be obtained by conventional colonoscopy. The time to create these movies was approximately 30 min for one direction. It quickly became apparent that if CTC was going to make an impact in colon carcinoma screening, the interpretation time would have to decrease. Now, most investigators are reviewing the individual slices in a two-dimensional scrolling fashion on dedicated workstations and reserving the limited three-dimensional views or multiplanar reconstructions to those confusing areas. By using this technique, interpretation times now are approximately 5–10 min (Fig. 4).

Results of CTC have improved since it was evaluated initially and now are very promising. Most studies are reporting greater than 80% sensitivities for the detection of polyps greater than 7–8 mm in size *(27–30)*. These results are superior to those reported in the literature for barium enema. Also, this exam is significantly shorter than an air-contrast barium enema (10–15 min in comparison to 30 min) and seems to be tolerated better by patients.

Much research is being performed to address the limitations of this technique. Adequate bowel preparations are necessary to cleanse the colon, as stool can mimic polyps. Too much fluid remaining in the colon can obscure polyps. Scanning patients in both the supine and prone positions has helped to overcome these limitations. Also, contrast agents are being developed that may be incorporated into the stool and thus act as a stool marker. A multislice CT will allow higher resolution scans to

Chapter 17 / Advanced Imaging Technology 281

be obtained, which may provide even greater sensitivities. New postprocessing techniques are being developed that will further decrease interpretation times and may also improve polyp conspicuity. One of these techniques, "virtual pathology," allows the computer to open the colon and display it in a straight line.

Most of the research using cross-sectional techniques to detect polyps has been done with CT; however, a few investigators are currently also evaluating MR. Each modality has advantages over the other and limitations unique to their technique.

Prostate Cancer

Currently, neither CT nor MRI has a role in the screening for prostate cancer. In local staging, MRI is the best imaging technique; however, its use is controversial because of various reports of accuracy in staging. Therefore, it has not been widely implemented, with the exception of certain institutions.

Technical developments in prostate MR include endoluminal coils that allow exquisite high-resolution images to be obtained of the prostate. Recently, MR spectroscopy has been evaluated and shown improved specificity in characterization of focal prostate abnormalities and improvement in the evaluation for extracapsular tumor extension. Currently, this technique is investigational and only performed at limited institutions *(31,32)*.

Female Pelvis

As with prostate MR, there is no current role for CT or MRI in the detection or screening of female pelvic malignancies. MR demonstrates the female organ anatomy exquisitely and is the preferred technique for local staging. MR is also useful as a problem-solving technique to determine the organ of origin of a mass when ultrasound is inconclusive. With its superior tissue contrast, it can characterize masses such as fibroids, adenomyosis, endometriomas, and teratomas. The use of MR in staging female malignancies is also controversial. In staging, MR has been shown to be useful in demonstrating parametrial extension of cervical cancer and showing deep myometrial invasion for endometrial carcinoma. Research is ongoing, evaluating MR to currently accepted clinical staging techniques to assess its potential clinical role.

SUMMARY

Several new imaging modalities have shown promising results in cancer screening; however, they are costly and are not widely available.

282   Part VIII / Future Prospects in Cancer Screening

If these modalities are to be implemented into widespread cancer screening programs, they must be cost-effective with high accuracy. Further work is required in several areas; these include improvement in the specificity and sensitivity, development of organ-specific contrast agents, and better software programs for three-dimensional display.

REFERENCES

1. Gaa J, Hatabu H, Jenkins R, et al. (1996) Liver masses: replacement of conventional T2-weighted spin-echo MR imaging with breath-hold MR imaging. *Radiology* 200:459–464.
2. Fulcher AS. (1997) HASTE MR cholangiography in the valuation of hilar cholangiocarcinoma. *Am J Roentgenol* 169:1501–1505.
3. Namimoto T, Yamashita Y, Sumi S, et al. (1997) Focal liver masses: characterization with diffusion-weighted echo-planar MR imaging. *Radiology* 204:739–744.
4. Piccoli CW, Greer JG, Mitchell DG. (1996) Breast MR imaging for cancer detection and implant evaluation: potential pitfalls. *RadioGraphics* 16:63–75.
5. Kuhl CK, Bieling HB, Gieseke, J, et al. (1997) Healthy premenopausal breast parenchyma in dynamic contrast-enhanced MR imaging of the breast: normal contrast medium enhancement and cyclical-phase dependency. *Radiology* 203:137–144.
6. Daniel BL, Yen Y, Glover, GH, et al. (1998) Breast disease: dynamic spiral MR imaging. *Radiology* 209:499–509.
7. Nunes LW, Schnall MD, Orel SG, et al. (1997) Breast MR imaging: interpretation model. *Radiology* 202:833–841.
8. Orel SG. (1998) High-resolution MR imaging for the detection, diagnosis, and staging of breast cancer. *RadioGraphics* 18:903–912.
9. Orel SG, Reynolds C, Schnall MD, et al. (1997) Breast carcinoma: MR imaging before re-excisional biopsy. *Radiology* 205:429–436.
10. Morris EA, Schwartz LH, Dershaw DD, et al. (1997) MR imaging of the breast in patients with occult primary breast carcinoma. *Radiology* 205:437–440.
11. Kuhl CK, Elevelt A, Leutner, CC, et al. (1997) Interventional breast MR imaging: clinical use of a stereotactic localization and biopsy device. *Radiology* 204:667–675.
12. Rusinek H, Naidich DP, McGuiness G, et al. (1998) Pulmonary nodule detection: low-dose versus conventional CT. *Radiology* 209:243–249.
13. Swensen SJ, Brown LR, Colby TV, et al. (1996) Lung nodule enhancement at CT: prospective findings. *Radiology* 201:447–455.
14. Chalasani N, Said A, Ness R, et al. (1999) Screening for hepatocellular carcinoma in patients with cirrhosis in the United States: results of a national survey. *Am J Gastroenterol* 94:2224–2229.
15. Bottelli R, Tibballs J, Hochhauser D, et al. (1998) Review ultrasound screening for hepatocellular carcinoma (HCC) in cirrhosis: the evidence for an established clinical practice. *Clin Radiol* 53:713–716.
16. Kelekis NL, Semelka RC, Worawattanakul S, et al. (1998) Hepatocellular carcinoma in North America: a multiinstitutional study of appearance on T1-weighted, T2-weighted, and serial gadolinium-enhanced gradient-echo images. *Am J Roentgenol* 170:1005–1013.
17. Oi H, Murakami T, Kim T, et al. (1996) Dynamic MR imaging and early-phase helical CT for detecting small intrahepatic metastases of hepatocellular carcinoma. *Am J Roentgenol* 166:369–374.

Chapter 17 / Advanced Imaging Technology   283

18. Kanematsu M, Oliver JH, Carr B, Baron RL. (1997) Hepatocellular carcinoma: the role of helical biphasic contrast-enhanced CT versus CT during arterial protography. *Radiology* 205:75–80.

19. Vogl TJ, Stupavsky A, Pegios W, et al. (1997) Hepatocellular carcinoma:Evaluation with dynamic and static gadobenate dimeglumine-enhanced MR imaging and histopathologic correlation. *Radiology* 205:721–728.

20. Yamashita Y, Mitsuzaki K, Yi T, et al. (1996) Small hepatocellular carcinoma in patients with chronic liver damage: prospective comparison of detection with dynamic MR imaging and helical CT of the whole liver. *Radiology* 200:79–84.

21. Murakami T, Baron RL, Peterson MS, et al. (1996) Hepatocellular carcinoma: MR imaging with mangafodipir trisodium (Mn-DPDP). *Radiology* 200:69–77.

22. Choi BI, Chung MJ, Han JK, et al. (1997) Detection of pancreatic adenocarcinoma: relative value of arterial and late phases of spiral CT. *Abdom Imaging* 22:199–203.

23. Ichikawa T, Haradome H, Hachiya J, et al. (1997) Pancreatic ductal adenocarcinoma: preoperative assessment with helical CT versus dynamic MR imaging. *Radiology* 202:655–662.

24. Irie H, Honda H, Kaneko K, et al. (1997) Comparison of helical CT and MR imaging in detecting and staging small pancreatic adenocarcinoma. *Abdom Imaging* 22:429–433.

25. Legmann P, Vignaux O, Dousset B, et al. (1998) Pancreatic tumors: comparison of dual-phase helical CT and endoscopic sonography. *Am J Roentgenol* 170:1315–1322.

26. Ariyama J, Suyama M, Satoh K, Wakabayashi K. (1998) Endoscopic ultrasound and intraductal ultrasound in the diagnosis of small pancreatic tumors. *Abdom Imaging* 23:380–386.

27. Fenlon HM, Nunes DP, Schroy III PC, et al. (1999) A comparison of virtual and conventional colonoscopy for the detection of colorectal polyps. *N Engl J Med* 341:1496–503.

28. Dachman AH, Kuniyoski JK, Boyle CM, et al. (1998) CT colonography with three-dimensional problem solving for detection of colonic polyps. *Am J Roentgenol* 171:989–995.

29. Royster AP, Fenlow HM, Clarke PD, et al. (1997) CT colonoscopy of colorectal neoplasms: two-dimensional and three-dimensional virtual-reality techniques with colonoscopic correlation. *Am J Roentgenol* 169:1237–1242.

30. Hara AK, Johnson CD, Reed JE, et al. (1997) Detection of colorectal polyps with CT colography: initial assessment of sensitivity and specificity. *Radiology* 205:59–65.

31. Kurhanewicz J, Vigneron D, Hricak H, et al. (1996) Three-dimensional H-1 MR spectroscopic imaging of the in situ human prostate with high (0.24-0.7-cm^3) spatial resolution. *Radiology* 198:795–805.

32. Scheidler J, Hricak H, Kurhanewicz J, et al. (1997) Combined MR imaging and H1-MR spectroscopic imaging in prostate cancer localization: correlation with step-section pathology [abstract]. *Radiology* 205(Suppl):150.

33. Sonnenberg A, Delco F, Bauerfeind P. (1999) Is virtual colonoscopy a cost-effective option to screen for colorectal cancer? *Am J Gastroenterol* 94:2268–2274.

34. Valev V, Wang G, Vannier MW. (1999) Techniques of CT colonography (virtual colonoscopy.) *Biomed Eng* 27(1&2):1–25.

18 Molecular Genetics and Cancer Screening:

Current Status and Future Prospects

Zhong Ling, MD, PhD, Khalid Aziz, MD, and George Y. Wu, MD, PhD

KEY PRINCIPLES

- Both intrinsic (genetic) and extrinsic (environmental) factors play important roles in cancer pathogenesis.
- Mutations in three major classes of genes (oncogenes, tumor suppressor genes, and DNA mismatch repair genes) predispose individuals to malignancy.
- Hereditary cancer accounts for only 5–10% of the total cancer burden in humans.
- Genetic testing is only currently available for familial cancer syndromes.
- Over 30 familial cancer syndrome genes have been identified and genetic tests are available for all of them.
- Effective prophylactic treatments are available only for carriers of some of these familial cancer genes.
- Ethical and legal issues are also important considerations in the application of genetic testing for cancer screening. Cancer gene carriers will have a potential threat of decreased health and life insurability and compromised employability.

INTRODUCTION

In 1953, Watson and Crick discovered the double-helical structure of DNA, the universal genetic material for almost all life-forms on earth

From: *Cancer Screening: A Practical Guide for Physicians*
Edited by: K. Aziz and G. Y. Wu © Humana Press Inc., Totowa, NJ

286 Part VIII / Future Prospects in Cancer Screening

(1). Only a half-century later, the entire human genome has been mapped and approx 100,000 human genes have been found.

In the near future, medical genetics will inevitably become an integral part of medical practice. It will influence every aspect of medicine, from disease screening and diagnosis to its treatment and prognosis. Furthermore, multiple new ethical and legal issues will surface along with it. The hereditary nature of gene defects has required a higher level of coordination in medical practice: coordination between practitioners caring for geographically separated family members and coordination between different subspecialists for the care of genetic diseases that typically affect multiple organ systems. The fact that the genetic information obtained by DNA testing may implicate one's future health requires a much higher and more stringent standard of confidentiality in handling this information. Many patients have a reasonable fear that the leakage of unfavorable genetic information will decrease their employability and medical or life insurability. As medical practitioners, we will offer genetic counseling, order and interpret the genetic test, and may prescribe genetic therapy in the very near future. Medical practitioners need to further learn some of the language of molecular biology and also become more adept at communicating these new diagnostic or therapeutic means to a variety of patients with different backgrounds of education *(2,3).*

One of the most studied areas in medical genetics is the molecular biology of cancer. There are 1,200,000 new cases of cancer in the United States and more than 500,000 lives are lost annually *(4,5).* Both intrinsic (genetic) and extrinsic (environmental) factors play important roles in the pathogenesis of cancer. In the case of some cancers, the environmental factors supersede the genetic factors (e.g., cigaret smoking and lung cancer). Classically, in cases of familial cancers, the genetic factors play a more critical role. The knowledge of factors affecting the pathogenesis of a particular type of cancer is crucial to the development of strategies related to its screening, risk reduction, and treatment. The most important intrinsic factor in carcinogenesis is the individual susceptibility determined by his/her unique genetic makeup.

Hereditary cancer accounts for approx 5–10% of all cancers. Biomedical research on the underlying genetic abnormalities for these hereditary cancer syndromes have been critical in providing insight into cell-cycle controls and the genetic basis of some sporadic cancers *(5).*

It is estimated that at least five different critical gene mutations are required for a given clonal expansion of cells to acquire a full carcinogenic phenotype *(4).* A multistep molecular carcinogenesis postulated by Vogelstein et al. in 1988 using colorectal carcinoma as a model has

Chapter 18 / Molecular Genetics and Cancer Screening 287

much support *(6)*. The stepwise progression from mucosal dysplasia to benign adenoma and eventually to malignant carcinoma is merely the manifestation of serial somatic mutations occurring in the epithelial cells. Patients with familial adenomatous polyposis carry a germline mutant *APC* gene in all cells, resulting in multifocal adenomas and an accelerated course of carcinogenesis. In these patients, the *APC* gene mutation, the initiating event, is followed by the activation of the *RAS* proto-oncogene, and followed by inactivation of tumor-suppressor genes such as *DCC* and *P53 (7)*.

Therefore, germline mutations, which predispose an individual to a specific type of cancer, in combination with somatic (acquired) mutations in the same or other genes result in the formation of a malignant neoplasm. The knowledge of both mutations is essential in the clinical management of cancer, including screening, diagnosis, treatment, and prognosis. Currently, however, genetic tests are only available for a small subset of cancers (hereditary cancer syndromes) that account for only 5–10% of the total cancer burden.

The recommendations of the American Society of Clinical Oncology (ASCO) with regard to a cancer predisposition test (genetic screening test for cancer) require that a test meet three criteria:

1. Reasonable probability of hereditary cancer syndrome (a strong family history or very early age of onset)
2. Existing genetic test(s) can be adequately interpreted (good sensitivity and specificity)
3. Results will influence the clinical management of the patient or family member *(4)*.

ONCOGENES, TUMOR-SUPPRESSOR GENES, AND DNA MISMATCH REPAIR GENES AND THEIR ROLES IN CARCINOGENESIS

Three major groups of genes have been implicated in the process of tumor pathogenesis including proto-oncogenes, tumor-suppressor genes, and DNA mismatch repair genes. Oncogenes are originally genes isolated from tumorogenic viruses capable of transforming the cells in culture into neoplastic cell lines. Subsequent studies have shown that many "viral" oncogenes were merely altered versions of normal human cellular genes, called proto-oncogenes. Furthermore, physiological function studies have demonstrated that many of these proto-oncogenes are involved in the regulation of cell proliferation and differentiation. Their protein products may be categorized into growth factors, receptors, signal transduction machinery, transcriptional regulators, and so

288 Part VIII / Future Prospects in Cancer Screening

forth. Classical examples of this group of genes are *RET* (multiple endocrine neoplasia type 2) and *RAS* (many cancers including colon, lung, and thyroid). The second group of genes, tumor-suppressor genes, is defined as genes that sustain the loss of function, resulting in the development or progression of neoplasm. They include cell-surface adhesion proteins, cell-cycle control proteins, transcriptional factors, and apoptosis (programmed cell death) and related proteins. Knudson's "two-hit" theory refers to the inactivation of both alleles of the tumor-suppressor gene, leading to clonal cancer development. One allele carries a germline mutation and the other allele acquires a somatic mutation *(8)*. Classical examples of tumor-suppressor genes include *RB* (retinoblastoma) and *P53* (colon, breast cancer). The physiological role of DNA mismatch repair genes is to maintain the fidelity of DNA molecules during DNA replication. Classical examples of this group of genes are *hMSH2/hMLH1* (hereditary nonpolyposis colorectal cancer) and *ATM* (ataxia telangiectasia) *(9,10)*.

Mutations resulting in the constitutive activation of proto-oncogenes or loss of function of tumor-suppressor genes may lead to unlimited cell cycling, resulting in cancer development. Loss of function of DNA mismatch repair genes will lead to DNA instability and an increase of somatic mutations during the cell cycle, which predispose an individual to malignant neoplasms.

COMMON CONCEPTS IN MOLECULAR BIOLOGY

Central Dogma: The Flow of Genetic Information

The genetic information flows from DNA, to RNA, to protein. Transcription refers to the synthesis of the RNA molecule by RNA polymerase using the DNA as a template. Translation refers to the synthesis of polypeptides by ribosomes using the genetic message encoded in mRNA. Both transcription and translation are tightly regulated processes.

Autosomal vs Sex-Link Genetic Disorders

There are a total of 46 pairs of chromosomes in each human cell, including 22 pairs of autosomes and 1 pair of sex chromosomes (chromosome X and/or Y). Genes on chromosome X and Y are inherited in a sex-linked manner, whereas genes on others chromosomes (autosomes) are not sex linked. For example, a genetic trait on the Y chromosome will only be expressed phenotypically in the male, because the normal female will not carry Y chromosome.

Chromosomal Abnormalities vs Monogenic Mutations

Chromosomal disorders involve a lack or excess of or an abnormal arrangement of chromosomes. Most are embryonically lethal, because

Chapter 18 / Molecular Genetics and Cancer Screening   289

they result in an enormous amount of deficient or excessive genetic material that affects normal expression and function of many different genes. Monogenic mutations affect only a single gene. They obey Mendelian law and usually display one of the three patterns of inheritance: (1) autosomal dominant, (2) autosomal recessive, and (3) X-linked.

Homozygosity, Heterozygosity, Genetic Polymorphism, and Genetic Heterogeneity

For each genetic locus, every individual has two alleles: one paternal and one maternal. Homozygosity indicates that the two alleles are identical, whereas heterozygosity indicates that they are different. It is known that many proteins exist in more than two forms in a population. Genetic polymorphism refers to the existence of multiple alleles at a single genetic locus coding for the same protein. From a medical genetic perspective, heterogeneity means that different genes may cause the same phenotype.

Dominant, Recessive, and Genetic Imprint

In most genetic loci, the two alleles are coexpressed. A dominant mutation is a mutation that will dictate the clinical phenotype in a heterozygous genotype. A recessive mutation will require homozygosity for the manifestation of its clinical phenotype. However, in some genetic loci, only one of the two alleles is expressed, with the other allele repressed. This genetic phenomenon is referred to as "genetic imprint." Because the gene is functionally homozygous, the dominant or recessive characteristics are not applicable in the imprinted locus. A mutation in the imprinted allele will always be expressed, whereas the mutation in the other will not.

Penetrance and Expressivity

Both penetrance and expressivity are genetic concepts frequently used for autosomal dominant disorders. Penetrance refers to the portion of individuals carrying a given genotype that presents with any phenotypical features of that disorder. In other words, the percentage of people with a specific disease gene will actually have the clinically diagnosable disease. A mutation with 100% penetrance means that everyone with that mutation will eventually develop the clinical disease. Expressivity, on the other hand, describes the range of clinical phenotypic effects in individuals carrying a given mutation. It is also termed *variability in clinical expression*. The explanations for penetrance and expressivity include (1) differences in the intrinsic genetic makeup in different individuals or the effects of the other genes and (2) the difference in extrinsic or environmental factors.

Germline vs Somatic Mutations

Germline mutations originate from the sperm or oocyte. They will be present in the genomic DNA of every single cell of the affected individual and will be passed from generation to generation. The mutations occurring in embryogenesis or later during development are referred to as somatic mutations. They only exist in the affected cells or tissue of an individual. They usually do not transmit to the offspring because they do not affect the germline.

Large Mutations vs Point Mutations

Point mutations, or base substitutions, refer to the single-base sequence changes in the coding region of a gene. Conversely, large mutations refer to segmental DNA insertions, deletions, inversions, or duplications.

Silent, Missense, Nonsense, and Frameshift Mutations

A silent mutation is a base substitution that does not lead to a change in its coding amino acid. A point mutation that results in a single-amino acid substitution in the protein is called a missense mutation, whereas one that results in the formation of a translation-terminating codon or other non-amino-acid corresponding codon is referred to as a nonsense mutation. A one or two bases insertion or deletion in the coding region of a gene is called frameshift mutation because it alters the reading frame of the triplet genetic code.

FREQUENTLY USED MOLECULAR GENETIC TECHNIQUES

Restriction Endonuclease and Molecular Cloning

Restriction endonucleases are enzymes purified from microorganisms that cut double-stranded DNA at specific sequences. Each enzyme recognizes a pallindromic DNA sequence, typically 4–8 bp. They are critical in recombinant DNA manipulations. DNA fragments of interest may be excised, purified, and inserted into a vector for manipulation and propagation, a process called molecular cloning. Once cloned, the gene and products may be produced in unlimited amounts for various purposes of scientific research, genetic diagnosis, and gene therapy.

Nucleic Acid Hybridizaton and Allele-Specific Oligonucleotides

The nature of DNA and RNA structures allows the base pairing and formation of the double-stranded helical structure between two complementary molecules of nucleic acid under proper conditions. This revers-

Chapter 18 / Molecular Genetics and Cancer Screening 291

ible process involves nucleic acid denaturation, separation of the two strands, and hybridization (reformation of the double-stranded hybrid). Oligonucleotides are short stretches of single-stranded DNA, typically 15–25 bp in length, synthesized in vitro. An oligonucleotide that perfectly matches the mutant sequence, allele-specific, may be used as a probe to detect the presence or absence of a particular mutant gene.

Southern Blot, Northern Blot, and Western Blot Analyses

All "blot" analyses consist of two steps: electrophoresis and transfer. Samples containing DNA (or RNA or protein) are subjected to gel electrophoresis that separates molecules according to their molecular weight. They are then transferred onto a cellulose paper and subjected to detection using a radioactive-isotope-labeled probe. For Southern blot analysis, the hybridization is between a DNA probe and a DNA sample. It may be used to detect gross rearrangements in the genomic DNA molecules. In Northern blot analysis, the hybridization is between a DNA probe and an RNA sample. It is usually used to assay the presence or absence of a mRNA molecule, assess the level of its expression, and approximate its size. In Western blot analysis, also called immunoblotting, the detection of a protein antigenic molecule is by a specific labeled antibody.

Polymerase Chain Reaction

The development of polymerase chain reaction (PCR) has revolutionized molecular diagnosis. PCR allows the amplification of a specific DNA or RNA segment between two selected oligonucleotide primers chosen. The sample DNA to be amplified is incubated with oligonucleotide primers in the presence of a thermostable DNA polymerase. A thermovariation cycle is require to complete the reaction. At denaturing temperature, typically 90–99°C, double-stranded DNA molecules are dissociated to single-stranded DNA. The annealing temperature, usually 50–60°C, allows the oligonucleotide primers to hybridize with target DNA molecules. At a polymerization temperature, typically 72°C, the thermostable DNA polymerase synthesizes a new strand-complementary DNA molecule using the target DNA as a template. Twenty to 30 or more thermovariation cycles will result in at least a 10^5-fold increase in the target DNA molecules, which allows the detection of a single gene molecule in a gross sample. Because of the combination of DNA molecular stability and PCR reaction simplicity, PCR may be performed with various easily obtainable samples: peripheral white blood cells (WBCs), dry blood, mouthwash, old tissue section, and so forth. PCR has become one of the principal tools in molecular diagnosis. PCR may be used in many different ways for molecular diagnosis:

the presence or absence of normal or pathognomonic PCR products, using the PCR product as a probe for Southern, Northern, or *in situ* analyses. The PCR product may even be directly sequenced to detect genetic abnormalities, and so forth.

Protein Truncation Assay

Amplified genomic DNA or cDNA is transcribed and translated in vitro. The protein products are then electrophoresed to detect truncated protein products. This assay will detect any mutation that results in premature termination of polypeptide synthesis: nonsense, frameshift, gene fragment deletion, and so forth.

Microsatellite Instability Test

Microsatellite DNA containing repeat units of two, three, or four nucleotides exist throughout the human genome. Their function is currently unknown. The fact that they comprise a large percentage of the human genome makes them a likely target for somatic mutations. The microsatellite instability test will be able to detect the existence of increased alterations in microsatellite DNA, which is an indication of malfunction(s) or loss of function in DNA mismatch repair genes.

Analysis of Unknown Mutations

There are multiple molecular biological methods used to detect mismatches in genomic DNA (e.g., single-strand conformational polymorphism [SSCP], denaturing gradient gel electrophoresis [DGGE], heteroduplex analysis, and so on). These tests are currently cumbersome to perform and are generally used as research tools. This may not be the case in the near future.

DNA Chip Arrays

The DNA chip is used to hold large arrays of oligonucleotides, in all possible sequences, on a miniaturized solid support for the analyses of target DNA sequence. Automated hybridization will make the comparison of thousands of genes possible. This technology may become one of the key components of molecular diagnosis in the near future.

CURRENT STATUS IN MOLECULAR GENETICS AND CANCER SCREENING

Hereditary Breast Cancer and BRCA1/BRCA2 *Genes*

Genes that predispose women to breast cancer are classified into two groups: major genes and polygenes. This concept may also be appli-

Chapter 18 / Molecular Genetics and Cancer Screening 293

cable for the pathogenesis of other neoplasms *(11)*. "Major genes" are associated with inherent or familial breast cancer. These germline mutant genes, which confer a high degree of breast cancer risk in disease families, include *BRCA1*, *BRCA2*, and *TP53*. They are relatively rare in the general population. Many other gene loci that confer a lower risk of breast cancer also exist in a much larger proportion of the general population. This group of genes, referred to as the "polygenes," is heterogeneous and includes *ATM*, *CYP1A1*, *CYP2D6*, *CYP2E1*, *GSTM1*, *HRAS1*, *NAT2*, and so forth *(11,12)*. *CYP* genes encode for cytochrome P450 variants, which are involved in chemical detoxification in the liver. They have been implicated either in the formation or elimination of environmental chemical carcinogens.

BRCA1 and *BRCA2* mutations account for the vast majority of hereditary breast cancer, 52 and 32%, respectively *(13)*. Women carrying either mutant *BRCA1* and *BRCA2* genes are at a very high risk for breast cancer, estimated to be 85% at age 70. They are also at greater risk for ovarian cancer, 50% risk for BRCA1 and 15% for BRCA2, respectively, at age 70. The *BRCA1* gene has been mapped to chromosome 17q21. It encodes a 220-kDa protein that may contain a "zinc-finger" domain, a known protein–protein or protein–DNA binding domain *(13)*. Gene transfer studies have shown that wild-type BRCA1 protein inhibits the growth of breast cancer both in vitro and in vivo. The putative physiologic function of BRCA1 includes (1) regulation of the initiation of the proliferating cycle through its interaction with P53 or (2) involvement in the DNA repair mechanism through binding with DNA *(12)*. The *BRCA2* has been mapped to chromosome 13q13. It has been cloned and sequenced, but its exact physiological function remains uncharacterized. Approximately 1% of Ashkenazi Jewish women carry a specific *BRCA1* frameshift mutation, the 185delAG (deletion of A and G at nucleotide position 185), and approx 1.4% carry a particular *BRCA2* frameshift mutation, 617delT. This means that the prevalence of two easily tested *BRCA* gene mutations in this subset of women approaches 1:40, making genetic screening beneficial in this group. In contrast, more than 1000 different variants of BRCA1 exist in the general population, of which 664 are associated with detrimental effects regarding tumorgenesis *(12)*. This has rendered routine genetic screening in the general population impractical *(12)*. However, more than 90% of all mutations in both *BRCA1* and *BRCA2* result in truncated proteins. New genetic tests that can identify various mutations in *BRCA* genes and possibly assay for the presence or absence of truncated BRCA1 and BRCA2 proteins still need development in order to make routine genetic screening both feasible and practical.

There are three potential clinical options in managing women that carry *BRCA1* and *BRCA2*: (1) intensive surveillance, (2) chemoprevention with tamoxifen, and (3) prophylactic mastectomy *(14)*. The efficacy of surveillance and chemoprevention in this subgroup of high-risk females has yet to be proven. Prophylactic mastectomy remains the most efficient method in breast cancer prevention.

Hereditary Ovarian Cancer and BRCA1/BRCA2 *Genes*

Hereditary ovarian cancer accounts for approx 10% of all ovarian cancers. Two genes, *BRCA1* and *BRCA2*, have been identified and are linked to hereditary ovarian cancer *(13,15)*. Best estimates of lifetime risk of ovarian cancer in women carrying *BRCA* mutations range between 15 and 60% *(13,15)*. Although the risk for breast cancer is comparable between the two groups, *BRCA1* carriers are at a much higher risk for ovarian cancer than *BRCA2* carriers. Different *BRCA1* variants have variable penetrance of breast and ovarian cancers. It has been suggested that mutations in the amino terminus giving rise to shorter truncated proteins results in a higher frequency of ovarian than breast cancers. Mutations of the carboxyl terminus give rise to longer truncated proteins and lead to more breast than ovarian cancers.

As in the case of breast cancer, three clinical options exist for *BRCA* carrier women: (1) early detection by vigilant screening, (2) chemoprevention with oral contraceptives, and (3) prophylactic oophorectomy *(15)*. In view of the high lethality of ovarian cancer, prophylactic oophorectomy would be a reasonable choice for women carrying *BRCA1* and *BRCA2* mutations. However, this may be delayed to allow childbearing because the risk for ovarian cancer does not increase until after age 40.

Hereditary Nonpolyposis Colorectal Cancer and hMSH2/hMLH1 *Genes*

A group of DNA mismatch repair genes has been identified as the cause of hereditary nonpolyposis colorectal cancer (HNPCC) *(9)*. These include *hMSH2* and *hMSH6* on chromosome 2p16, *hMLH1* on chromosome 3p21, *hPMS1* on chromosome 2q31, and *hPMS2* on chromosome 7q11 *(16)*. Two of these mutations, *hMSH2* and *hMLH1*, are thought to account for the majority of HNPCC cases *(10)*. However, the genetic tests for *hMSH2* and *hMLH1* using in vitro translation or DNA sequencing are very costly ($750 to $2600 per test) *(10)*.

The function of these mismatch repair genes is to maintain the fidelity of DNA during DNA replication in cell division. A positive microsatellite instability (MSI) test indicating defects in the DNA mismatch repair machinery may be used instead of primary genetic screening for

Chapter 18 / Molecular Genetics and Cancer Screening   295

HNPCC. A MSI test is sensitive but fairly nonspecific and costs approx $350 *(10)*.

Hereditary Colorectal Cancer Syndromes and APC

Germline nonsense and frameshift mutations in the *APC* (adenomatous polyposis coli) gene are known to be associated with familial adenomatous polyposis (FAP) and attenuated familial adenomatous polyposis. FAP is an autosomal dominant disorder that carries 100% risk of colon cancer. The *APC* gene mapped to chromosome 5q21 encodes a 2843-amino-acid cell-adhesion molecule, which is involved in signal transduction. Mutations in APC genes typically result in truncated protein products *(16)*. The clinical APC genetic test, a protein truncation assay, is now commercially available at $750/test *(17)*. It has a sensitivity of about 80% *(16)*.

One specific *APC* missense mutation I1307K is found in 6% of the Ashkenazi Jewish population and confers a 20% lifetime risk of colorectal cancer. I1307K genetic testing by allele-specific oligonucleotide PCR is extremely sensitive and specific and costs about $200 *(16)*.

Hereditary Melanoma and CDKN2A/CDK4 Genes

Three genetic loci (*CMM1*, *CMM2*, and *CMM3*) have been associated with hereditary melanoma and dysplastic nevi syndromes *(18)*. *CMM1* is located on chromosome 1p36, but the candidate gene remains to be identified. CMM2 is located on chromosome 9p21. Genetic linkage analysis has provided strong evidence for an autosomal dominant inheritance with partial penetrance *(19)*. The penetrance for melanoma is estimated to be 53% by age 80 in the carriers of CMM2 *(20)*. Families carrying germline mutations in *CDKN2A* have a higher incidence of pancreatic carcinoma. The *CMM2* gene, identified as *CDKN2A*, encodes a 16-kDa (P16) protein that binds and inhibits the cyclin-dependent kinases CDK4 and CDK6, a group of key regulators in cell proliferation *(21,22)*. *CMM3* is located on chromosome 12q14. Ironically, the *CMM3* gene proved to be CDK4 itself. The mutant *CDK4* gene product was unable to bind to or inhibit itself by P16, resulting in unregulated kinase activity.

Of the two known genes related to hereditary melanoma, *CDKN2A* and *CDK4*, commercial genetic testing is only available for *CDKN2A* *(21,22)*. The sensitivity and specificity of the *CDKN2A* test are unstudied. Furthermore, its clinical benefit is uncertain at this point because the test result would not affect the clinical management of these family members. Yet, this may not be always true in the future, especially if gene therapy may be able to alter the natural course of the disease.

Multiple Endocrine Neoplasia and MEN1/RET Genes

Both multiple endocrine neoplasia (MEN) type 1 and type 2 are highly penetrant autosomal dominant disorders characterized by tumors involving multiple endocrine organs. In MEN1, tumors typically affect the parathyroid, endocrine pancreas, anterior pituitary, and adrenal glands. The *MEN1* gene located on chromosome 11q13 has recently been cloned *(23)*. It functions as a tumor-suppressor gene and encodes a 610-amino-acid nuclear protein, menin. Its physiological function remains unclear. More than 200 different germline mutations in the *MEN1* gene have been identified *(7,23)*. *MEN1* gene screening is a powerful tool in the presymptomatic diagnosis of MEN1 and should be offered to the family members of patients with MEN1 *(7,23)*. Mutant MEN1 gene carriers, identified by genetic testing, require vigilant biological monitoring for early detection and treatment of endocrine tumors *(23)*.

Common tumors of MEN2 include medullary thyroid carcinoma (MTC), parathyroid tumor, and pheochromocytoma. MTC is the most consistently occurring tumor in all subtypes of MEN2 (90% lifetime risk) and is the most common cause of death *(24)*. The gene responsible for MEN2 (*RET*) is also identified. It is a proto-oncogene that encodes a transmembrane tyrosine-kinase receptor that is involved in cell-cycling control through the signal transduction mechanism *(24)*. Multiple mutations have been identified in the coding region of *RET* either at the ligand-binding domain (MEN2A and familial MTC) or intracellular catalytic domain (MEN2A, MEN2B, and FMTC) of the protein *(23)*. *RET* mutation analysis is now available. Prophylactic thyroidectomy may be a valid option for mutant *RET*s carriers at very young age because it carries only minimal morbidity and virtually no mortality *(23)*.

Von Hippel–Lindau Syndrome and VHL Gene

Von Hippel–Lindau (VHL) syndrome is an autosomal dominant disorder characterized by hemangioblastomas of the central nervous system. The *VHL* gene has been mapped to chromosome 3p25 and has been identified as a tumor-suppressor gene *(25–27)*. Clear-cell renal cell carcinoma (RCC) occurs in up to 70% of patients with *VHL* mutation. Pheochromocytoma has also been associated with the *VHL* gene. The *VHL* gene encodes a 30-kDa protein that regulates the transcription elongation step, which has been shown to suppress RCC tumor formation in the nude mice-xenograft assay *(28)*.

Germline mutations in the *VHL* gene include large deletions (20%), missense mutations (27%), nonsense and frameshift mutations (27%) *(25)*. Various mutation analyses confirming nonsense, missense, or

Chapter 18 / Molecular Genetics and Cancer Screening 297

deletions in the VHL gene currently exist. Their sensitivities and specificities have not been studied systematically.

Medical, Legal, and Ethical Issues in Molecular Genetics and Cancer Screening

With the development of molecular genetic testing, there exists an accurate way of predicting the individual risk of or predisposition to a specific medical illness. For the majority of these diseases, especially malignancies, there is no curative therapy. For some of these diseases, there is not even a prophylactic therapy. From the commercial insurance industry's perspective, the carriers of genetic mutations would be undesirable candidates for life, health, and employment insurance. From the employer's perspective, they would be less fit subjects for employment. Thus, genetic discrimination may become a major complicating factor in the practice of genetic screening for cancer (29,30). The US Congress is considering many bills targeting genetic privacy by limiting access to and use of genetic information, including the proposed Genetic Confidentiality and Nondiscrimination Act (29,31). As with any other medical screening tool, guidelines for the genetic testing and screening of specific cancer need development. First, the tests developed must fulfill the prerequisite of a screening test. Furthermore, the physicians, researchers, insurers, employers, and the general public must reach a consensus on the meaning of, need for, and access to the genetic information (29).

There are two additional medicolegal issues regarding genetic testing for cancers that require specific attention: (1) the pretest informed consent and (2) the posttest genetic counseling (31). Some of the benefits of cancer genetic testing include (1) reassurance/emotional relief, (2) opportunity for vigilant surveillance and risk-reducing behaviors, (3) chance for chemical or surgical prophylaxis, (4) chance for close relatives to undergo genetic testing, and (5) knowledge accumulated for future medical practice (31). Some risks and harms include (1) psychological stress for the patient and their close relatives, (2) strained family relationships, (3) and basis for genetic discrimination with regard to life and health insurance and employability (31). The pretest and posttest genetic counseling are crucial. Patients must comprehend the statistical concepts of susceptibility and probability because a "positive test" does not always equal the "development of disease" and a "negative test" is not "disease-proof." Misinterpretation or misunderstanding of the genetic test result is an invitation for lawsuit.

With the systemic accumulation of genetics information in a statistical manner, the prevalence of "bad genes" in a specific ethnic group will soon be available. This might serve as a basis for ethnic discrimination.

Table 1

Genes in Common Hereditary Cancer Syndromes

Gene	Chromosome	Principal cancers	Prophylactic surgery
BRCA1	17q21	Breast, ovarian	Mastectomy
BRCA2	13q13	Breast, pancreatic	Mastectomy
hMSH2	2p16	Colorectal, endometrial, ovarian	Colectomy
hMLH1	3p21	Colorectal, endometrial, ovarian	Colectomy
APC	5q21	Colorectal	Colectomy
CDK4	12q14	Melanoma, pancreatic	None
CDKN2A	9p21	Melanoma	None
MEN1	11q13	Pancreatic islet	None
RET	10q11	Medullary thyroid	Thyroidectomy
VHL	3p25	Central nervous system hemangioma, renal cell	None

SUMMARY AND FUTURE PERSPECTIVES

Cancer currently remains the second leading cause of death in the United States. With the gradual fall in mortality from cardiovascular disease, it may soon supersede the former as the leading cause of death. The interaction between genetic predisposition and environmental factors is the key in cancer pathogenesis. With the rapid expansion of the body of knowledge in medical genetics, molecular bases of many hereditary and sporadic cancers have been identified. Medical genetics will have a great impact in the medical practice from cancer screening and diagnosis to its treatment and prognosis.

Genetic tests are currently only available for the familial cancer syndromes, which account for 5–10% of all cancers. More than 30 hereditary cancer syndromes are known and genetic testing is now available for most of them. Table 1 summarizes the most common hereditary cancers and their genetic tests. They include hereditary breast/ovarian cancer (*BRCA1* and *BRCA2* genes), hereditary nonpolyposis colorectal cancer (*hMSH1* and *hMLH2* genes), familial adenomatous polyposis (*APC* gene), hereditary melanoma (*CDKN2A* and *CDK4* genes), multiple endocrine neoplasia (*MEN1* and *RET* genes), and Von Hippel–Lindau syndrome (*VHL* gene).

There are many issues that need resolution with regard to the clinical application of routine genetic screening for the general population,

Chapter 18 / Molecular Genetics and Cancer Screening 299

including high cost, imperfect sensitivity and specificity, the psychological impact on the patient, and legal issues regarding potential employment and insurance discrimination. Genetic testing is not likely to completely replace current clinical protocols for common cancer screening. Rather, this technique, like any other newly developed medical techniques, will become an integral part of the whole array of tools used by clinicians. Clinical genetic testing will assume multiple roles. It may identify genetically predisposed individuals to direct vigilant conventional screening and follow-up, chemoprevention, or prophylactic surgery. It may confirm a specific diagnosis at the molecular level after a positive result from routing screening. Genetic testing for sporadic mutations may serve as a useful tool for cancer treatment monitoring. It will also have important prognostic value for cancer patients.

REFERENCES

1. Watson JD, Crick FHC. (1953) A structure for deoxyribose nucleic acid. *Nature* 171:737,738.
2. Neuhausen S. (1999) Ethnic differences in cancer risk resulting from genetic variation. *Cancer* 86(8):1755–1762.
3. Webb MJ. (1998) Symposium: genetic testing and management of the cancer patient and cancer families. *J Am Coll Surg* 187(4):449–456.
4. Weitzel JN. (1999) Genetic cancer risk assessment. *Cancer* 86(8):1663–1672.
5. Lynch HT, et al. (1999) Clinical impact of molecular genetic diagnosis, genetic counseling, and management of hereditary cancer. *Cancer* 86(8):1629–1636.
6. Gelehrter TD, et al. (1998) *Principles of Medical Genetics.* Baltimore, MD: Williams and Wilkins.
7. Heppner C, Reincke M, Agarwalsk, et al. (1999) MEN1 gene analysis in sporadic adrenocortical neoplasms. *J Clin Endo Meta* 84(1):216–219.
8. Knudson AG. (1996) Hereditary cancer: Two hits revisited. *J Cancer Res Clin Oncol* 122(3):135–140.
9. Leach FS, Nicolaides NC, Papadopoulos N, et al. (1993) Mutation of a MutS homologue in hereditary non-polyposis colorectal cancer. *Cell* 75:1215–1225.
10. Nystrrom-Lahti M, Parson R, Sistonen P, et al. (1994) Mismatch repair genes on chromosome 2p and 3p account for a major share of hereditary non-polyposis colorectal cancer families evaluated by linkage. *Am J Hum Genet* 55:659–665.
11. Rebbeck TR. (1999) Inherited genetic predisposition in breast cancer-a population-based perspective. *Cancer* 86(8):1673–1681.
12. Gauthier-Villars M, et al. (1999) Genetic testing for breast cancer predisposition. *Breast Cancer Manag* 79(5):1171–1187.
13. Gayther SA, et al. (1995) Germline mutations of the BRCA1 gene in breast and ovarian cancer families provide evidence for genotype-phenotype correlation. *Nat Genet* 11:428–433.
14. Hughes KS, et al. (1999) Prophylactic mastectomy and inherited predisposition to breast carcinoma. *Cancer* 86(8):1682–1696.
15. Berchuck A, et al. (1999) Managing hereditary ovarian cancer risk. *Cancer* 86(8):1697–1704.
16. Petersen GM, et al. (1999) Genetic testing and counseling for hereditary forms of colorectal cancer. *Cancer* 86(8):1720–1730.

300 Part VIII / Future Prospects in Cancer Screening

17. Powell SM, et al. (1993) Molecular diagnosis of familial adenomatous polyposis. *N Engl J Med* 329:1982–1987.
18. Green MH. (1999) The genetics of hereditary melanoma and nevi. *Cancer* 86(8):1644–1657.
19. Cannon-Albright IA, et al. (1994) Localization of the 9p melanoma susceptibility locus (MLM) to a 2-cM region between D9S726 and D9S171. *Genomics* 23:265–268.
20. Cannon-Albright IA, et al. (1994) Penetrance and expressivity of the chromosome 9p melanoma susceptibility locus (MLM). *Cancer Res* 54:6041–6044.
21. Kamb GA, et al. (1994) A cell cycle regulator potentially involved in genesis of many tumor types. *Science* 264:436–440.
22. Wolfel HT, et al. (1995) A p16^{INK4a} insensitive CDK4 mutant targeted by cytotoxic T-cells in a human melanoma. *Science* 269:1281–1284.
23. Calender A. (1998) genetic testing in multiple endocrine neoplasia and related syndromes. *Forum* (Genova) 8(2):146–159.
24. Wohllk N, et al. (1996) Application of genetic screening information to the management of medullary thyroid carcinoma and multiple endocrine neoplasia type 2. *Endo Metabol Clin* 25(1):1–25.
25. Ilipoulos KO, et al. (1995) Tumor suppressor by the human von Hippel-Lindau gene product. *Nat Med* 1:822–826.
26. Duan, DR, et al. (1995) Inhibition of transcriptional elongation by the VHL tumor suppressor protein. *Science* 269:1402–1406.
27. Seizinger BR, et al. (1988) von Hippel Lindau disease maps to the region of chromosome 3 associated with renal cell carcinoma. *Nature* 332:268,269.
28. Friedrich CA. (1999) von Hippel Lindau syndrome—a pleomorphic condition. *Cancer* 86(8):1658–1662.
29. Bondy M, et al. (1997) Ethical issues of genetic testing and their implications in epidemiological studies. *Ann Epidemiol* 7:363–366.
30. Parker LS, et al. (1996) Standards of care and ethical concerns in genetic testing and screening. *Clin Obstet Gynnocol* 9(4):873–884.
31. White MT, et al. (1999) Genetic testing for disease susceptibility: social, ethical and legal issues for family physicians. *Am Fam Physician* 60(3):748–755.

IX MEDICOLEGAL ASPECTS OF CANCER SCREENING

19 Medicolegal Issues in Cancer Screening

Charlotte Brooks, BS, RN

KEY PRINCIPLES

- Physicians should have an understanding of what the legal system defines as malpractice.
- Primary care physicians are responsible for informing patients regarding both general and high-risk screening.
- There are four types of cancer for which physicians are at highest risk to be sued for delayed diagnosis if timely screening is not done: breast, cervical, colorectal, and prostate.
- Even if timely screening is done, lawsuits may still arise from breakdowns in communication in various ways.

DEFINITION OF A MERITORIOUS MALPRACTICE CASE

Medical malpractice is defined by law as a departure from the standard of care. The standard of care is the same throughout the country, regardless of whether the physician practices privately or in an academic setting, in a big city or small town. In order for a potential malpractice case to have merit, it also is necessary that it be proven more likely than not (51% probability) that the departure from the standard of care caused the damage that the patient or patient's family is complaining about. Lawyers refer to this as proximate cause or causation.

In some states, death cases do not require proximate cause, but rather recognize the doctrine of lost chance of survival. This means that a physician can be sued if a delayed diagnosis results in a further reduction of the patient's odds for survival, even if those odds were less than 50% to start. The ultimate outcome could be the same with or without the

From: *Cancer Screening: A Practical Guide for Physicians*
Edited by: K. Aziz and G. Y. Wu © Humana Press Inc., Totowa, NJ

304 Part IX / Medicolegal Aspects of Cancer Screening

delayed diagnosis. In 1994, the doctrine was recognized in 26 states and the District of Columbia *(1)*. The doctrine of lost chance of survival has come about as the result of state supreme court decisions, not by legislation.

Lawyers have successfully extended this concept not only to death cases but to others as well. A delay in diagnosis or improper treatment, for example, could mean a less successful outcome, a shorter life expectancy, or loss of a limb or other body part. The lost chance doctrine has increased the number of malpractice suits filed in the states where it is recognized.

Sometimes, evidence of both negligence and proximate cause are in question, but the case will still have a successful outcome for the plaintiff. In an Ohio case, a gynecologist was sued for failing to do a digital rectal exam at the first prenatal visit on a 19-yr-old pregnant woman who was diagnosed with colon cancer 8 mo after delivery. Gynecological experts disagreed as to whether a rectal exam was the standard of care for young women having their first prenatal exams. Surgical experts differed in opinions regarding whether it was more likely than not that the tumor would have been large enough and low enough to have been felt by a digital rectal exam 15 mo prior to diagnosis. An arbitration panel was not convinced that a rectal exam at the first prenatal visit was the standard of care, but they found for the physician on the grounds that even if he had done the exam at that time, it had not been proven more likely than not that he could have felt the mass. The panel's ruling was not binding and the case was eventually settled for a considerable amount of money so that the defendant could avoid a jury trial. The patient died after the arbitration panel hearing, but her videotaped deposition was taken while she was near death in the hospital and would have been played at trial. She left a beautiful 4-yr-old daughter who had been seen by the arbitrators at the hearing and no doubt would have been seen by jurors at trial. In deciding to settle the case, two of the factors that defense attorneys took into consideration were that jurors would see both the child and the deposition of the mother.

According to the U.S. Department of Justice's Bureau of Justice Statistics, national statistics are not kept regarding numbers of medical malpractice cases filed in this country that involve issues of cancer screening. The best available statistics on medical malpractice cases are from 1996 and include only those cases that went to trial in the 75 largest counties of the country. Of 1195 trial verdicts in these counties, 23.4% resulted in plaintiff verdicts. Most of these, 1112 of the verdicts, resulted from jury trials, but 53 were a result of cases tried to a judge. It is interesting to note that juries awarded a million dollars or more in 22% of these plaintiff verdicts, whereas judges, despite finding for plaintiffs

Chapter 19 / Medicolegal Issues in Cancer Screening   305

in a greater percentage of cases than did juries, never awarded that large an amount *(2)*.

FAILURE TO SCREEN

Probably the major cause of medical malpractice cases having to do with cancer screening is failure of physicians to screen patients on a time line that is accepted as the standard of care. Organizations such as the American Cancer Society and the American College of Preventive Medicine publish guidelines and policy statements regarding exams and testing to help with early detection for a variety of malignancies. Indeed, if published guidelines are not carefully followed by physicians whose patients or their families end up suing them, one can be certain that attorneys for these plaintiffs will be using the guidelines as Exhibit A in a courtroom.

There are two categories of screening to be considered: general and high risk. For the most part, primary care physicians (PCPs) are concerned with general screening which includes mammograms, Pap or other cervical cytological smears, blood tests such as prostate-specific antigen (PSA), fecal occult testing, and other procedures suggested earlier in this book. Digital rectal exams, breast palpation, ovarian palpation during pelvic exams, and examination of the skin for suspicious lesions also are included in general screening.

More intensive screening for patients who are at higher risk for cancer, by either patient or family history, may be performed by specialists. Nevertheless, the PCP should make necessary referrals and instruct and remind patients to follow through with these procedures. For example, patients with a history of inflammatory bowel disease, being at higher risk for colon cancer, will need periodic colonoscopies, which will usually be performed by gastroenterologists. Asymptomatic patients may go years without seeing specialists, so it is useful for PCPs to remind their patients of the need for follow-up in regard to preventive screening measures.

TYPES OF CANCER AND WHICH PHYSICIANS ARE AT RISK TO BE SUED

Breast Cancer

High on the list of medical malpractice lawsuits are cases alleging failure to diagnose breast cancer. In a 20-yr review of causes of breast cancer litigation, 45 cases that went to trial were identified and all involved a delayed diagnosis. There were no treatment-related cases. The number of physicians sued ranged from 1 to 4 in each of 42 cases.

306   Part IX / Medicolegal Aspects of Cancer Screening

Obstetrician-gynecologists were involved in the greatest number of cases (50%), followed by family practitioners and internists (41%), general surgeons (28%), and radiologists (10%) *(3)*.

Delay of diagnosis lawsuits arise both from mammograms that are incorrectly read by radiologists and from palpable lumps that are not dealt with appropriately by either primary care physicians or surgeons to whom the patients are referred. A patient may have a discrete mass and a negative mammogram, but something still must be done about the mass. Some PCPs might do fine-needle aspiration. Others may choose to send the patient to a surgeon for further evaluation. But something must be done, both for the sake of the patient and the protection of the doctor.

In a Kentucky malpractice case, a family practitioner was found negligent by a jury for failure to address a marble-sized lump in a 46-yr-old woman with a negative mammogram. The patient, who had found the lump herself, had not been to a physician for many years. Although neither an ultrasound nor a needle biopsy was done, the doctor told the patient the lump was a cyst, and if it started to grow, it could be drained. When she returned 19 mo later with the idea of having drainage of what she believed was then a large cyst, she was seen by a different doctor in the office and referred to a surgeon. A diagnosis was made of infiltrating ductal carcinoma with six out of eight positive lymph nodes. The tumor was so large by the time of diagnosis that presurgical chemotherapy and radiation were required before a mastectomy was performed. The treating surgeon's testimony was that a lumpectomy would have sufficed, in all probability, if the patient had been treated 19 mo sooner. A highly respected pathologist testified for the defense that the tumor responded so well to presurgical treatment that he doubted the delay had changed the patient's prognosis. Regardless of the pathologist's testimony, the jury found for the plaintiff on the basis that the delay in diagnosis had necessitated a mastectomy rather than a lumpectomy. The lesson to be taken from this case is that discrete breast lumps must not be ignored and that more than a mammogram, if it is negative, needs to be done for evaluation.

The evaluation of lumps can be more difficult than usual in patients with long histories of fibrocystic breast disease who have had multiple biopsies, given the scarring that undoubtedly exists. An illustrative case in Arizona involved a 56-yr-old woman who had a 19-yr history of fibrocystic breast disease with multiple biopsies of both breasts. She found a new lump and her primary care physician ordered a mammogram that was negative. After the patient made several calls to the PCPs office over a period of 2–3 mo to complain that the lump was enlarging,

Chapter 19 / Medicolegal Issues in Cancer Screening 307

the doctor "aspirated the cyst," but obtained no fluid. Five months later, he referred the patient to a surgeon who made a diagnosis of infiltrating ductal carcinoma with two positive lymph nodes.

The delay in diagnosis in this case was almost 8 mo. A pathologist who reviewed it concluded this did not change the outcome and therefore a lawsuit was not filed. However, a highly experienced cancer surgeon who reviewed the case believed the PCP was negligent for not referring the patient to a surgeon as soon as he identified a new solid mass. His belief is that regardless of negative mammograms in a postmenopausal woman with a solid breast lump, excision is the correct procedure.

Cervical Cancer

Lawsuits arising from delayed diagnosis of cervical cancer are aimed predominately at pathologists and laboratories for inaccurate reading of cervical cytological (CC) smears. The Papanicolaou (Pap) smear has been a highly successful CC cancer screening test, reducing the death rate from cervical cancer in the United States by about 70% since 1943, when the procedure first came into use. However, failures in early diagnosis can and do occur. The International Academy of Cytology acknowledges that problem laboratories and cytology practitioners exist (4). The majority of CC smears are read by cytotechnologists, with pathologists only seeing the ones found to be abnormal. Errors in interpretation will possibly be reduced with the introduction of new CC smear tests—some including automated reading—but that remains to be seen.

Primary care physicians are at risk to be sued in cases of delayed diagnosis for several reasons. These include failure to offer cervical screening, failure to adequately warn the patient of the risk she is taking if she refuses screening, or failure to inform the patient of an abnormal smear report and arrange follow-up care. Another potential area of liability for the PCP is improper collection or preservation of the smear. If the laboratory determines that the specimen is inadequate and the PCP is informed of this, he or she must notify the patient to return to the office for another smear. Providing the laboratory with a complete history of risk factors (e.g., prior positive smears or human papilloma virus) also is expected. This information is directly relevant to the screening process and, if not provided, opens an area of potential liability for the physician. It should go without saying that properly labeled identification of the CC smear by the PCP is crucial both for the sake of the patient and the physician if the smear proves to be positive.

One attorney in the state of Washington, who has had considerable experience in litigating these cases, believes that a woman who consis-

308 Part IX / Medicolegal Aspects of Cancer Screening

tently has had CC tests over a period of years and who subsequently develops cervical cancer, probably has a valid medical malpractice claim for delayed diagnosis against either her physician or the laboratory that interpreted her smear slides *(5)*. This is because the development of cervical cancer is a slow process that starts with atypical cells and progresses through stages of dysplasia to carcinoma *in situ* before becoming invasive. Theoretically, there should be time to prevent invasive carcinoma and effect a 100% cure if the patient's CC smear slides have been correctly read and if follow-up care is attended to when abnormalities are observed.

If a woman is faithful in getting annual CC smears and an error is made in one year, there still may be time to rectify the situation the following year. However, there can be sequential errors made in interpreting the smears on the same patient. In an Ohio case that was settled out of court, a 21-yr-old woman allegedly had three successive false-negative Pap smears. By the time of diagnosis, her cancer had progressed to the point where a hysterectomy was required, rather than a less radical procedure. Her physician said her prognosis was excellent, but a significant financial settlement was reached because her ability to bear children had been taken away.

Colorectal Cancer

Physicians at risk of being sued for delayed diagnosis of colorectal (CRC) cancer include primary care doctors, gastroenterologists, and radiologists. Radiologists have been sued either for failure to make the diagnosis by barium enema or for alleged improper performance of such an exam if perforation should occur *(6)*.

Gastroenterologists also may be sued when perforation occurs during an endoscopic procedure, even though this is a known complication. If the perforation is suspected and diagnosed quickly and morbidity is kept to a minimum, the physician may avoid a lawsuit or have a successful defense if one is filed. Another reason for lawsuits against gastroenterologists is failure to find the malignancy because of doing a sigmoidoscopy rather than a colonoscopy as a screening procedure, thereby missing a lesion that is above the sigmoid colon. This is not considered malpractice if the patient is asymptomatic and does not have risk factors. However, if either symptoms or risk factors are present, the gastroenterologist may be sued for not detecting the malignant lesion.

When an asymptomatic patient over age 50 who has been seen at least annually by his or her PCP is diagnosed with rectal or colon cancer that is beyond an early stage, an attorney may be consulted to determine if there is a basis for a medical malpractice suit. The office records of the

Chapter 19 / Medicolegal Issues in Cancer Screening 309

physician will be closely examined to see if recommended screening was done. If annual fecal occult blood testing has been done and is documented to have been negative and if flexible sigmoidoscopies have been recommended at least every 5 yr or a colonoscopy every 10 yr, the PCP will probably not be sued.

Closer surveillance is the standard of care for patients with significant risk factors, among which are a personal history of CRC, adenomatous polyps, or chronic inflammatory bowel disease. A family history of polyps or CRC syndromes, including familial adenomatous polyposis (FAP) or hereditary nonpolyposis colon cancer (HNPCC), also constitute significant risk factors. Primary care physicians have been sued successfully for failure to adhere to the guidelines advised by the American Cancer Society in these situations.

Interestingly, numerous cases involving children of patients who have died from FAP or HNPCC have been adjudicated successfully for offspring who have developed CRC and claimed that they should have been advised and educated by their parents' physicians about the importance of surveillance for themselves. In one such case, a daughter, who had been 10-yr-old at the time of her father's death from FAP, was herself diagnosed with FAP at age 36. She filed a claim of negligence against the estate of her father's surgeon. The suit was dismissed by the trial court based partly on its opinion that the physician had no doctor–patient relationship with the daughter. This ruling was reversed by the appeals court, whose opinion was that the physician must take action to make available the genetic knowledge of the hereditary disease to those who are likely to be affected (7). In this type of lawsuit, there is no reason to think that attorneys would not include primary care physicians who have an ongoing relationship with the patient and family.

Prostate Cancer

There is considerable controversy regarding whether or not population screening for prostate cancer is beneficial. The guidelines among various organizations differ on the subject. The PSA is an imperfect test and the digital rectal exam misses very small tumors. Nevertheless, the American Cancer Society recommends that both should be offered annually to men age 50 and older who have at least 10 yr of life expectancy (8). The U.S. Preventive Services Task Force and the Congressional Office of Technology Assessment recommend against screening. The American College of Physicians and American Academy of Family Physicians believe the decision to screen should be individualized and made with the input of the patient after he has been advised of the potential benefits and harms of the screening process. The American ological Association takes a similar position, believing patients should be given the option to participate in screening *(9)*.

Primary care physicians have been sued for alleged delay in diagnosis when PSA testing has not been done. No statistics are available on the numbers of these cases, according to the American Urological Association and the U.S. Department of Justice's Bureau of Justice Statistics. Many physicians feel compelled to screen to avoid litigation and "the widespread use of PSA has created a standard of care that many clinicians are reluctant to ignore" *(9)*. In fact, attorneys have no trouble finding PCPs and urologists to testify in courts of law that PCA testing and digital rectal examination are the standard of care, despite the controversy over the value of PSA.

BREAKDOWNS IN COMMUNICATION

The importance of keeping legible and complete medical records cannot be emphasized enough. Doctors must document the screening procedures they do, whether the findings are positive or negative. "If it is not recorded, it was not done" is the mantra of plaintiff attorneys when litigating a malpractice case. If a physician wishes to correct something in a record, the correct procedure is to put a line through what he or she wishes to delete and then write the appropriate word or words. Scribbling through something that had been written so that it is then illegible makes the record appear to have been changed. Records should never be rewritten or altered if a doctor is sued. This almost invariably is discovered and causes a jury to be very suspicious of the defendant, even if there is no merit to the case.

Another area of crucial importance in avoiding malpractice suits is making certain that the patient is advised of results of abnormal screening procedures so that follow-up care can be arranged. Communication of results either by phone call or letter must be documented in the record. In some offices, phone logs are kept separately from the patients' records and may not be available to attorneys when the medical record is being reviewed. It is far more preferable to keep this information with patients' charts, but if this is not done, phone logs must be saved and must be made available to patients and their attorneys upon request. The same goes for letters and faxes between doctors' offices.

There can be misunderstandings between physicians and patients regarding who is in charge of a case once the patient has been referred to a specialist. In a Pennsylvania case, a patient with a significantly elevated PSA was referred by his internist to a urologist. A prostatic needle biopsy was benign, but 2 yr later, when the PSA again was high,

Chapter 19 / Medicolegal Issues in Cancer Screening 311

a repeat needle biopsy was positive for prostate cancer. In the intervening year between these biopsies, the patient had a transurethral resection of the prostate (TURP) with benign findings, although without needle biopsy. The patient chose to change urologists after his cancer was diagnosed and a radical prostatectomy was done by another physician. The patient's PSA continued to be elevated postoperatively and metastasis was assumed, although a site was never identified. The patient sued the first urologist, claiming that the first biopsy had yielded an inadequate amount of prostatic tissue to make a correct diagnosis and the biopsies from the TURP were not taken from deep enough into the gland. The allegation was that diagnosis and treatment had been delayed by 2 yr. He also sued the internist, stating that the doctor had promised him he would oversee his care and treatment and had failed in this duty. The internist claimed he had told the patient he would continue to be his PCP, but at no time did he hold himself out to be an expert in diagnosing or treating prostate cancer.

Another complaint against the internist was that he should have felt the tumor on a digital rectal exam done $1^1/_2$ yr before referral to the urologist, which was the patient's last office visit prior to the referral visit. The record clearly documented a normal rectal exam at that time. The judge refused to let the internist out of the case before it was tried to a jury. He had to endure a 2-wk trial, along with the urologist, before the internist's lawyer was permitted to make a successful argument to the judge that his client should be let out of the case. The jury verdict was for the plaintiff and the urologist's insurance company bore the burden of paying the entire award.

Physicians must not forget that they are ultimately responsible for the actions of their auxiliary personnel. These include physician assistants and nurse practitioners, who may be seeing patients independently, and secretaries and nursing staff, who may be responsible for making sure test results are entered into the record. A comment about test results should be noted at the time of the subsequent office visit after testing is done, unless the test produces immediate results that should be recorded contemporaneously with the testing. It is surprising how often abnormal test results are not even mentioned in records, let alone recorded as having been discussed with patients. Although this can happen with results of cancer screening tests, it is more common with blood work, such as liver enzymes or lipid profiles.

When a medical record is requested by a patient (or the executor of his or her estate in a death case), the entire record, including laboratory and X-ray results as well as all correspondence and phone calls should be provided. This saves time for everyone in the long run, including the _ysician, and enables the attorney to make a decision more quickly as _ whether or not the potential case has merit. It is important to remember that when a patient or family alleges physician negligence to a lawyer, the lawyer must have all the facts to make an intelligent decision regarding the merits of the case. Most of the time, reviewed cases are found not to be meritorious and the physician can breathe a sigh of relief.

PATIENTS' RIGHTS

- Right to be advised regarding when screening procedures should be done.
- Right to have procedures explained and done correctly and accurately.
- Right to be informed of screening procedure results. In some states, this is required in writing for certain procedures (i.e., mammograms and Pap smears).
- Right to be advised regarding follow-up care when necessary.

RECOMMENDATIONS FOR PHYSICIANS

- Keep cancer screening procedures in mind even if you are seeing patients for a medical problem. Patients may not come in for annual physicals. A checklist of which procedures should be done for general screening is a good idea.
- Get a good patient and family history to be aware of patients at increased risk for cancer who will need additional screening.
- Document when you inform patients of recommended procedures. Be sure to record their refusals if applicable.
- Look at procedure results and make sure they get put into the medical record. If something needs to be repeated, such as an inadequate Pap smear, do it!
- Have a certain method of communicating results to patients and record that the information has been given.
- Refer patients as necessary when results are positive.
- Keep legible and complete records, including copies of letters to and from other physicians and notes of phone calls.
- Do not alter records. If requested by the patient, provide the complete and unaltered record.
- Educate your office staff as to the importance of all of the above. Their work is your responsibility.

SUMMARY

Liability issues in cancer screening primarily have to do with the failure of physicians to recommend and/or perform accepted screening procedures on a timely basis. Types of cancer for which recommenda-

Chapter 19 / Medicolegal Issues in Cancer Screening

tions are generally accepted and should be complied with in order to benefit patients and protect physicians are breast, cervical, colorectal, and prostate. A patient who attempts to sue his physician for delayed diagnosis of cancer must prove that there was a departure from the standard of care in the failure to screen and that this departure led to damages that would not have otherwise occurred. A persuasive case of this proof must be made to the defense in order to settle the case without trial, or to a judge or jury if a trial takes place. Physicians should be very careful in keeping accurate and legible records and in educating their office staffs as to the importance of all communication, both written and verbal, being entered into medical records. Patients must be informed of test results and of the importance of follow-up when abnormal results occur.

REFERENCES

1. Heland KV, Rutledge P. (1994) Medicolegal issues. *Ob-Gyn Clin North Am* 21:781–788.
2. DeFrances CJ, Litras MFX. (1999) Civil trial cases and verdicts in large counties, 1996. *Bureau of Justice Statistics Bulletin* September 1999, NCJ 173426, pp. 1–24.
3. Kern AK. (1992) Causes of breast cancer malpractice litigation. *Arch Surg* 127:542–546.
4. Frable J, et al. (1998) Medicolegal affairs IAC task force summary. *Acta Cytologica* 42(1):76–119.
5. Perey R. (1998) Cervical cancer and the misdiagnosed smear. *Acta Cytologica* 42(1):123–127.
6. Barloon TJ, Shumway J. (1995) Medical malpractice involving radiologic colon examinations: a review of 38 recent cases. *Am J Roentgenol* 165(2):343–346.
7. Lynch HT, et al. (1999) Failure to diagnose hereditary colorectal cancer and its medicolegal implications. *Dis Colon Rectum* 42(1):31–35.
8. Von Eschenbach A, et al. (1997) American Cancer Society guidelines for the early detection of prostate cancer. *Cancer* 80(9):1805–1807.
9. Woolf S, Rothemich SF. (1999) Screening for prostate cancer: the roles of science, policy, and opinion in determining what is best for patients. *Annu Rev Med* 50:207–221.

Index

A

Aflatoxin, hepatocellular carcinoma risks, 116, 243
AFP, *see* Alpha-fetoprotein
Alcohol,
    hepatocellular carcinoma risks, 116
    oropharyngeal cancer risks, 132
Allele-specific oligonucleotide, definition, 291
Alpha-fetoprotein (AFP), assays, 248
    hepatocellular carcinoma screening, 119, 120, 245, 246, 248, 249
    testicular mass work-up, 167
a1-Antitrypsin deficiency, hepatocellular carcinoma risks, 115
APC, *see* Familial *adenomatous polyposis*
Atrophic gastritis, stomach cancer risks, 256, 257
Autosomal disorder, definition, 288

B

Barium enema, colon cancer screening, 96
Barium X-ray, stomach cancer screening, 259, 260, 262
Barrett's esophagus,
    age at diagnosis, 213, 214
    chemoprevention, 222, 223
    endoscopy,
        chromoendoscopy, 217, 218
        cost-effectiveness of screening, 220, 221
        endoscopic ultrasound, 218, 219
        screening, 215, 216
        surveillance, 216, 217, 219–221
    esophageal cancer,

length of Barrett's esophagus and adenocarcinoma, 214, 215
    pathogenesis, 215
    risks, 213–215
    gastroesophageal reflux disease role, 213
    prevalence, 213
    referral indications, 223
    sex differences, 214
    transnasal balloon cell sampling, 217
    treatment,
        mucosal ablation, 222
        surgery, 221, 222
Basal cell carcinoma (BCC),
    see Skin cancer
BCC, *see* Basal cell carcinoma
Betel nut, chewing and oropharyngeal cancer risk, 131
BRCA1
    breast cancer genetic testing, 19, 20, 293, 294
    functions, 293
    locus, 293
    ovarian cancer,
        genetic testing, 53, 294
        mutations, 45, 294
BRCA2
    breast cancer genetic testing, 19, 20, 293, 294
    locus, 293
    ovarian cancer,
        genetic testing, 53, 294
        mutations, 45, 294
Breast cancer,
    ethnicity in epidemiology, 14
    genes, major genes vs polygenes, 292–293
    hormone replacement therapy risks, 21, 22
    incidence, 13, 14
    malpractice lawsuits, 305–307

316   Index

metastasis, 16
mortality, 13, 14
natural history, 16
prognostic factors, 13, 14
risk factors, 14, 15
screening,
  algorithms, 16, 17
  breast examination, 18
  complementarity of tech-
    niques, 19
  controversies, 21, 22
  cost-effectiveness, 20
  genetic testing, 19–21,
    292–294
  magnetic resonance imaging,
    19, 275, 276
  mammograms, 16, 18, 21
  rationale, 4, 6
  self-examination, 19
  surgeon referral indications,
    20, 21
  ultrasound, 19
tamoxifen benefits, 75

C

CA 125
  cost-effectiveness of screening, 54
  levels by tumor type, 49, 50
  ovarian cancer screening, 47,
    49–50, 54
Cancer screening,
  communication breakdowns,
    310–312
  failure to screen and malpractice
    lawsuits, 305
  goals, 3, 4
  patient rights, 312
  program,
  recommendations for physicians,
    312
  requirements for success, 4–6,
    117–119, 148–150
Carcinogenesis,
  genetic control, 287, 288
  multistep mechanisms, 286–288
Cervical cancer,
  colposcopy, 35, 37, 38
  epidemiology, 28

human immunodeficiency virus
  infection association, 39
human papilloma virus role,
  28–31
infectious agents in etiology, 29
malpractice lawsuits, 307, 308
mortality trends, 7, 8
oncoproteins, 30, 31
preinvasive lesions,
  Bethesda system, 31, 36, 37
  glandular lesions, 31, 32
  progression, 28, 29, 35
  squamous lesions, 31
  treatment options, 38, 39
risk factors,
  age, 29, 30
  contraceptive methods, 30
  smoking, 30
  socioeconomic status, 30
screening, *see also* Papanicolaou
  smear,
  access, 41
  algorithm, 37
  cervicography, 36
  human papilloma virus
    typing, 35, 36
  prospects,
    automated cytologic screen-
      ing, 40
    fluid-based technology, 40
    genetic testing, 40
  types, 28
Chest X-ray, lung cancer screening,
  197–200
Chromoendoscopy, Barrett's esophagus and esophageal cancer
  screening, 217, 218
Chromosomal disorder, definition,
  288, 289
Cirrhosis, hepatocellular carcinoma
  risks, 115
Clomiphene, ovarian cancer risks,
  45
Cloning, overview, 290
Colonoscopy, colon cancer screening, 95, 101
Colorectal cancer,
  adenoma natural history, 88, 89

Index

age at diagnosis, 87, 88
ethnicity factors, 88
incidence, 87, 88
malpractice lawsuits, 308, 309
mortality, 87
screening,
  algorithms, 101, 102
  barium enema, 96
  colonoscopy, 95, 101
  combined fecal occult blood
    testing and sigmoidos-
    copy, 94, 95
  comparison of methods, 100
  computed tomographic
    colonography, 96, 97,
    279–281
  cost-effectiveness, 89, 99, 100
  fecal occult blood testing, 90–
    92, 97
  genetic testing, 97–99
  high-risk patients, 101–104
  participation rates, 100, 101
  rationale, 89
  recommendations, 104, 105
  sigmoidoscopy, 92–94
Colposcopy, cervical cancer, 35,
  37, 38
Computed tomography (CT),
  colonography, 96, 97, 279–281
  costs, 274
  fluoroscopy, 272
  hepatocellular carcinoma screen-
    ing, 120, 121, 277, 278
  historical advances, 271, 272
  lung cancer screening, 200–202,
    206, 276, 277
  multislice detectors, 272, 273
  pancreatic cancer, 279
  spiral computed tomography, 272
  testicular mass work-up, 167
Cost-effectiveness, *see* Economics
Cryptorchidism, testicular cancer
  risks, 162

CT, *see* Computed tomography
Cutaneous malignant melanoma,
  see Skin cancer

D

DNA chip array, definition, 292
DNA mismatch repair, defects in
  cancer, 288
Dominant mutation, definition, 289

E

Economics,
  cost-effectiveness of screening
    programs,
    Barrett's esophagus, 220, 221
    breast cancer, 20
    colorectal cancer, 99, 100
    endometrial cancer, 74
    esophageal cancer in China,
      238
    hepatocellular carcinoma, 121–
      123, 249–251
    ovarian cancer, 54
    overview, 6, 9, 10
    prostate cancer, 156, 157
    skin cancer, 188
    stomach cancer in Japan, 263,
      264
  screening impact, 4
Endometrial cancer,
  age at diagnosis, 63
  clinical features, 67, 68
  ethnicity factors, 65
  hereditary nonpolyposis colorectal
    cancer association, 72, 73
  heredity, 66
  incidence, 63, 65
  obesity in diagnosis, 65, 67
  pathogenesis, 64, 67
  prevention, 77–79
  prognosis, 79
  prophylactic surgery, 73, 74
  risk factors, 64–66
  screening,

318   Index

algorithm, 72–74
biopsy, 69, 70, 75, 76
cost-effectiveness, 74
genetic testing, 72
Papanicolaou smear, 68, 69
recommendations, 68, 79
referral indications, 76, 77
sonohysterogram, 71, 75
tamoxifen patients, 74–76
ultrasound, 70, 71, 75
staging, 67
Endoscopy,
Barrett's esophagus,
China experience, 236, 237
chromoendoscopy, 217, 218
cost-effectiveness of screening, 220, 221
endoscopic ultrasound, 218,
219
screening, 215, 216
surveillance, 216, 217,
219–221
colon cancer, *see* Colon cancer
Epiluminescence microscopy, skin
cancer screening, 187
Esophageal cancer,
China,
epidemiology, 227, 228
etiology,
deficiencies in diet, 230,
231
fungal invasion, 231
hot food and beverages, 231,
232
miscellaneous factors, 232
nitrosamines in diet, 229,
230
historical perspectives, 227
public education, 237
screening,
algorithm, 233, 234
Chinese balloon cytology,
233, 234

cost-effectiveness, 238
endoscopy, 236, 237
government programs, 237,
238
Japanese sponge cytology,
234, 235
occult blood bead detector,
235, 236
chromoendoscopy, 217, 218
classification of countries by
risk, 229
early diagnosis and prognosis,
212
ethnicity factors, 212
geographic distribution, 227,
228
incidence trends, 223, 228
mortality, 211, 212, 228
natural history, 232, 233
pathogenesis, 232, 234
risk factors, *see* Barrett's
esophagus; Gastroe-
sophageal reflux disease
sex differences, 214
transnasal balloon cell sampling, 217
types of tumors, 212
Expressivity, definition, 289

F

False-negative test,
definition, 5
implications, 7
False-positive test,
definition, 5
implications, 6, 7
Familial adenomatous polyposis
(FAP),
APC mutations, 98, 295
colorectal cancer screening
recommendations, 101–104
genetic testing, 97, 98, 295
FAP, *see* Familial adenomatous polyposis
Fecal occult blood testing (FOBT),
bleeding of colorectal cancers, 90
combined with sigmoidoscopy,
94, 95

Index

cost-effectiveness, 100
dietary influences, 90, 91
efficacy of colorectal cancer
screening, 91, 92
follow-up, 101
immunochemical tests, 97
peroxidase test and limitations,
90, 91
sensitivity, 92
specificity, 92
Finasteride, effects on prostate-
specific antigen levels, 154,
155
FOBT, *see* Fecal occult blood testing

G

Gastric cancer, *see* Stomach cancer
Gastroesophageal reflux disease
(GERD),
Barrett's esophagus risks, 213
endoscopic screening, 215, 216
esophageal cancer risks, 213
treatment, 221
Genetic imprint, definition, 289
Genetic screening,
American Society of Clinical Oncology recommendations, 287
BRCA mutations, 19, 20, 53, 293,
294
breast cancer, 19–21, 292–294
cancer genes and test availability,
298
cervical cancer, 40
colorectal cancer, 97–99
counseling, 297
endometrial cancer, 72
familial adenomatous polyposis, 97,
98, 295
hereditary cancer prevalence, 286
hereditary nonpolyposis colorectal
cancer, 97–99, 294, 295
informed consent, 297
melanoma, 187, 188, 295
multiple endocrine neoplasia, 296
ovarian cancer, 53, 294
privacy issues, 297
role in cancer screening, 298, 299
GERD, *see* Gastroesophageal reflux
disease
Germline mutation, definition, 290

Glycogen storage diseases, hepatocellular carcinoma risks, 115, 116

H

HBV, see Hepatitis B virus
HCC, *see* Hepatocellular carcinoma
HCG, *see* Human chorionic gonadotropin
HCV, *see* Hepatitis C virus
Helicobacter pylori, stomach cancer
role, 256, 257
Hepatitis B virus (HBV), hepatocellular carcinoma,
genetic factors, 251, 252
risks, 113, 114, 242, 243
Hepatitis C virus (HCV), hepatocellular carcinoma risks, 114,
242, 243
Hepatocellular carcinoma (HCC),
chemoprevention, 125
China,
epidemiology, 241, 242
risk factors,
aflatoxin, 243
contaminated water, 243
hepatitis B virus, 242, 243,
251, 252
hepatitis C virus, 242, 243
screening,
algorithm, 249
alpha-fetoprotein, 245,
246, 248, 249
cost-effectiveness of tests
and program, 249–251
efficacy, 247
high-risk populations, 248
historical perspective, 244,
245
interval for screening, 249
referral indications, 251
ultrasound with alpha-fetoprotein, 246, 249
ethnicity factors, 113
etiology factors,
alcoholism, 116
a1-antitrypsin deficiency, 115
cirrhosis, 115

320

Index

glycogen storage diseases, 115, 116
hepatitis B virus infection, 113, 114
hepatitis C virus infection, 114
hereditary hemochromatosis, 115
membranous obstruction of inferior vena cava, 116
porphyria, 116
toxins, 116
tyrosinemia, 116
Wilson's disease, 116
geographic distribution, 112, 252
incidence, 241, 242
interferon therapy, 125
mortality, 111, 241
natural history, 243, 244
screening,
alpha-fetoprotein, 119, 120
biopsy, 121
combination of techniques, 121
computed tomography, 120, 121, 277, 278
cost-effectiveness, 121–123
magnetic resonance imaging, 120, 121, 277, 278
rationale, 117–119, 244, 245
recommendations, 124, 125
referral indications, 124
ultrasound, 120, 121
sex differences, 112, 113
staging and prognosis, 243, 244
Hereditary hemochromatosis, hepatocellular carcinoma risks, 115
Hereditary nonpolyposis colorectal cancer (HNPCC),
colorectal cancer screening recommendations, 101–104
endometrial cancer risks, 72, 73
genes,
DNA mismatch repair function, 294
mutations, 45, 72, 99, 294
genetic testing, 97–99, 294, 295

Herpes simplex virus (HSV), oropharyngeal cancer risks, 133
Heterozygosity, definition, 289
HIV, *see* Human immunodeficiency virus
HNPCC, *see* Hereditary nonpolyposis colorectal cancer
Homozygosity, definition, 289
Hormone replacement therapy (HRT),
breast cancer risks, 21, 22
endometrial cancer risks, 65, 66, 77
ovarian cancer risks, 45, 46
HPV, *see* Human papilloma virus
HRT, *see* Hormone replacement therapy
HSV, *see* Herpes simplex virus
Human chorionic gonadotropin (HCG), testicular mass workup, 167
Human genome, mapping, 286
Human immunodeficiency virus (HIV), cervical cancer association, 39
Human papilloma virus (HPV),
cervical cancer role, 28–31
oncoproteins, 30, 31
types and typing, 29, 35, 36

L

Lead-time bias, implications, 7
Lung cancer,
incidence trends, 195
mortality, 196
primary care physician role,
literature surveillance and awareness, 204, 205
prevention, 203
referral to specialists, 205
risk recognition, 203, 204
risk reduction, 204
screening practices, 199, 204
prognosis, 195, 196

Index

risk factors, 195, 186
screening,
chest X-ray, 197–200
computed tomography, 200–202, 206, 276, 277
historical perspective, 197–199
rationale, 197
sputum cytology, 197–199, 202, 203
sex differences, 196
treatment, 196

M

Magnetic resonance imaging (MRI),
breast cancer screening, 19, 275, 276
coils, 273
costs, 274
female malignancy staging, 281
hepatocellular carcinoma screening, 120, 121, 277, 278
pancreatic cancer, 279
prospects, 274
prostate cancer, 281
pulse sequences, 273, 274
testicular mass work-up, 166
Malpractice,
case studies by cancer type,
breast cancer, 305–307
cervical cancer, 307, 308
colorectal cancer, 308, 309
prostate cancer, 309–311
communication breakdowns, 310–312
failure to screen, 305
patient rights, 312
recommendations for physicians, 312
statistics, 304, 305
Mammogram,
breast cancer mortality impact, 16
surgeon referral indications, 20
timing, 18, 21
utilization rates, 22
views, 16, 18
Medical malpractice, *see* Malpractice
Melanoma, *see* Skin cancer
MEN, *see* Multiple endocrine neoplasia
Metastasis,
breast cancer, 16

ovarian cancer, 46, 47
prevention as goal of cancer screening, 4
skin cancers, 175, 177
Microsatellite instability test, overview, 292
Missense mutation, definition, 290
Monogenic mutation, definition, 289
MRI, *see* Magnetic resonance imaging
Multiple endocrine neoplasia (MEN),
gene mutations, 296
genetic testing, 296
types, 296

N

Nonsense mutation, definition, 290
Northern blot, definition, 291
Nucleic acid hybridization, overview, 290, 291

O

Occult blood bead detector, esophageal cancer screening, 235, 236
Oncogene, carcinogenesis role, 287, 288
Oral cancer, *see* Oropharyngeal cancer
Oral contraceptives,
endometrial cancer protection, 65
ovarian cancer protection, 54, 55
Oropharyngeal cancer,
cytology, 135
incidence, 130
lymphoma, 133
prognosis, 130
risk factors, 130
salivary gland tumors, 133
screening,
algorithm, 135
follow-up, 15
rationale, 133, 134
referral indications, 136
visual examination, 134, 135
squamous cell carcinoma,
alcohol risks, 132
betel nut chewing risk, 131

Index

epidemiology, 130, 131
genetics, 132
herpes simplex virus risks, 133
immunosuppressed patients, 133
tobacco risks, 131, 132
types of malignancies, 130
Ovarian cancer,
clinical features, 47
gene mutations, 45
incidence, 43
metastasis, 46, 47
mortality, 43
natural history, 46, 47
pathogenesis, 46
prevention, 54, 55
prophylactic surgery, 55
risk factors, 44–46
screening,
algorithm, 56
CA 125 levels, 47, 49, 50
cost-effectiveness, 54
difficulty, 8, 9
effects on outcome, 9
family history, 48
genetic testing, 53, 294
multimodal screening, 51, 52
pelvic examination, 49
rationale, 47, 48
recommendations, 52, 53, 55–57
ultrasound, 49–52
staging and survival, 47, 48

P

Pancreatic cancer,
computed tomography, 279
magnetic resonance imaging, 279
Papanicolaou smear, *see also* Cervical cancer,
abnormal smear management with colposcopy, 35, 37, 38
access, 8
automated cytologic screening, 40
cervical cancer mortality impact, 7, 8
endometrial cancer screening, 68, 69
fluid-based technology, 40
frequency recommendations, 35

malpractice lawsuits, 307, 308
quality control, 8
sensitivity, 35
specificity, 35
PCR, *see* Polymerase chain reaction
PDT, *see* Photodynamic therapy
Penetrance, definition, 289
Pepsinogen, stomach cancer screening, 262, 263
Pharyngeal cancer, *see* Oropharyngeal cancer
Photodynamic therapy (PDT),
mucosal ablation of Barrett's esophagus, 222
Point mutation, definition, 290
Polymerase chain reaction (PCR),
overview, 291, 292
Polymorphism, definition, 289
Porphyria, hepatocellular carcinoma risks, 116
Primary liver cancer, *see* Hepatocellular carcinoma
Progesterone challenge test,
endometrial cancer risk patients, 77, 78
Progestin, endometrial cancer prevention, 78, 79
Prostate cancer,
age of diagnosis, 142
diagnostic algorithm, 153–155
ethnicity effects, 142
growth rate, 148
incidence and trends, 141–144
magnetic resonance imaging, 281
malpractice lawsuits, 309–311
mortality and trends, 144–146
prognostic factors,
age, 146, 147
Gleason score, 146, 147
tumor volume, 148
screening,
controversies, 157, 158
cost-effectiveness, 156, 157
digital rectal examination, 150, 151, 154
impact, 142–144
prostate-specific antigen,
see Prostate-specific antigen

Index

rationale, 148–150
Prostate-specific antigen (PSA),
  aging effects on levels, 153
  assays, 152
  bloodstream release, 152
  cost-effectiveness of screening,
    156, 157
  finasteride effects on levels, 154,
    155
  impact on prostate cancer epide-
    miology, 142–144
  interpretation of levels, 154
  positive predictive value, 152,
    153
  protein complexes, 152, 153
  rising levels, 155
  sensitivity, 152, 153
  specificity for prostate cancer,
    151–153
  tumor volume correlation, 148
Protein truncation test, overview,
  292
PSA, see Prostate-specific antigen

R

Recessive mutation, definition, 289
Restriction endonuclease, definition,
  290

S

SCC, see Squamous cell carcinoma
Sensitivity, definition, 5, 6
Sex-linked disorder, definition, 288
Sigmoidoscopy,
  combined with fecal occult blood
    testing, 94, 95
  cost-effectiveness, 100
  efficacy of colorectal cancer
    screening, 94
  flexible vs rigid sigmoidoscopes,
    92, 93
  recommendations, 93, 94
  sensitivity, 94
  specificity, 94
Silent mutation, definition, 290
Skin cancer,
  differential diagnosis, 179
  incidence by type, 173, 174
  melanoma,

ABCD diagnostic criteria, 187
  early detection importance,
    178
  hereditary gene mutations and
    genetic testing, 187,
    188, 295
  incidence trends, 174, 175
  mortality, 177
  pigmented lesion clinics, 189
  relative risk factors, 176
pathogenesis, 177, 178
prognosis by type, 175, 177
risk factors, 175
screening,
  cost-effectiveness, 188
  epiluminescence microscopy,
    187
  genetic screening, 187, 188
  overview of methods, 178,
    179
physical examination,
    positive predictive value,
      180–184, 186, 187
    sensitivity, 180–184, 186,
      187
    specificity, 180–184, 186,
      187
    total-body vs partial exami-
      nation, 180
  rationale, 178
  referral indications, 188, 189
  total-body photography, 187
Smoking, see Tobacco
Somatic mutation, definition, 290
Sonohysterogram, endometrial
  cancer screening, 71, 75
Southern blot, definition, 291
Specificity, definition, 5
Sputum cytology, lung cancer
  screening, 197–199, 202, 203
Squamous cell carcinoma (SCC),
  see Esophageal cancer; Oropha-
    ryngeal cancer; Skin cancer
Stomach cancer,
  adenocarcinoma classification,
    257, 258

324   Index

atrophic gastritis risks, 256, 257
diagnosis, 258, 259
geographic distribution, 255
Helicobacter pylori role, 256, 257
Japan,
  epidemiology, 256, 257, 263
  screening,
    algorithm, 265
    barium X-ray, 259, 260, 262
    cost-effectiveness, 263, 264
    overview, 256
    pepsinogen in serum, 262,
     263
    rationale, 263, 265
pathogenesis, 257, 258
staging and prognosis, 258, 259
types of tumors, 257
Survival, improvement as goal of
  cancer screening, 3

T

Tamoxifen,
  breast cancer benefits, 75
  endometrial cancer,
    risks, 66, 74
    screening recommendations,
     74–76
Testicular cancer,
  cisplatin therapy, 161
  classification, 162, 163
  clinical features by cell type, 163,
   164
  incidence, 161, 162
  prognosis, 161, 166, 167
  risk factors, 162
  screening,
    algorithm, 165
    testicular examination,
     average-risk population,
      164–166
     high-risk population, 166
     self-examination, 168
  work-up of testicular mass,
    alpha-fetoprotein, 167
    computed tomography, 167
    human chorionic gonadotropin,
     167

magnetic resonance imaging,
  166
referral indications, 167
ultrasound, 166
Tobacco,
  cervical cancer risks, 30
  lung cancer risks, 195, 196
  oropharyngeal cancer risks, 131,
   132
  smoking,
    cessation supports, 204
    trends, 196
Transnasal balloon cell sampling,
  Barrett's esophagus and esophageal cancer screening, 217
Tumor suppressor gene, definition,
  288
Tyrosinemia, hepatocellular carcinoma risks, 116

U

Ultrasound,
  Barrett's esophagus and esophageal cancer screening, 218,
   219
  breast cancer screening, 19
  endometrial cancer screening, 70,
   71, 75
  hepatocellular carcinoma screening, 120, 121, 246, 249
  ovarian cancer screening, 49–52
  testicular mass work-up, 166

V

VHL syndrome, *see* Von Hippel–
  Lindau syndrome
Von Hippel–Lindau (VHL) syndrome, gene mutations, 296,
  297

W

Western blot, definition, 291
Wilson's disease, hepatocellular carcinoma risks, 116